Radiographic Neuroanatomy
A Working Atlas

NOTICE

Medicine is an ever-changing science. As new research and clinical experience broaden our knowledge, changes in treatment and drug therapy are required. The author and the publisher of this work have checked with sources believed to be reliable in their efforts to provide information that is complete and generally in accord with the standards accepted at the time of publication. However, in view of the possibility of human error or changes in medical sciences, neither the author nor the publisher nor any other party who has been involved in the preparation or publication of this work warrants that the information contained herein is in every respect accurate or complete. Readers are encouraged to confirm the information contained herein with other sources. For example and in particular, readers are advised to check the product information sheet included in the package of each drug they plan to administer to be certain that the information contained in this book is accurate and that changes have not been made in the recommended dose or in the contraindications for administration. This recommendation is of particular importance in connection with new or infrequently used drugs.

Radiographic Neuroanatomy
A Working Atlas

Harry W. Fischer, M.D.

Former Professor of Radiology and
Chairman, Department of Radiology
University of Rochester School of Medicine and Dentistry;
Former Chief of Radiology
Strong Memorial Hospital
Rochester, New York

Leena Ketonen, M.D., Ph.D.

Visiting Assistant Professor of Radiology
University of Rochester Medical Center
Strong Memorial Hospital
Rochester, New York

McGraw-Hill, Inc.
Health Professions Division

New York St. Louis San Francisco Colorado Springs Auckland Bogotá Caracas
Hamburg Lisbon London Madrid Mexico Milan Montreal New Delhi Paris San Juan
São Paulo Singapore Sydney Tokyo Toronto

Radiographic Neuroanatomy: A Working Atlas

International Edition 1991

2 3 4 5 6 7 8 9 0 KKP 9 8 7 6 5 4 3 2

ISBN 0-07-021101-9

This book was set in Optima by York Graphic Services, Inc.; the editors were William Day and Peter McCurdy; the production supervisor was Robert R. Laffler; the book and its cover were designed by José Fonfrias.

Library of Congress Cataloging-in-Publication Data

Fischer, Harry W.

Radiographic neuroanatomy: a working atlas/Harry W. Fischer, Leena Ketonen.

p. cm.

ISBN 0-07-021101-9

1. Neuroanatomy—Atlases. 2. Central nervous system—Imaging—Atlases.

I. Ketonen, Leena. II. Title.

[DNLM: 1. Central Nervous System—anatomy & histology—atlases. 2. Central Nervous System—radiography—atlases. WL 17 F529r]

QM451.F57 1990

611'.8'0222—dc20

DNLM/DLC

for Library of Congress 90-13247

CIP

When ordering this title use ISBN 0-07-112615-5

Printed in Singapore

To the Scandinavian Radiologists
who have contributed greatly
to the department at Rochester. HWF

To my three young daughters
Irene, Laura, and Emilia,
whose encouragement and patience
contributed so much to this work. LK

CONTENTS

PREFACE

The study of the central nervous system is founded on mastery of its anatomy. It is on that foundation that a true understanding of physiology, biochemistry, pharmacology, and pathology can be built. After mastering neuroanatomy through the study of cadaver dissections and cross-sectional demonstrations, students must learn to correlate their knowledge of gross anatomy with its representation by modern imaging technology.

As this atlas is an aid to learning and reviewing normal anatomy, pathologic conditions are not illustrated. To enhance its usefulness as a tool for self-study and self-assessment, the images themselves are not labeled. Our format lets the images speak for themselves without intervening text.

Plain radiographic images of the skull and spine are of course included in the book, but the majority of the images come from angiography and myelography and from computed tomography and magnetic resonance. Nuclear medicine and ultrasound illustrate gross neuroanatomy suboptimally and therefore are not included. Sagittal and frontal plane images afforded by MR are included as well as MR cross-sectional images.

Readers seeking an affordable atlas of general radiographic anatomy should see *Radiographic Anatomy: A Working Atlas* by Harry W. Fischer (McGraw-Hill, 1988).

ACKNOWLEDGMENTS

Alyce Norder and John J. Allen of Lakeshore Graphic Arts made all the drawings of the neural structures. We are indebted to them for their excellent work and full and prompt cooperation.

Most of the images came from the daily case material of Strong Memorial Hospital and some came from the teaching files of the Department of Radiology of the University of Rochester School of Medicine and Dentistry.

William Smith and Michael Malerk of the medical illustration services of the medical school were most helpful to us in making the photographs. Scott Yohe and Dr. Maury Blumenfeld of the General Electric Company provided the MR angiographic images of the head and neck. Oili Salonen, M.D., Ph.D. (Helsinki, Finland), provided some of the myelograms and arteriograms.

This picture collection could not have been completed without the excellent help of Aileen MacKay and Daniel Prosser and other members of the MRI laboratory and CT staff, to whom we would like to express our thanks.

INTRODUCTION

In radiography of the living man, identification of the images is based on the path taken by the central x-ray as it passes through the body part. A *posterior-anterior (PA) view* is one in which the x-ray enters from the posterior surface of the body part, passes through the body part, exits from the anterior or front surface, and then reaches the x-ray cassette, which holds intensifying screens and film. The x-rays striking the intensifying screens interact with the crystals of the screen, producing light which exposes the photosensitive film emulsion. The emulsion is then developed chemically to bring out the image. In a PA view, the central ray coming from the x-ray tube is perpendicular to the film and is centered on the center of the part being examined (Fig. 1). An *anterior-posterior (AP) view* is one in which the central x-ray enters from the anterior surface of the body part, exits from the posterior surface, and then reaches the film (Fig. 2). A *lateral view* is one in which the central ray enters one side of the body part and exits from the opposite side (Fig. 3). These three projections, PA, AP, and lateral, suffice for the majority of x-ray images in clinical practice. In an *oblique view,* the central x-ray passes through the body part at an angle approximately halfway between that of a PA and a lateral view (Fig. 4).

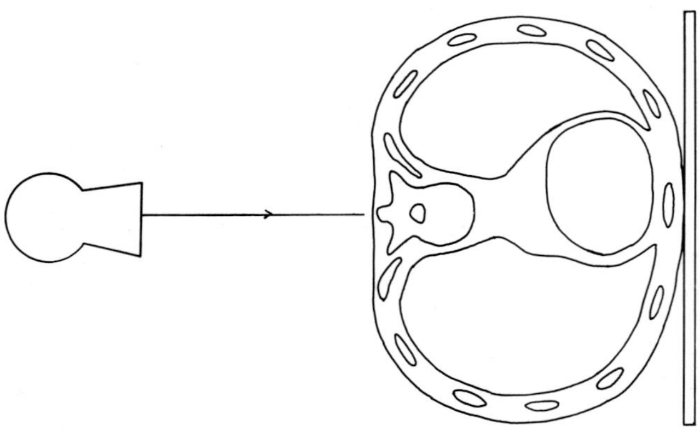

Fig. 1 PA view of the chest.

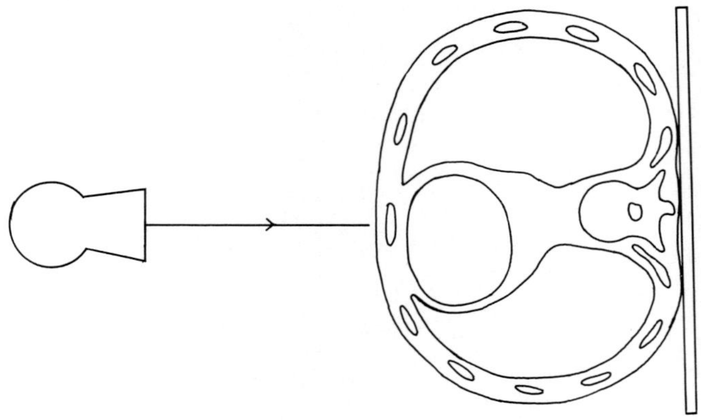

Fig. 2 AP view of the chest.

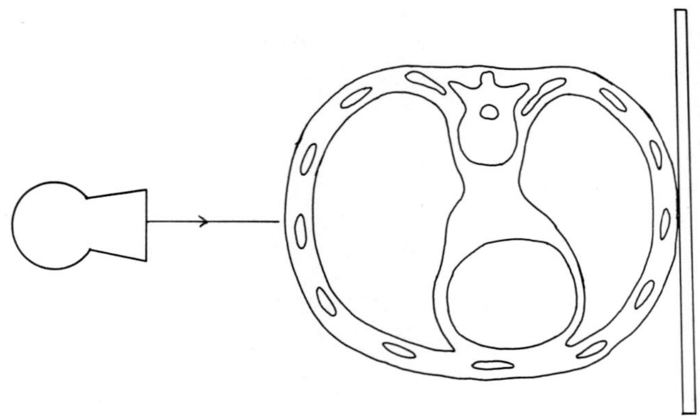

Fig. 3 Lateral view of the chest.

For the skull, a number of different views employ different orientations of the skull in relation to the central ray and the x-ray film. The PA view of the skull, sinuses, or facial bones has the central ray angled 15° to the orbital-meatal line (Fig. 5). The lateral view has the patient's head turned to the side and positioned against the film, while the central ray is directed perpendicular to

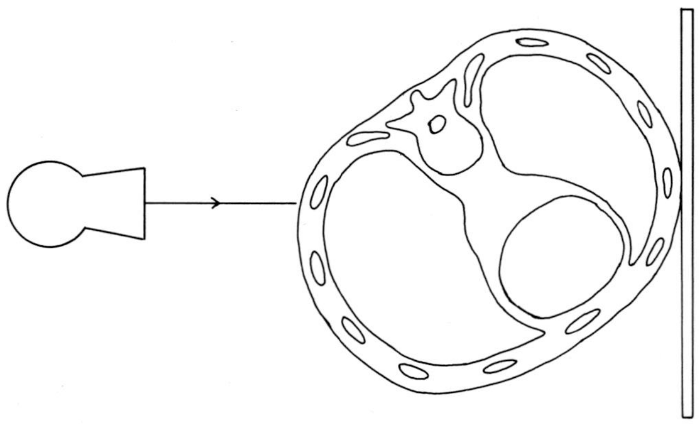

Fig. 4 Left anterior oblique view of the chest.

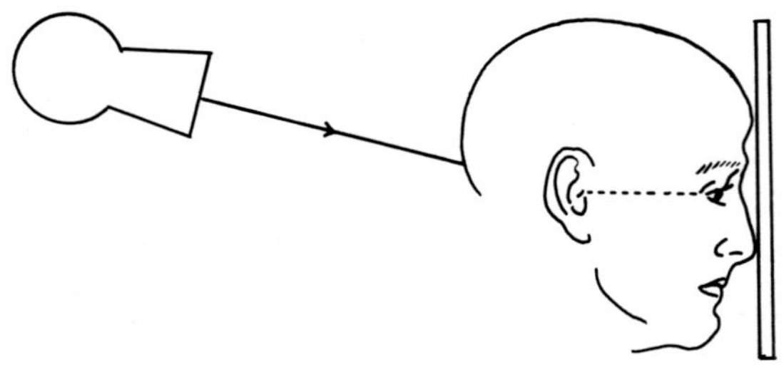

Fig. 5 PA view of the skull [→—: represents the central ray; - - - - - - -: represents the orbital-meatal (OM) line, from the angle of the eye to the external meatus of the ear.]

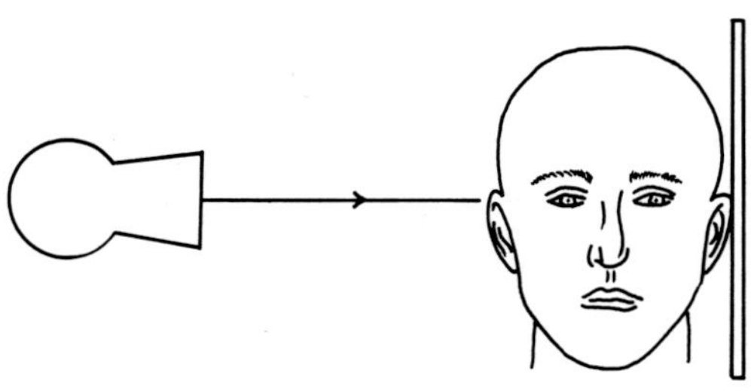

Fig. 6 Lateral view of the skull.

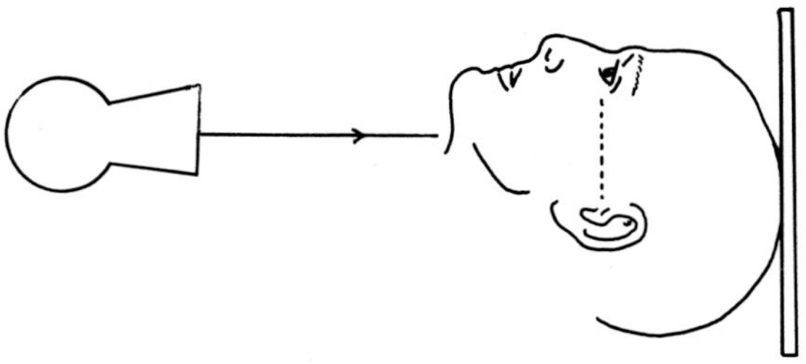

Fig. 7 Basal view of the skull (see Fig. 5 for key).

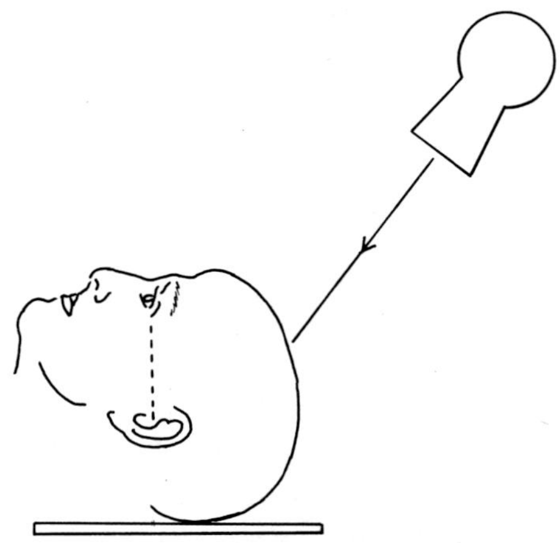

Fig. 8 Occipital (Towne) view of the skull (see Fig. 5 for key).

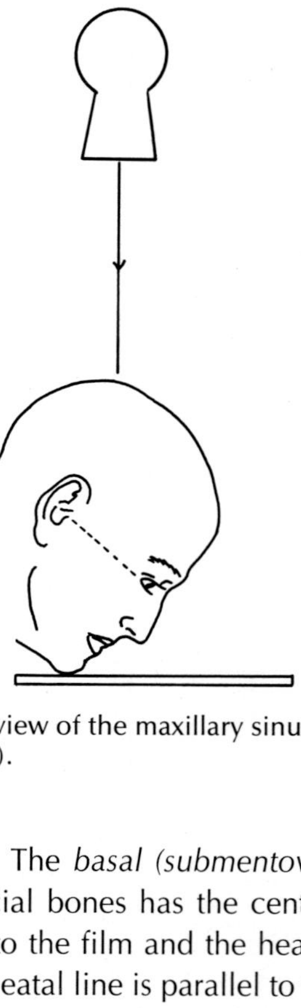

Fig. 9 PA (Waters) view of the maxillary sinus and facial bones (see Fig. 5 for key).

the film (Fig. 6). The *basal (submentovertical) view* of the skull and facial bones has the central ray directed perpendicularly to the film and the head tilted back so that the orbital-meatal line is parallel to the film (Fig. 7). The *occipital,* or *Towne, view* of the skull and mastoids has the patient supine, with the back of the head against the film and chin tucked down on the chest. The central ray is directed 37° to the feet (Fig. 8). The *Waters view* is a PA view of the maxillary sinuses and facial bones in which the prone patient's chin is against the film, with the nose elevated about 1.5 cm from the film so that the orbital-meatal line makes an angle of 37° with the plane of the film. The central ray is directed perpendicularly to the film (Fig. 9).

For the mastoids there are special views. The *Stenvers view* has the central ray angled 12° to the head of the patient while the prone patient's head is turned 45° to the film (Fig. 10). The *Law view* has the central ray angled 15° to the patients feet and 10 to 15° to the face,

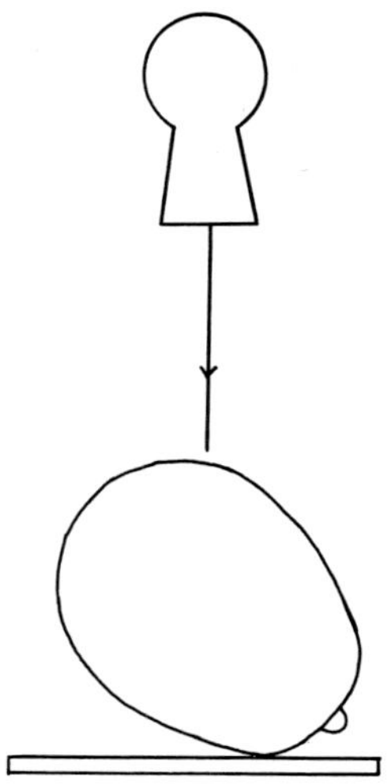

Fig. 10 Stenvers view of the mastoid.

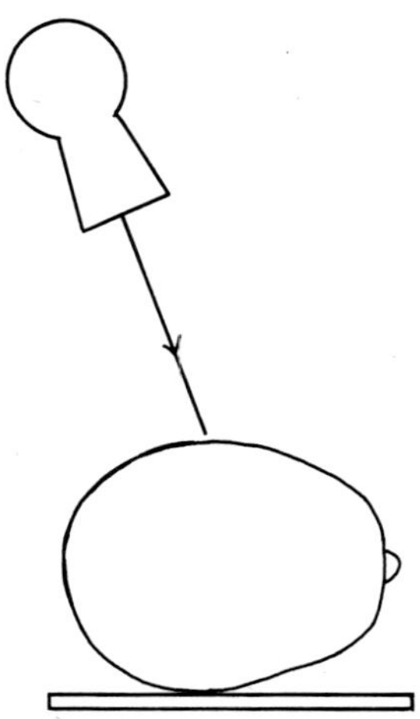

Fig. 11 Law view of the mastoid.

while the prone patient has the side of the head against the film (Fig. 11).

A view to better visualize the atlas, axis, and the odontoid process of the upper cervical spine is obtained by directing the central ray through the open mouth in the AP projection.

Imaging Modalities

Angiography

Angiography in radiology is based on the rapid injection of a volume of water-soluble organic iodide compound (the contrast median) into an artery supplying the circulation of the part to be examined. For the brain and head, injection is made into the carotid and vertebral arteries. Multiple exposures are made as the radiopaque solution flows through the arteries, the capillaries, and the veins.

Myelography

Myelography, or cisternography, in radiography is based on the injection of water-soluble organic iodide compound into the subarachnoid space by lumbar or cervical (C-1–C-2) puncture. Multiple exposures are made as the fluoroscopic table is tilted, which allows the contrast medium to flow around and define the spinal cord and spinal nerve roots or to fill the cisterns in the head. The water-soluble medium is removed from the body by renal excretion. Air can be used as a contrast medium to define the spinal cord or brain structures, but with the coming of CT and MR, the performance of pneumoencephalography (air cisternography) has practically disappeared from clinical practice. Water-soluble, intravenously administered contrast medium is employed to enhance the vessels in computed tomography. In the normal central nervous system, that is, in those with an intact blood-brain barrier, the contrast medium does not pass from the vessels into the brain or spinal cord tissue. In the remainder of the body the contrast medium passes quickly from the vessels into the extravascular spaces.

The only FDA-approved contrast medium employed thus far in magnetic resonance imaging is gadolinium-DTPA, which is used to enhance lesions. When administered intravenously it does not penetrate into normal brain or spinal cord due to an intact blood-brain barrier. In this feature, gadolinium-DTPA behaves like the water-soluble organic iodides in x-ray angiography and CT enhancement. Gadolinium-DTPA enhancement on MR is not entirely the same as iodinated contrast enhancement on CT. Enhancement of the large blood vessels, falx, tentorium, and dura is not nearly as prominent on contrast MR scan as on contrast CT. However, the cavernous sinus, pituitary stalk, and choroid plexus enhance markedly with contrast. Moderate enhancement is seen in the durea, pituitary gland, and in the small cortical veins.

CT Images

Computed tomography images are cross-sectional and defined by the thickness of the slice taken, which is usually 1.5, 3.0, 5.0, or 10.0 mm wide. Gaps between the slices are usually not employed. For the skull and its contents the standard planes of the slices are parallel to the supraorbitomeatal line (25° to Reid's anthropologic baseline), and all slices are parallel to each other. The radiologist may select slices of the skull and brain at other angles to the base of the skull. Slices in the anterior-posterior plane or frontal plane are used particularly for visualization of abnormalities of the facial bones, orbits, and the pituitary gland.

Magnetic Resonance Images

Magnetic resonance, in addition to producing excellent cross-sectional images, also provides sagittal and parasagittal and frontal plane images at the selection of the radiologist. Intervals between slices along with the slice thickness can be varied. The illustrations in the book are picked mainly from daily clinical material. The choice of image plane varies not only because of limitations imposed by patient positioning, but also because special planes are used for ideal demonstration of specific anatomic structures.

Pulse Sequence

The choice of a pulse sequence requires explanation. One single technique will not display all the anatomy in the optimal way. There are various MR techniques which produce very different appearances of the same structures, depending on the clinical needs.

A pulse sequence consists of one or more pulses of radiowaves. The most commonly used pulse sequence is *spin echo (SE),* which is defined as a series of alternating 90 degree and 180 degree pulses. The time between the 90 degree pulses is called *repetition time (TR).*

The intrinsic tissue characteristics, such as proton density, T1- and T2-relaxation times and movement (blood flow) can be displayed in many different ways, depending on the clinical need. For example, the CSF can be demonstrated as high signal (bright) or low signal (dark) intensity on the T2-weighted images. By the choice of TR and TE the SE pulse sequence may be either T1- or T2-weighted. Typically, the SE pulse sequence with short TR and short TE produces T1-weighted images. In these images, CSF, cortical bone and rapidly flowing blood appear as black areas (negligible signal). However, fat (orbit, bone marrow, and subcutaneous areas) appears as bright areas (high signal).

The other commonly used sequences in the clinical setting is long TR with short or long TE. The combination of long TR, short TE (for example 2000/30 msec) produces an image where the signal intensity is related primarily to proton density. In this image CFS has dark signal, fat has bright, and gray and white matter have intermediate intensities. The combination of long TR, long TE (for example 2000/90 msec) produces an image that has a signal intensity related to the T2 values of the tissues. In the T2-weight image, CSF has a bright signal relative to the dark signal from gray and white matter. Cortical bone and rapidly flowing blood have a negligible signal (dark). Fat has a less intense signal than in the proton density image.

Grass imaging (gradient-recalled acquisition in steady state) is a fast scanning technique widely used in spine and head studies.

Radiographic Neuroanatomy

A Working Atlas

PART I

THE SKULL

1/Skull, Paranasal Sinuses, Facial Area, and Orbit □ Skull

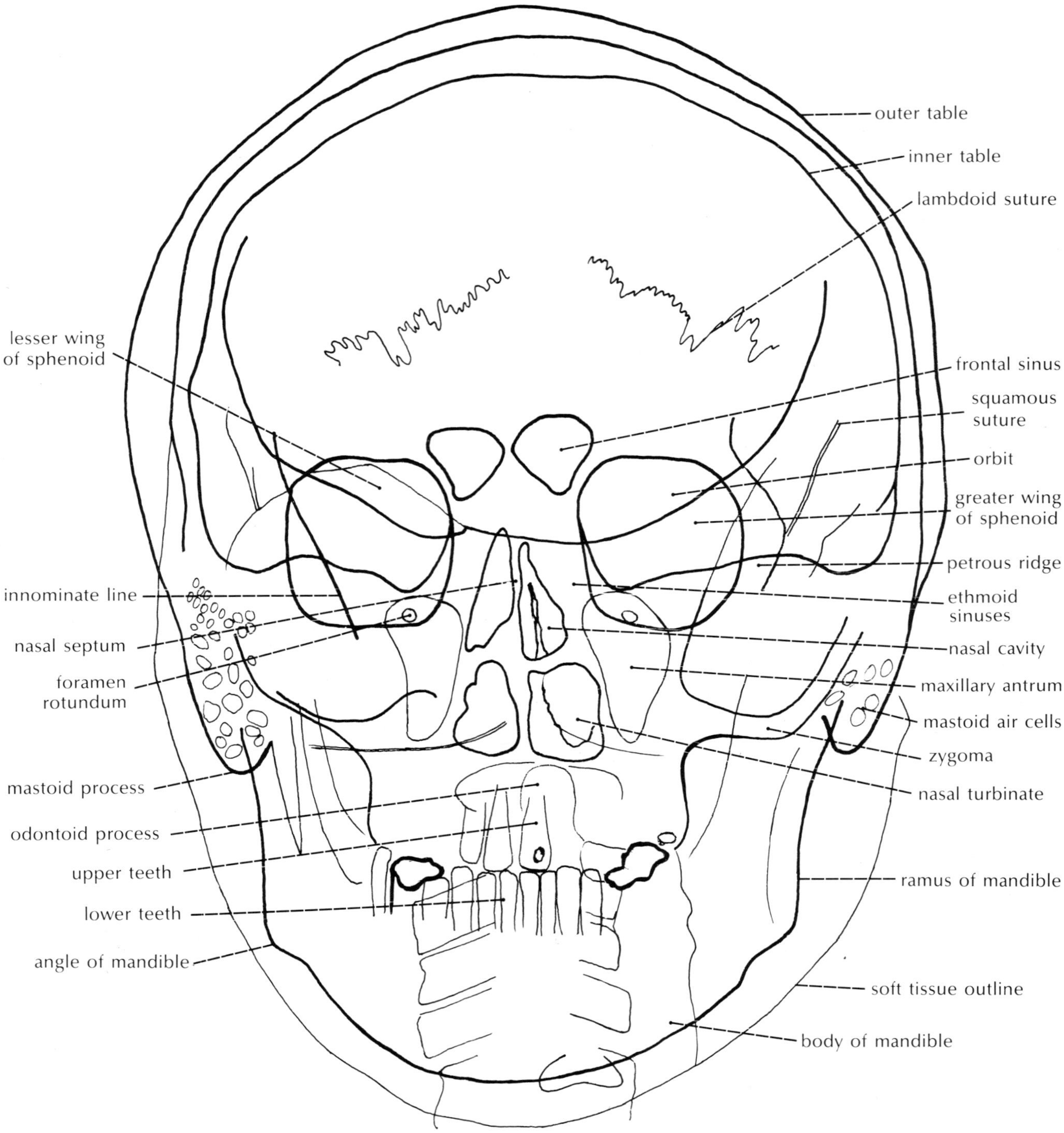

1/Skull, X-Ray

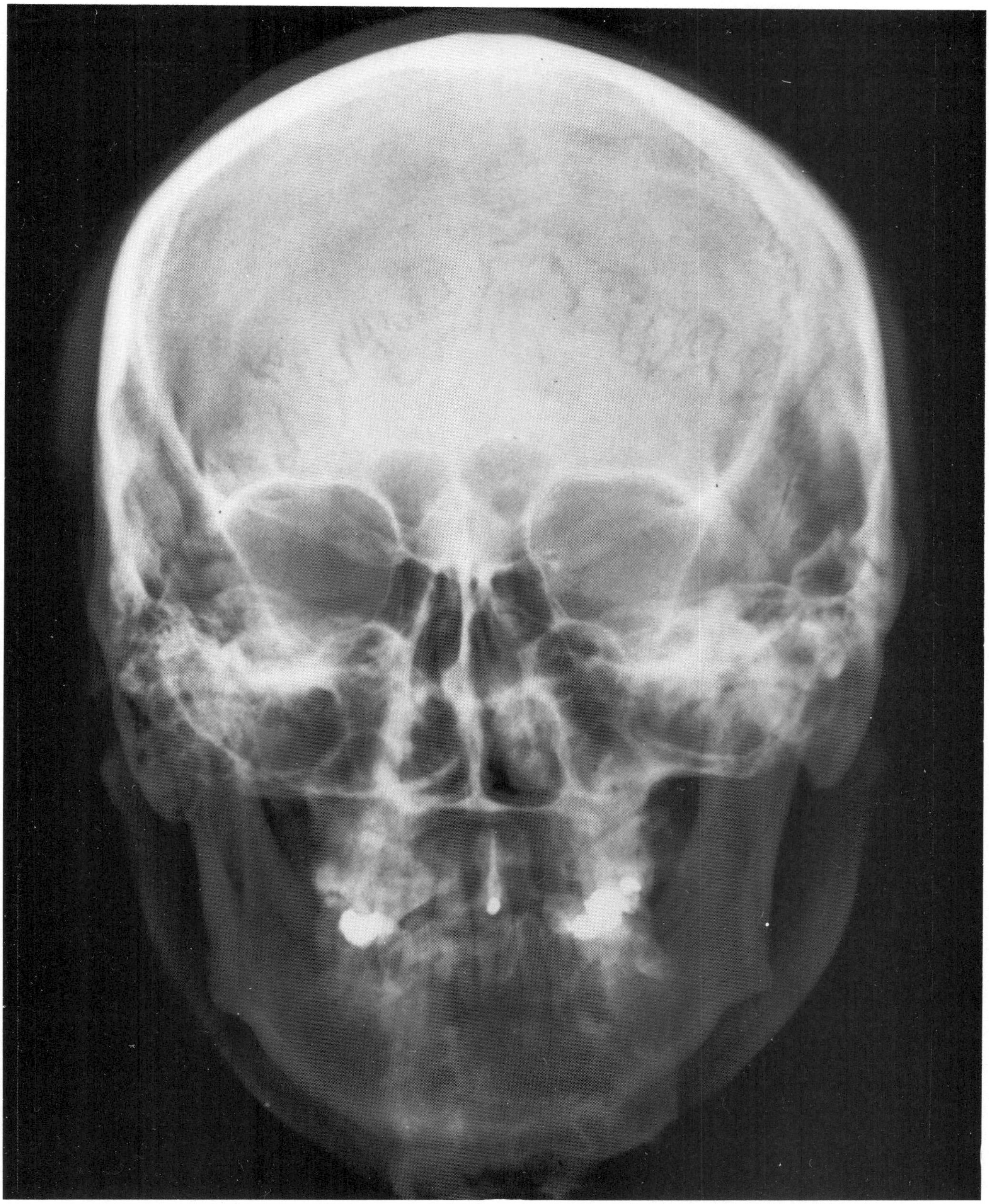

1-1 Skull, PA view.

1/Skull, X-Ray

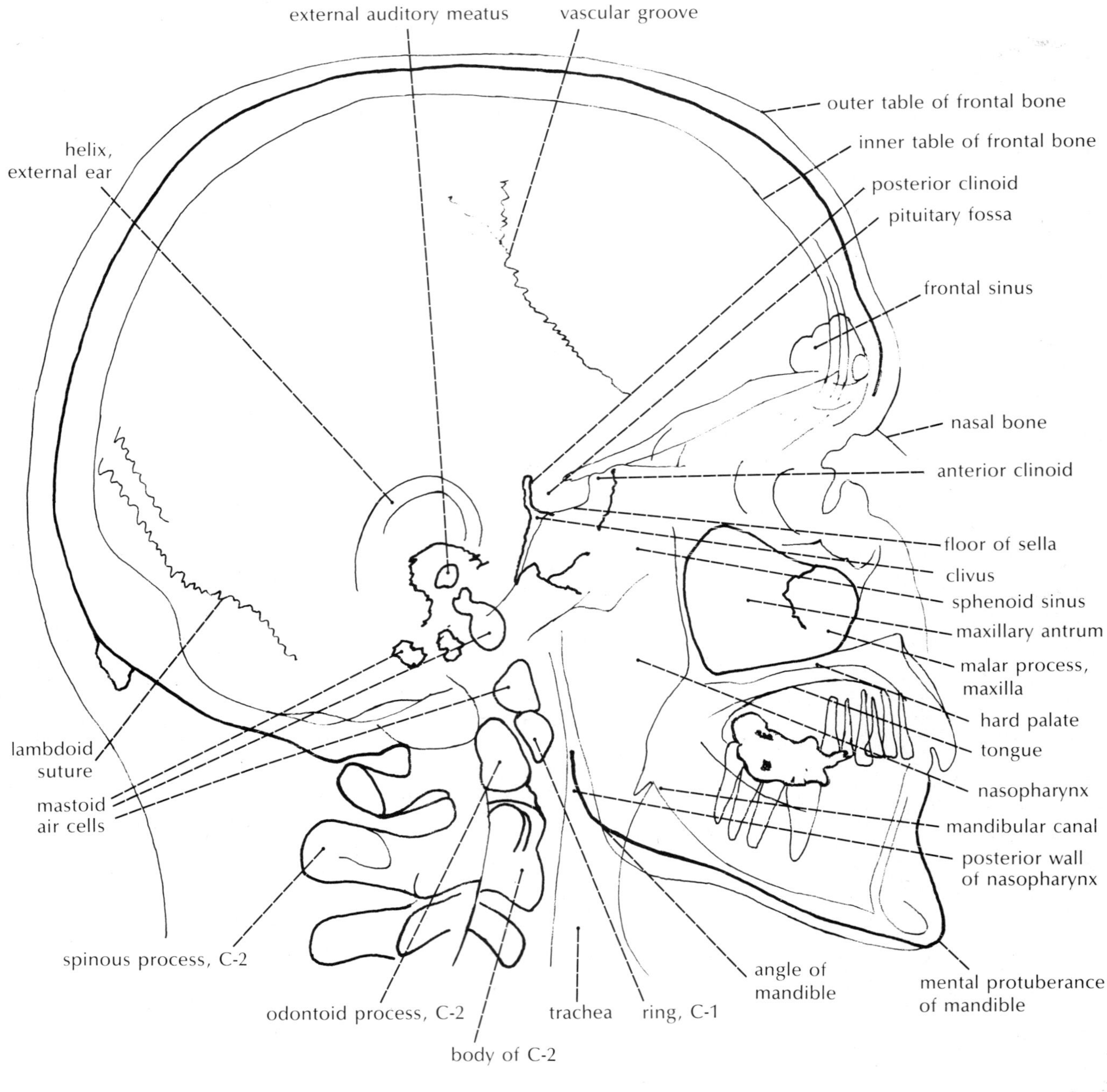
external auditory meatus
vascular groove
outer table of frontal bone
inner table of frontal bone
posterior clinoid
pituitary fossa
helix,
external ear
frontal sinus
nasal bone
anterior clinoid
floor of sella
clivus
sphenoid sinus
maxillary antrum
malar process,
maxilla
hard palate
tongue
lambdoid
suture
nasopharynx
mastoid
air cells
mandibular canal
posterior wall
of nasopharynx
spinous process, C-2
angle of
mandible
mental protuberance
of mandible
odontoid process, C-2
trachea
ring, C-1
body of C-2

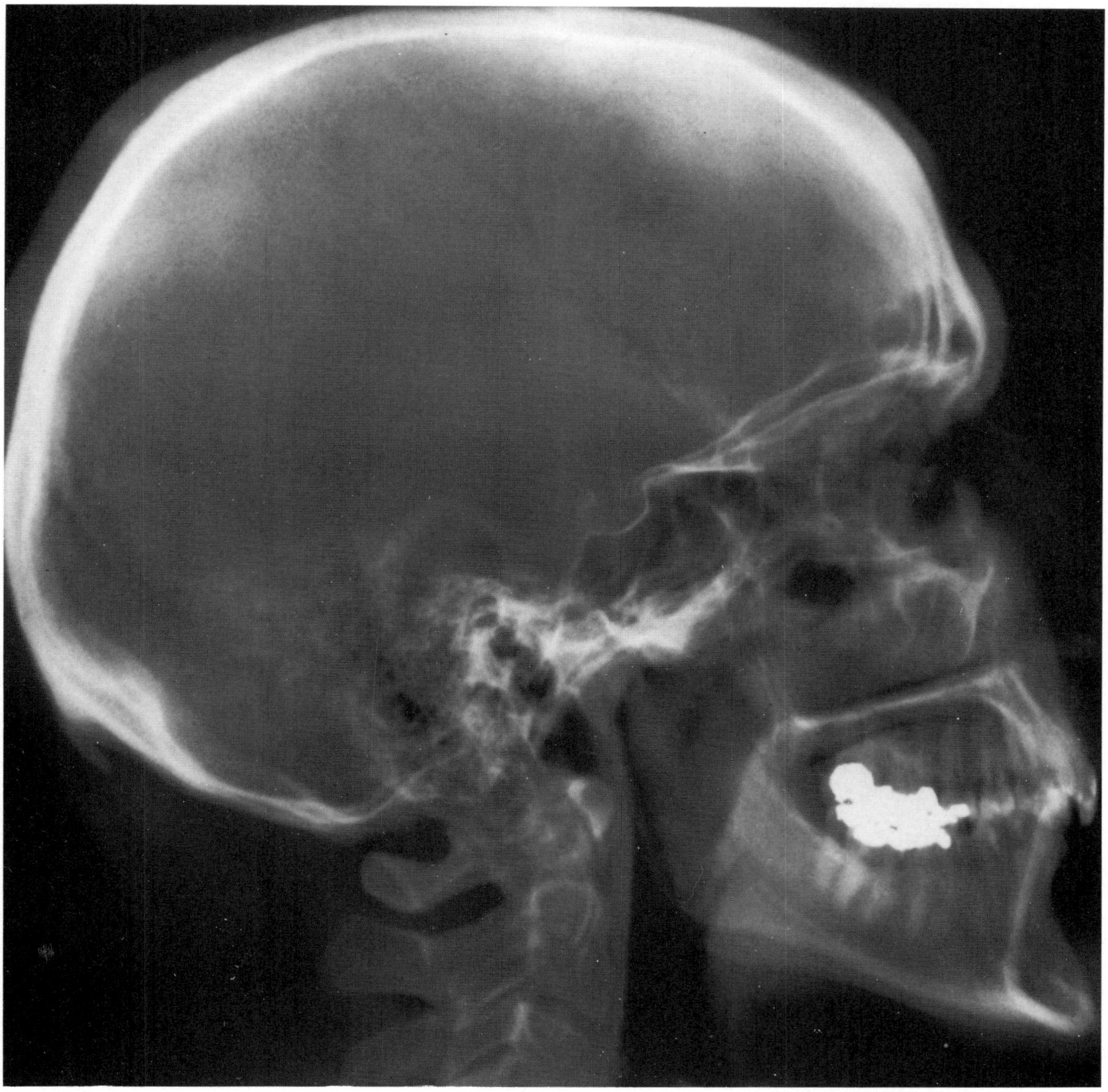

1-2 Skull, lateral view.

1/Skull, X-Ray

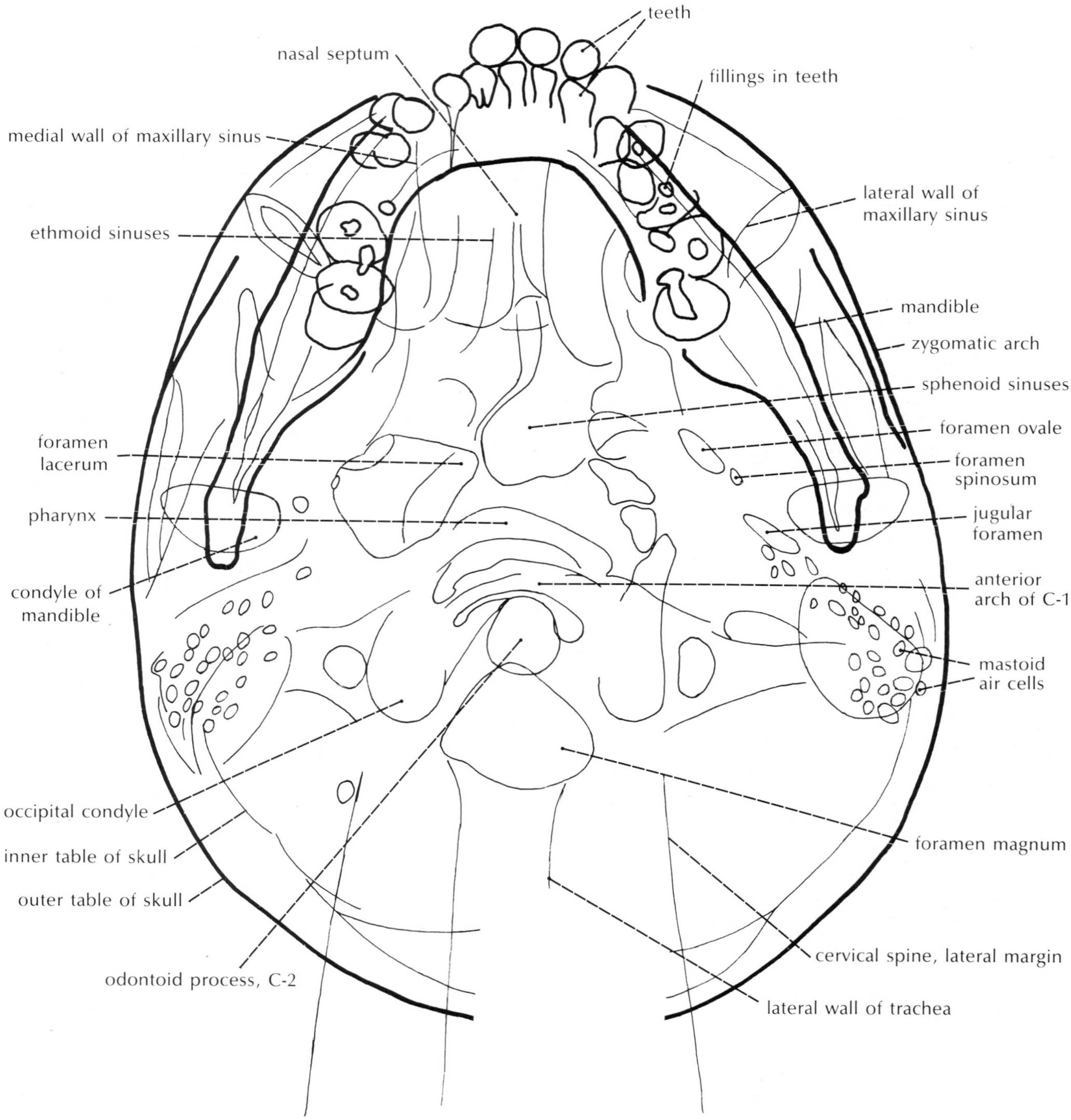
teeth
nasal septum
fillings in teeth
medial wall of maxillary sinus
lateral wall of maxillary sinus
ethmoid sinuses
mandible
zygomatic arch
sphenoid sinuses
foramen ovale
foramen lacerum
foramen spinosum
pharynx
jugular foramen
condyle of mandible
anterior arch of C-1
mastoid air cells
occipital condyle
foramen magnum
inner table of skull
outer table of skull
cervical spine, lateral margin
odontoid process, C-2
lateral wall of trachea

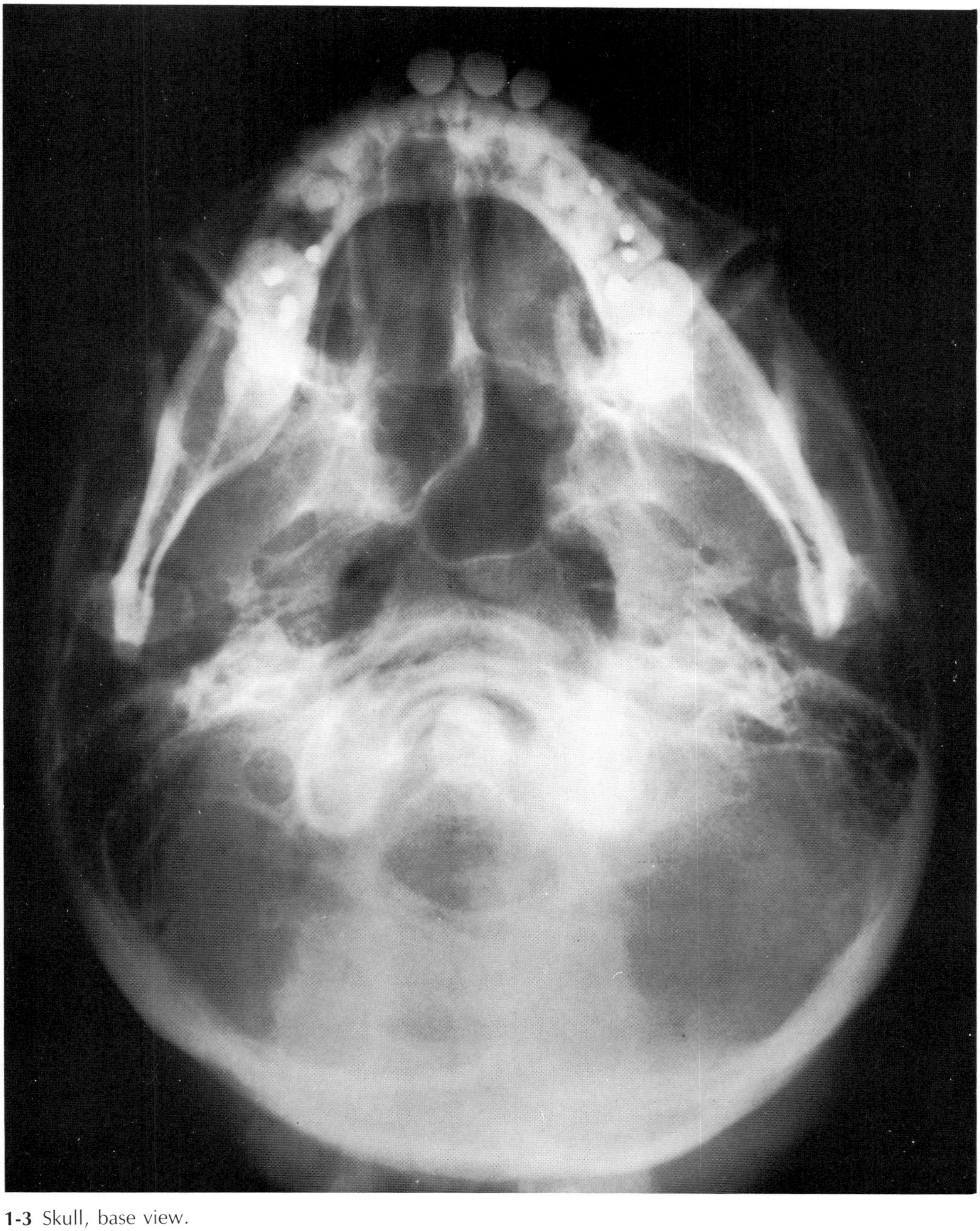

1-3 Skull, base view.

1/Skull, X-Ray

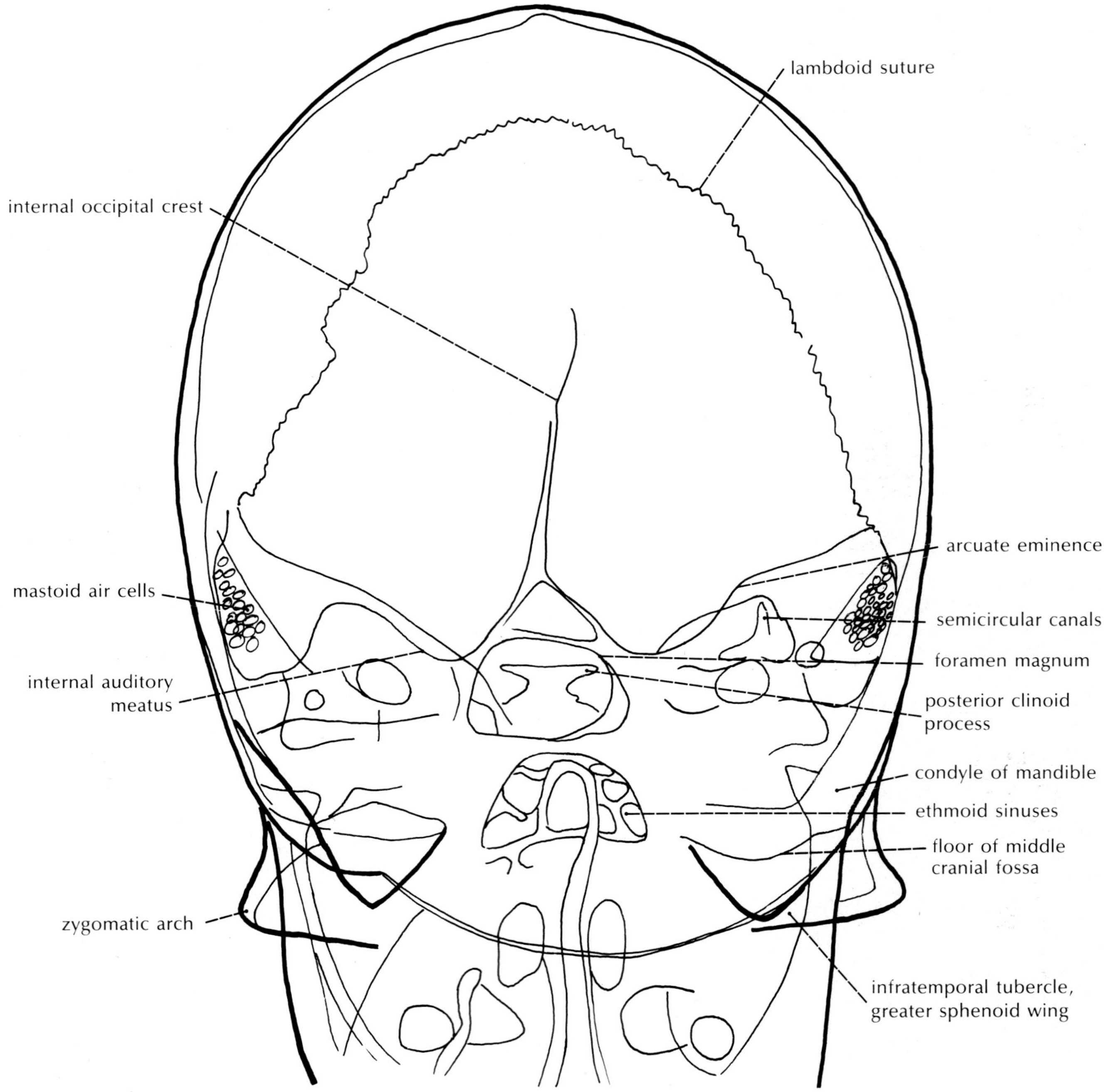
lambdoid suture
internal occipital crest
arcuate eminence
mastoid air cells
semicircular canals
foramen magnum
internal auditory meatus
posterior clinoid process
condyle of mandible
ethmoid sinuses
floor of middle cranial fossa
zygomatic arch
infratemporal tubercle, greater sphenoid wing

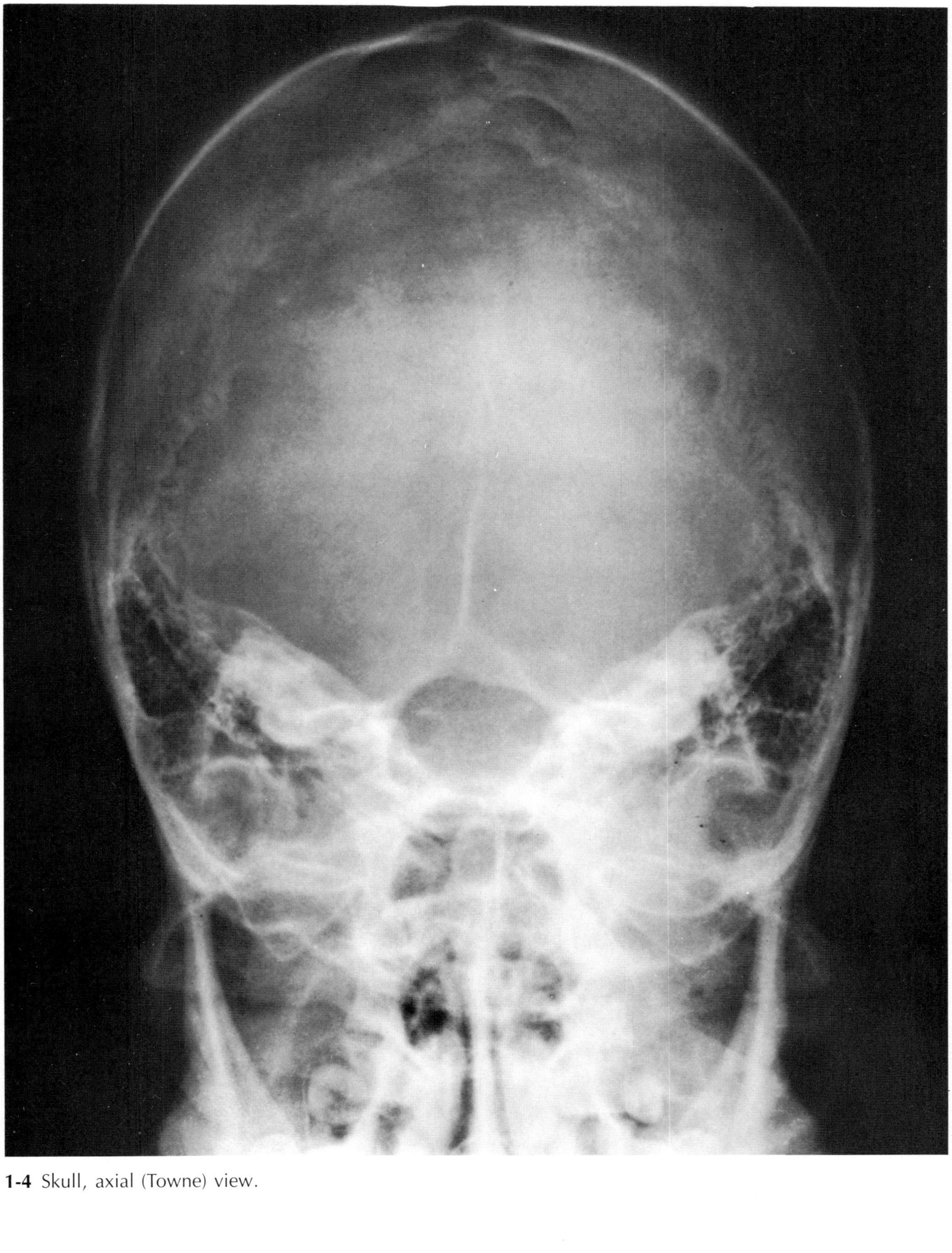

1-4 Skull, axial (Towne) view.

1/Skull, X-Ray

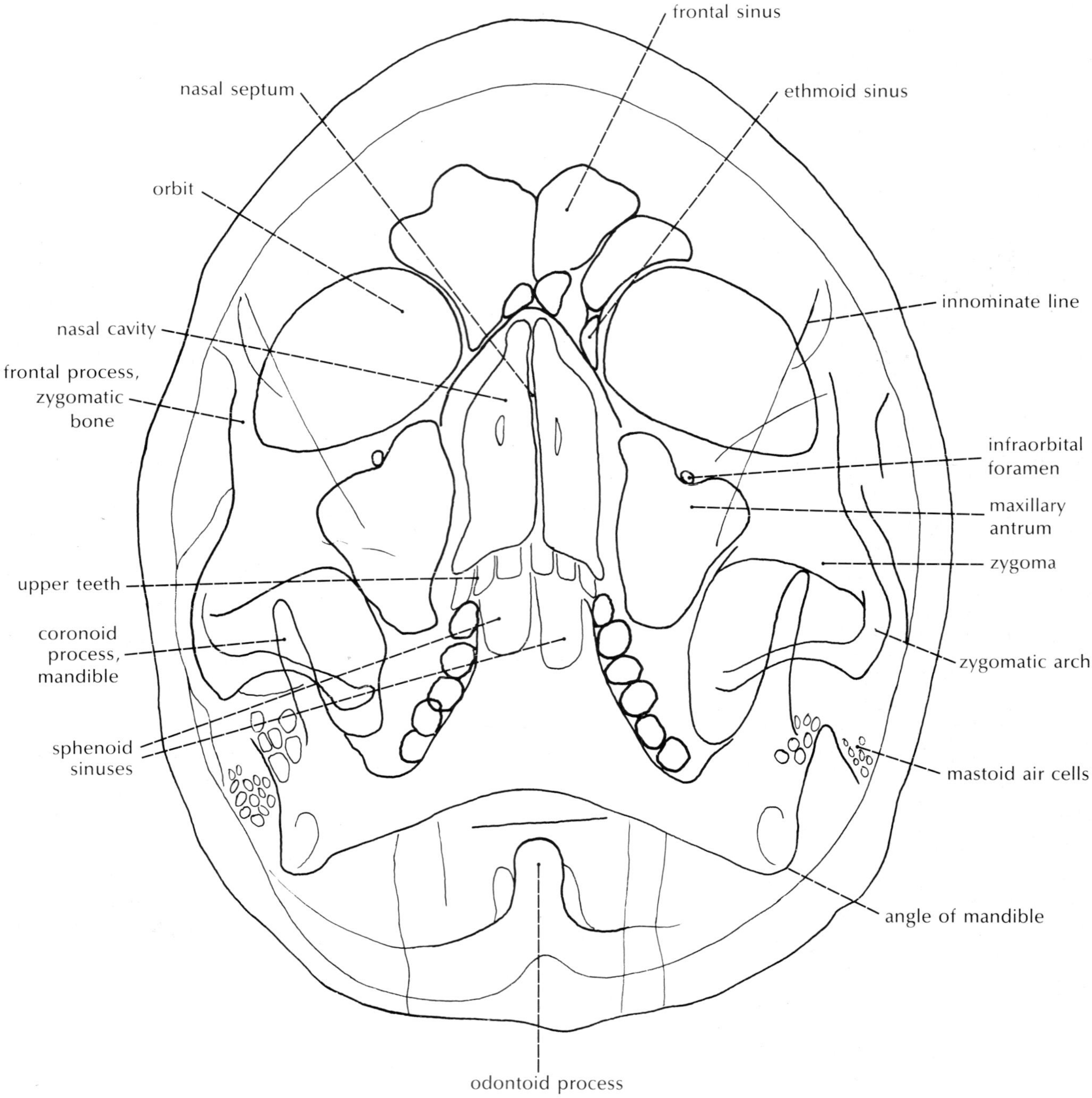
frontal sinus
nasal septum
ethmoid sinus
orbit
innominate line
nasal cavity
frontal process, zygomatic bone
infraorbital foramen
maxillary antrum
zygoma
upper teeth
coronoid process, mandible
zygomatic arch
sphenoid sinuses
mastoid air cells
angle of mandible
odontoid process

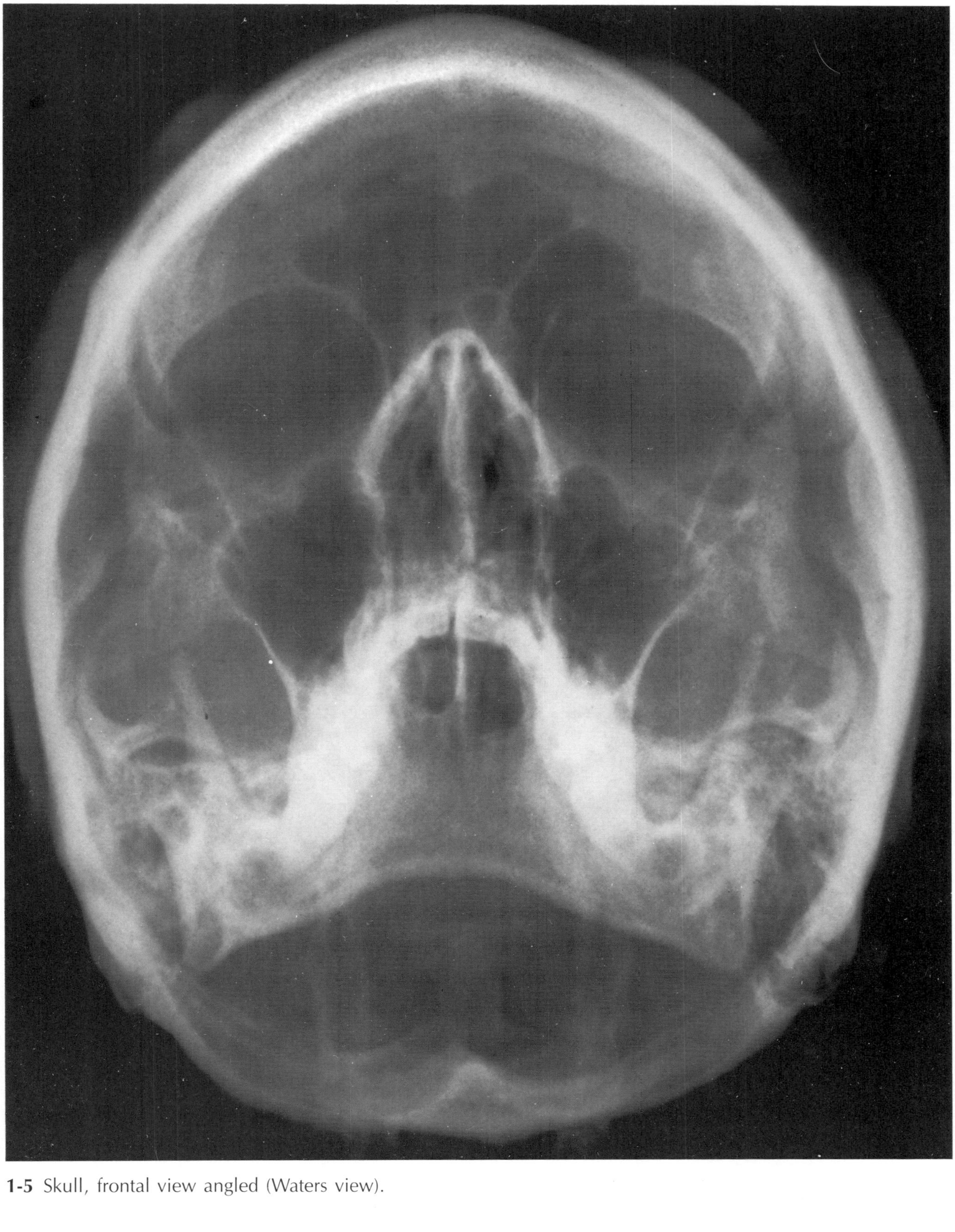

1-5 Skull, frontal view angled (Waters view).

1/Skull Base, Sagittal Scout and Axial CT

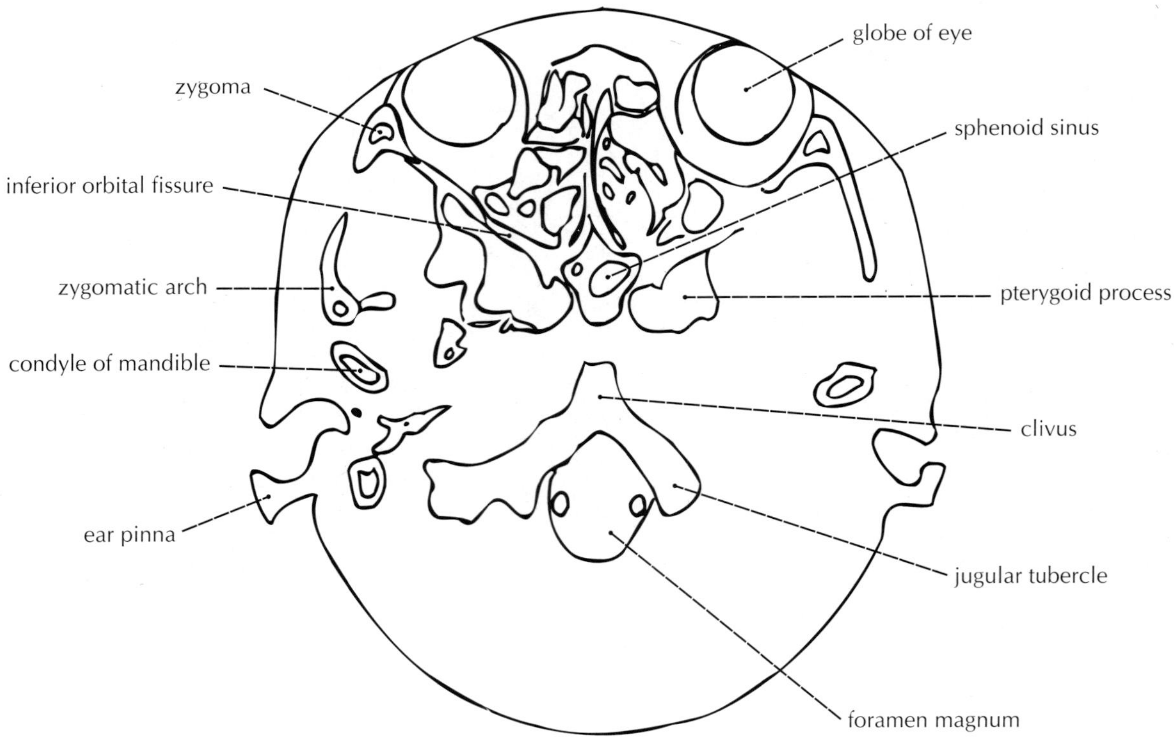

1/Skull Base, Sagittal Scout and Axial CT

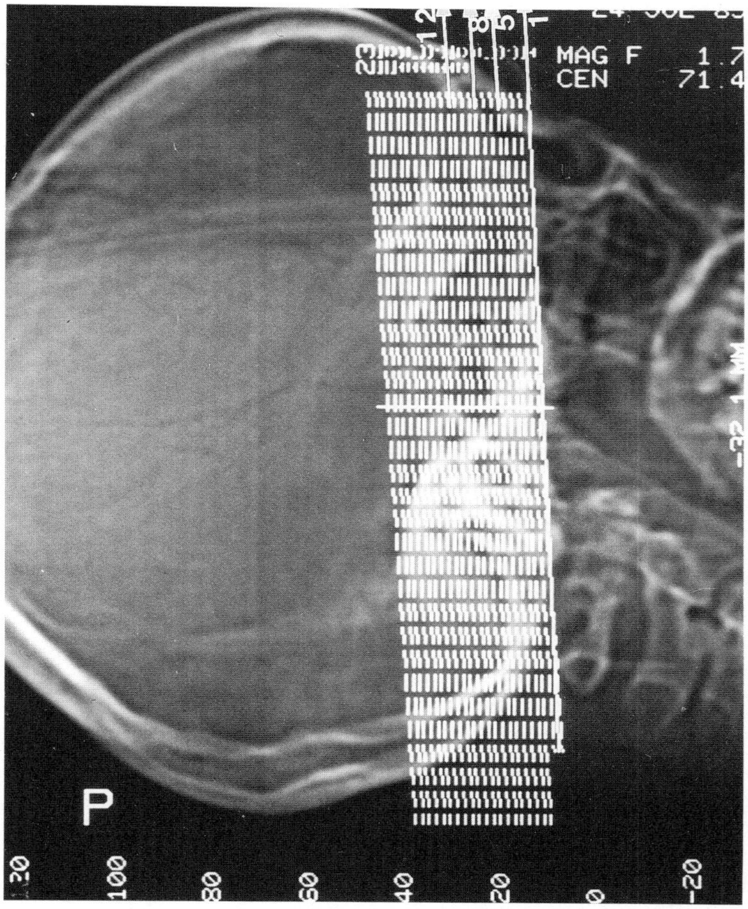

1-6 A sagittal scout CT scan used for demonstrating the location of selected axial CT scans of the skull base.

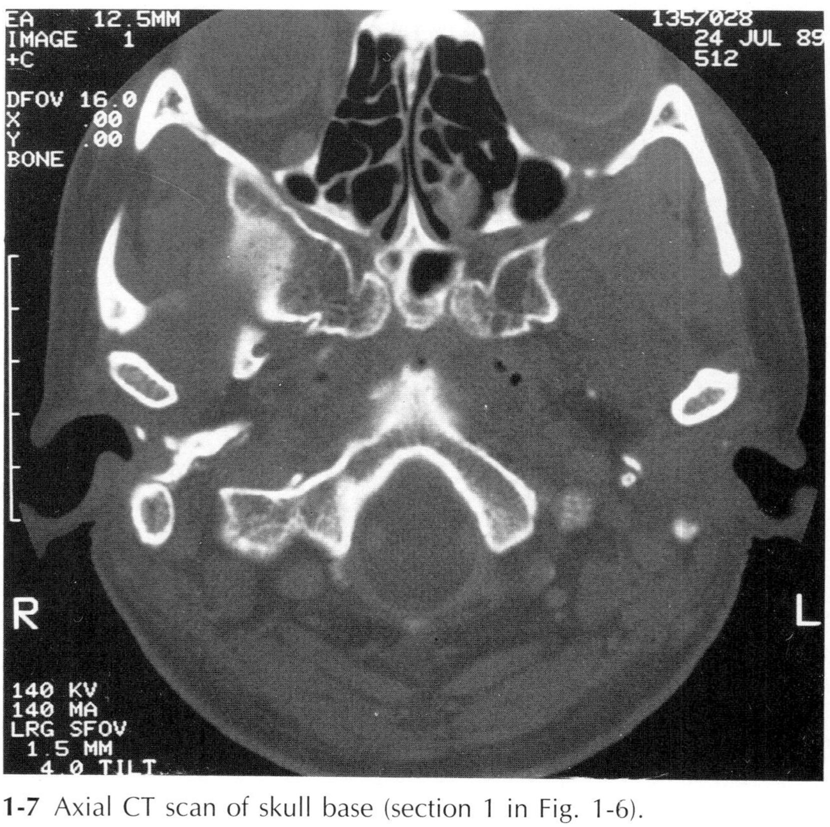

1-7 Axial CT scan of skull base (section 1 in Fig. 1-6).

1/Skull Base, Axial CT

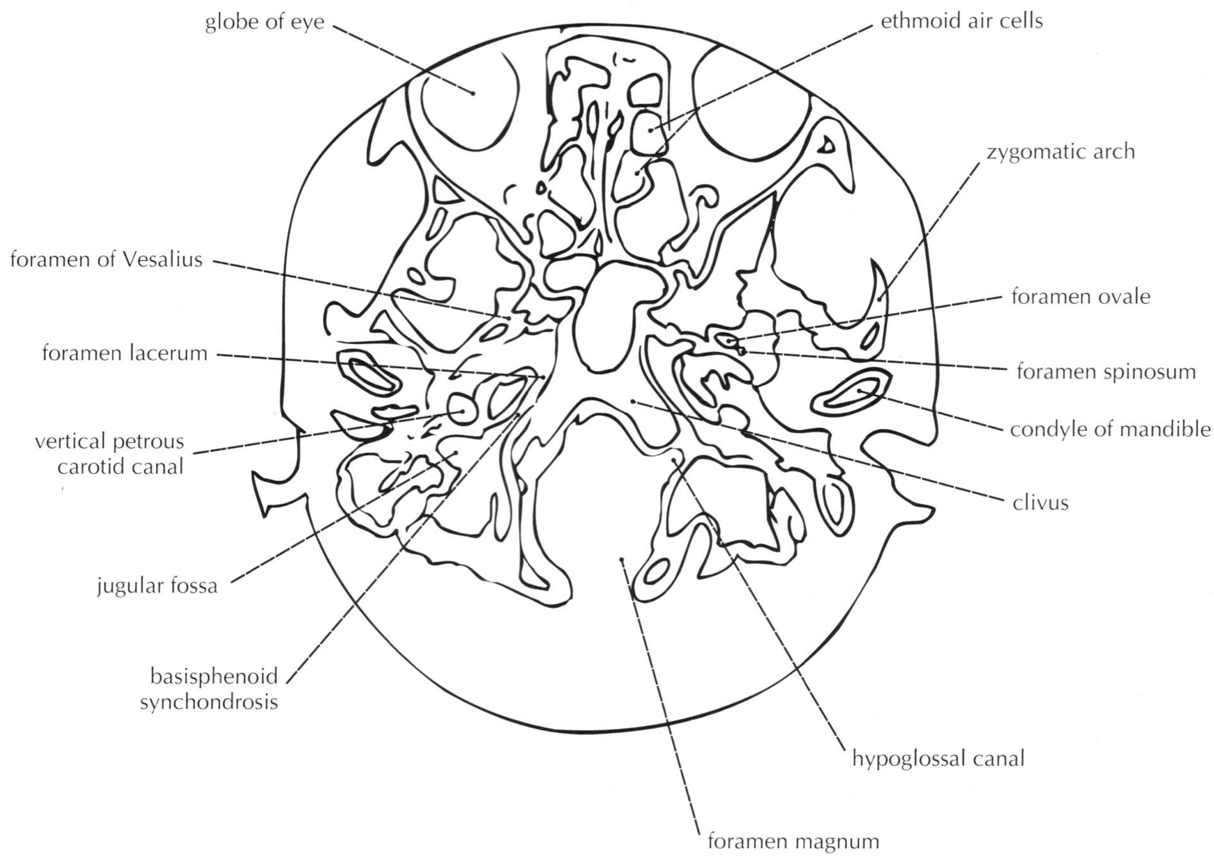

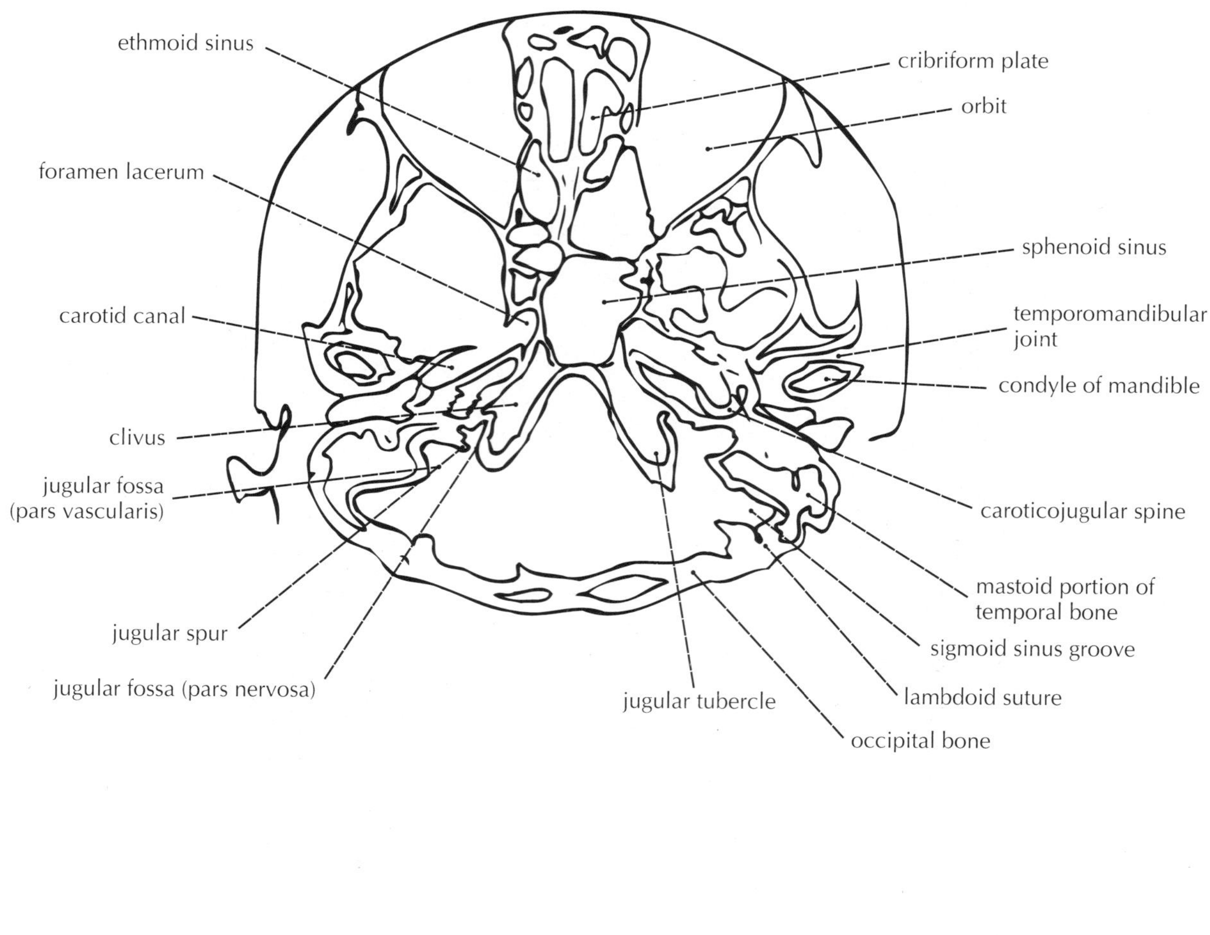

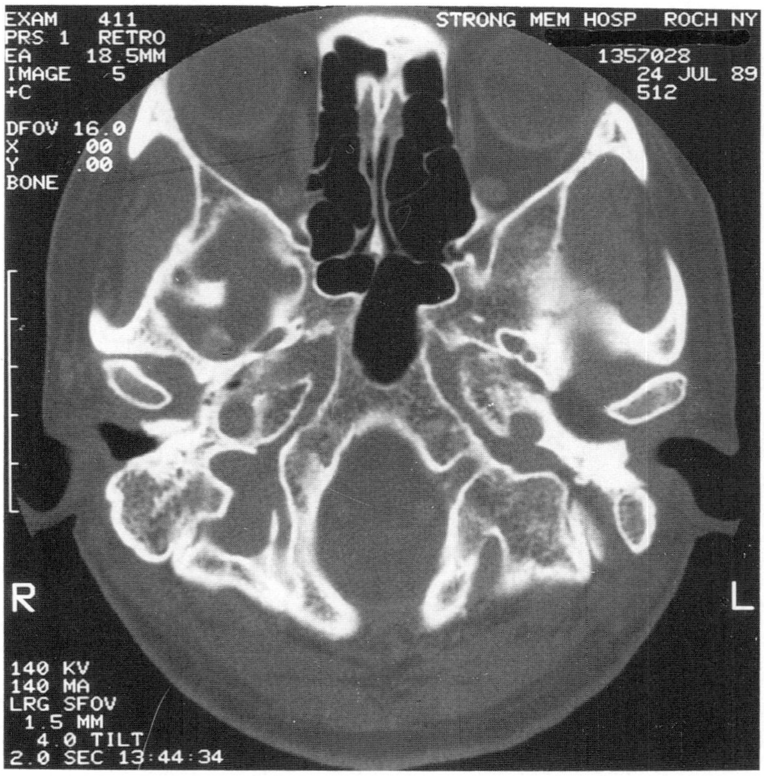

1-8 Axial CT scan of skull base (section 5 in Fig. 1-6).

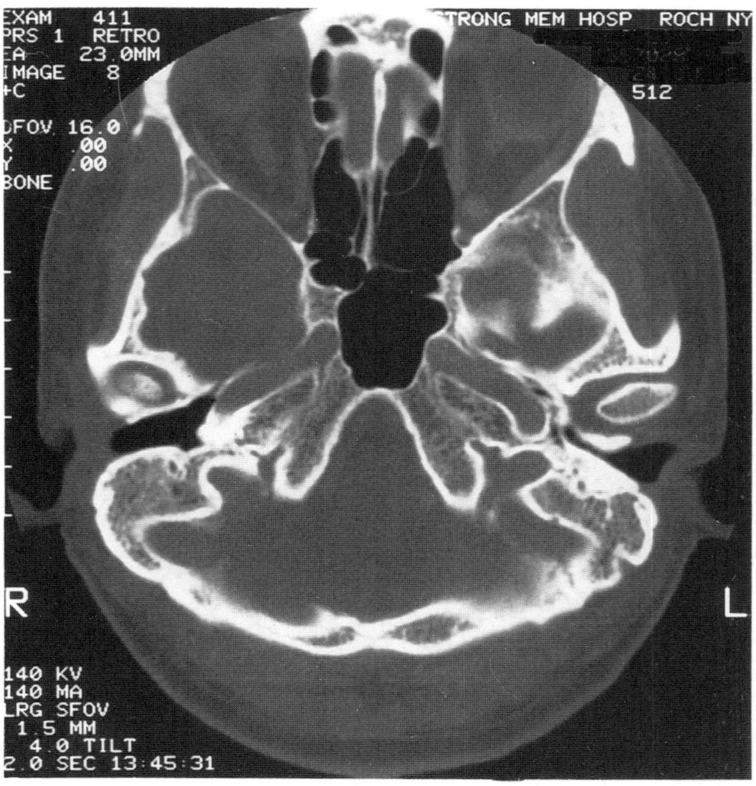

1-9 Axial CT scan of skull base (section 8 in Fig. 1-6).

1/Skull Base, Axial CT

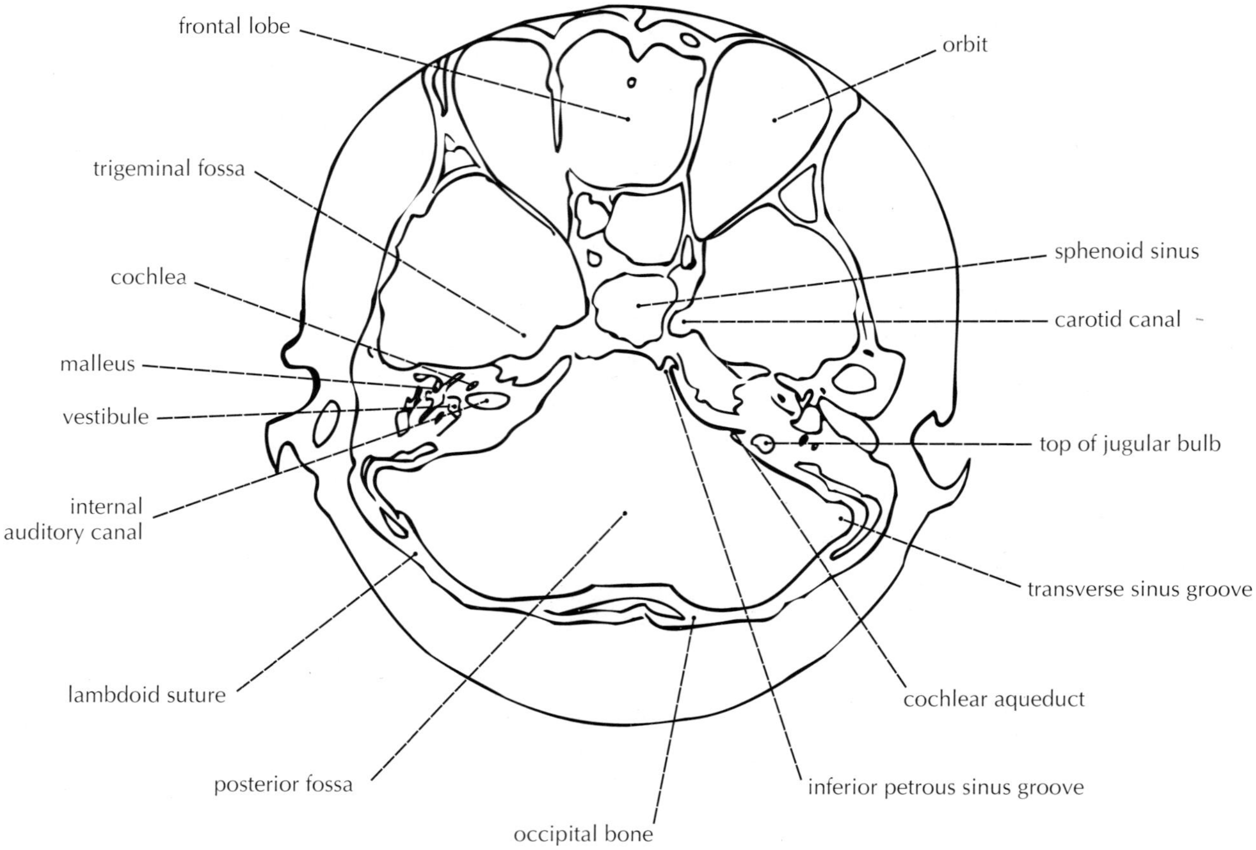

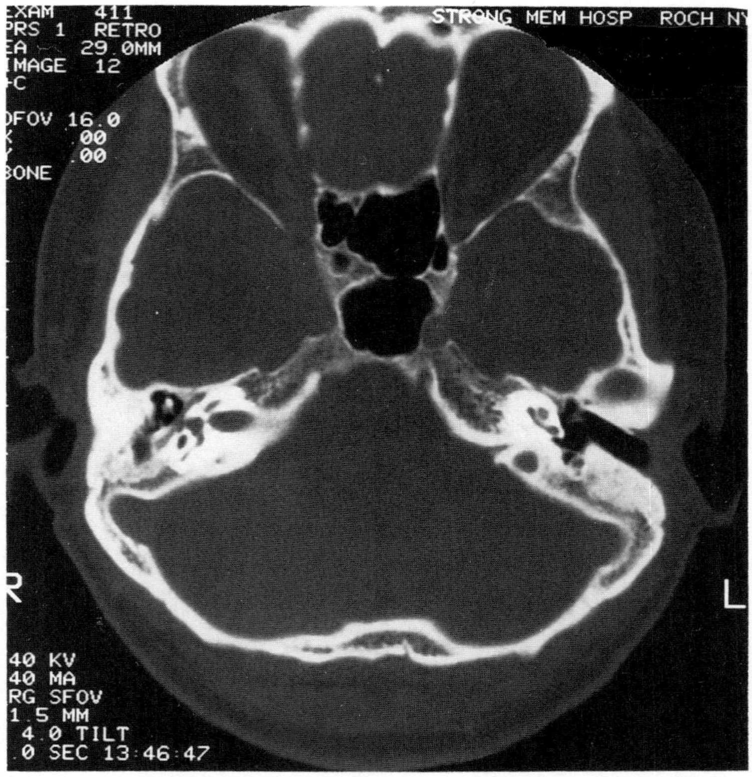

1-10 Axial CT scan of skull base (section 12 in Fig. 1-6).

1/Skull Base, Sagittal Scout and Coronal CT

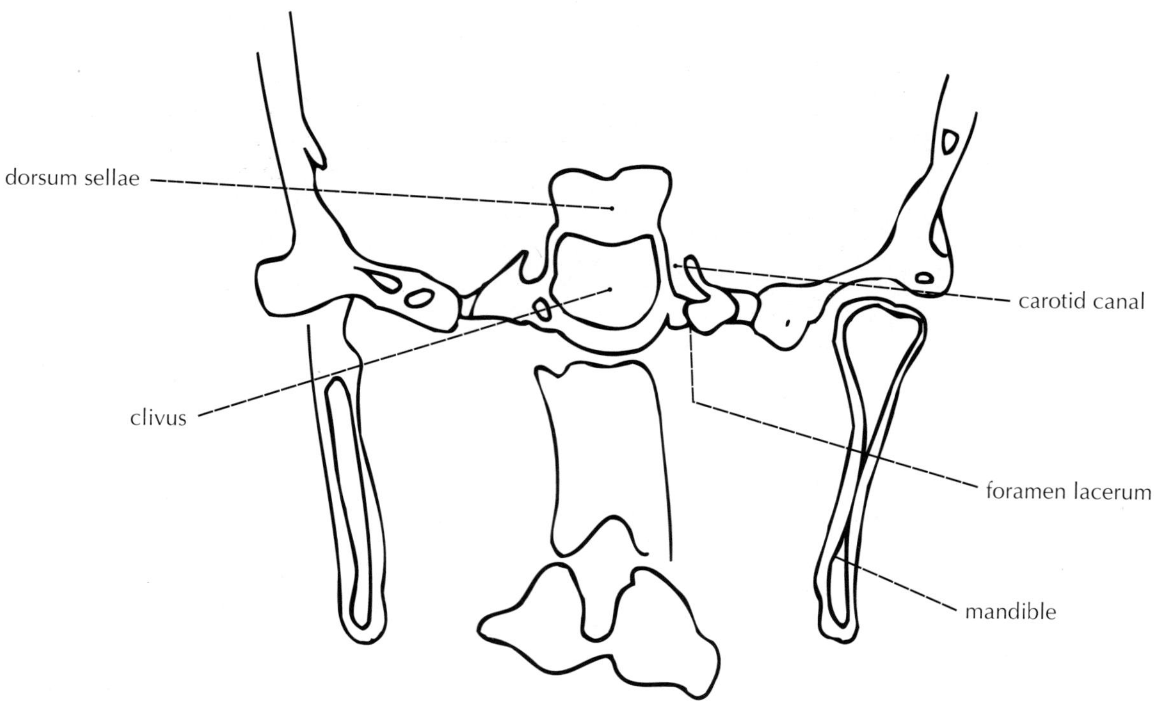

1/Skull Base, Sagittal Scout and Coronal CT

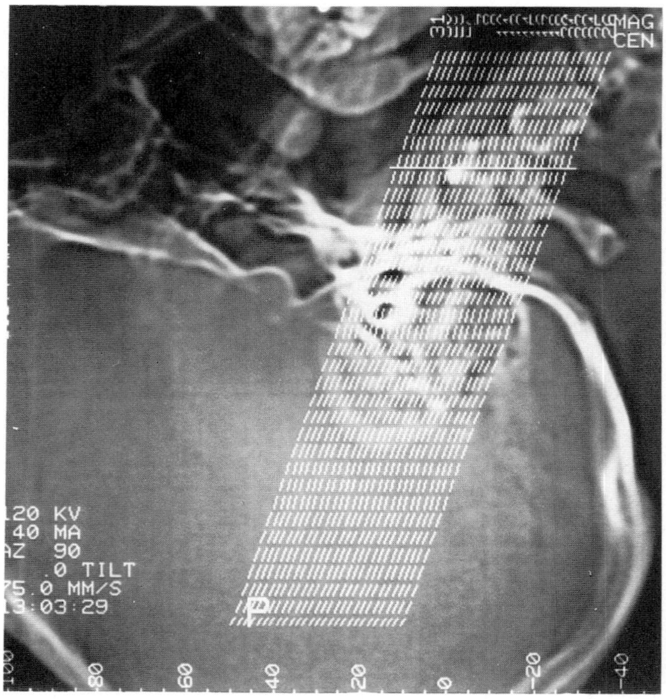

1-11 A sagittal scout CT scan used for demonstrating the orientation of selected coronal CT scans of the skull base.

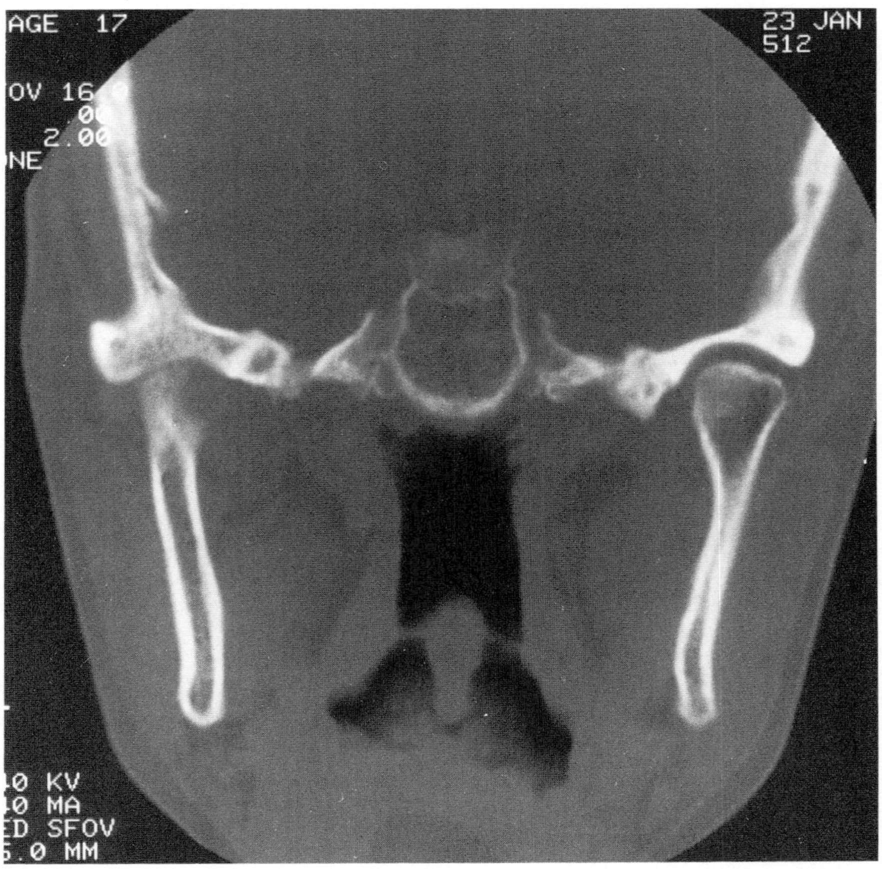

1-12 Coronal CT scan through skull base. This image is located anterior to section 31 in Fig. 1-11.

1/Skull Base, Coronal CT

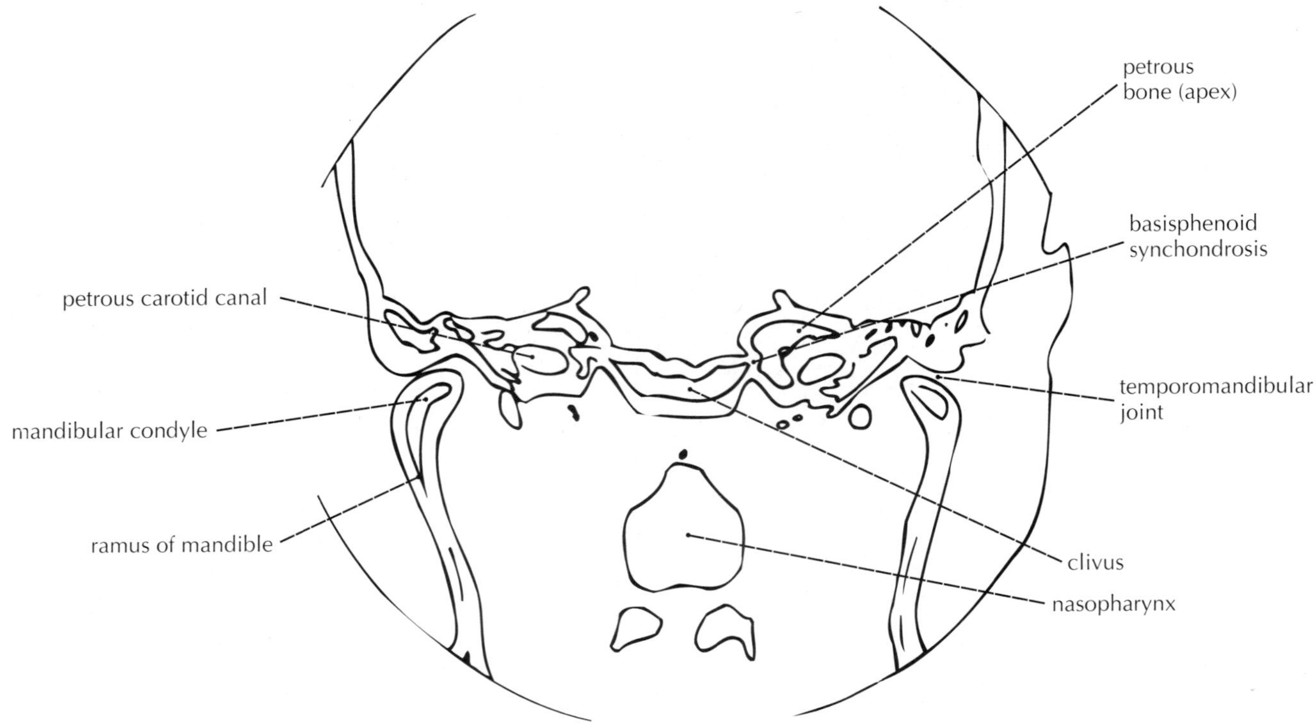

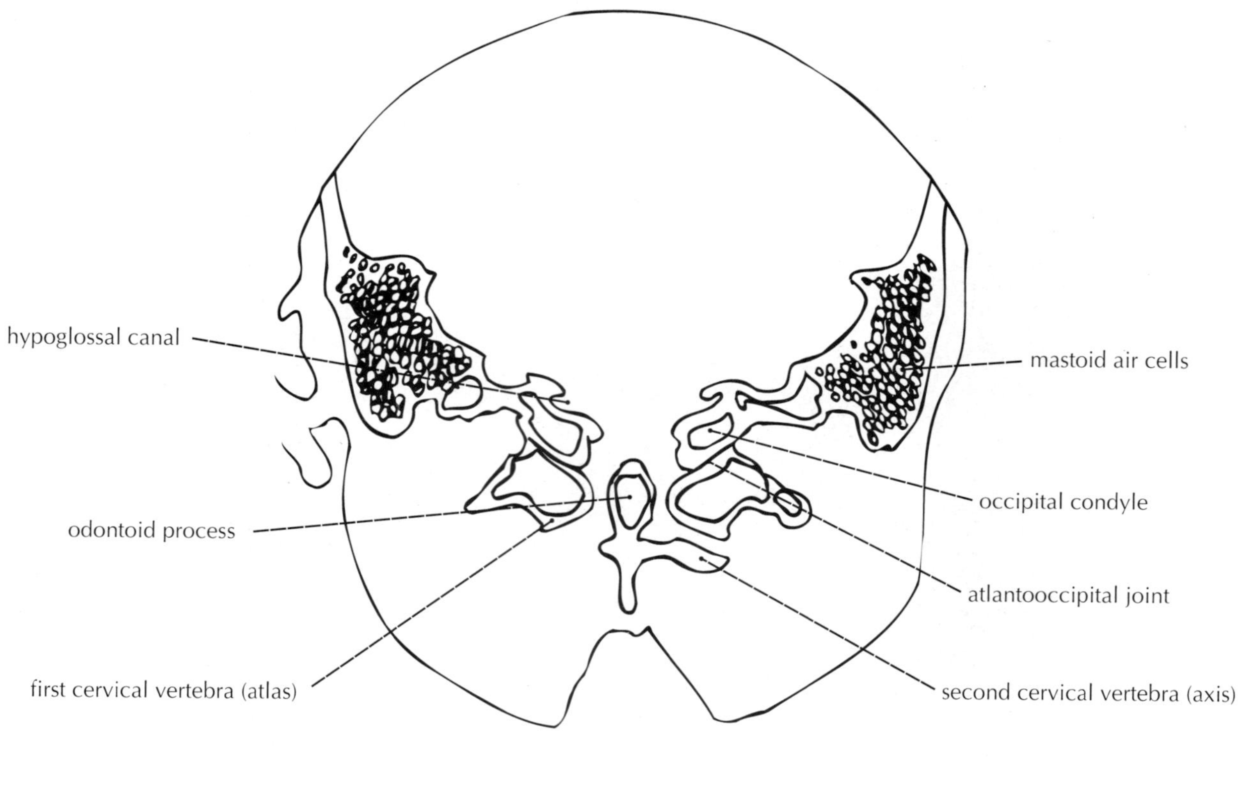

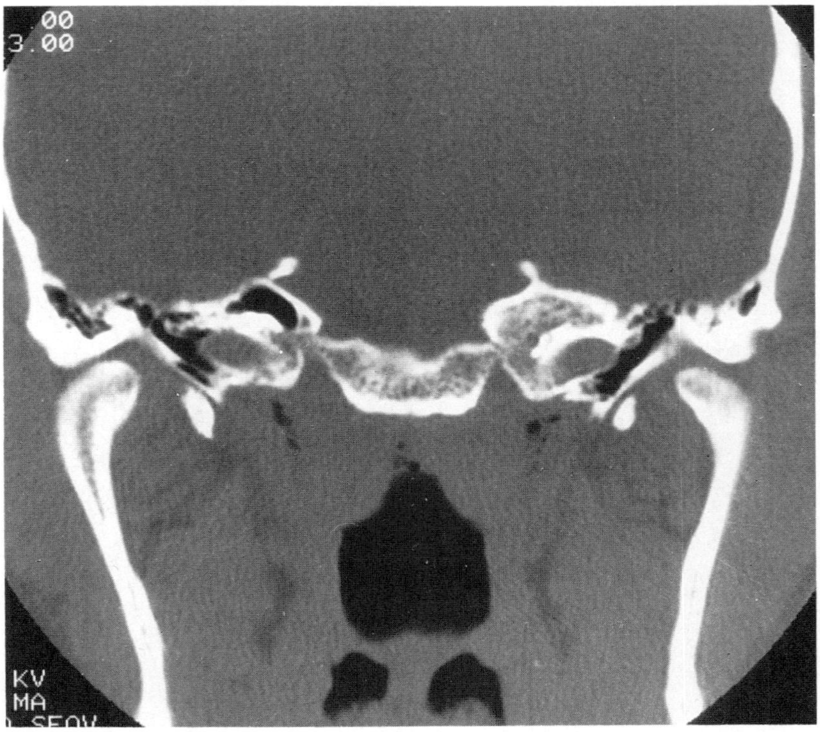

1-13 Coronal CT scan through skull base (section 30 in Fig. 1-11).

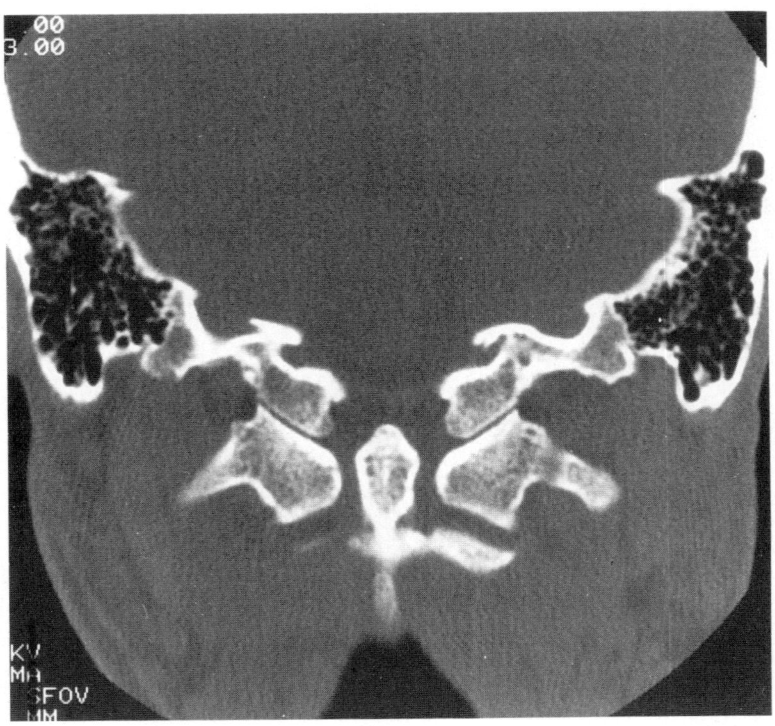

1-14 Coronal CT scan through skull base (section 17 in Fig. 1-11).

1/Skull Base, Coronal CT

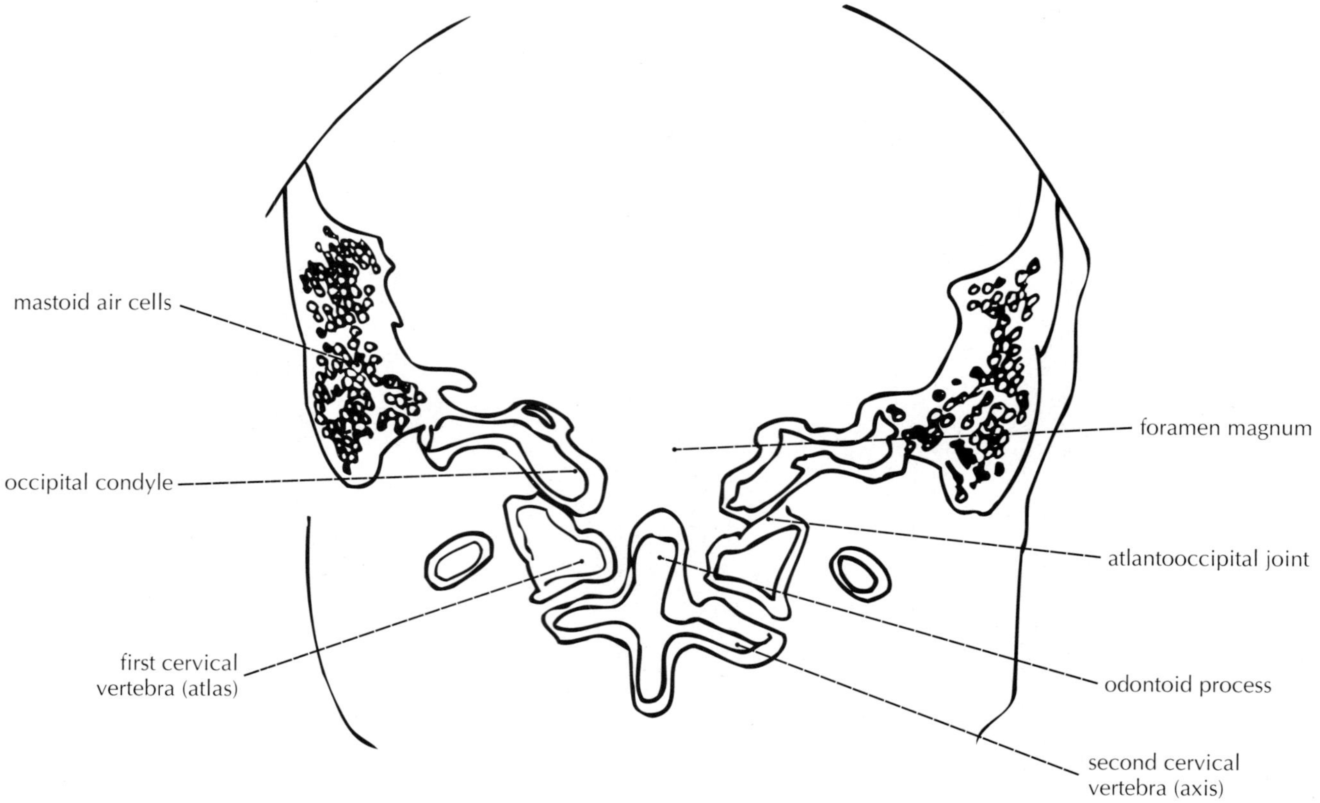

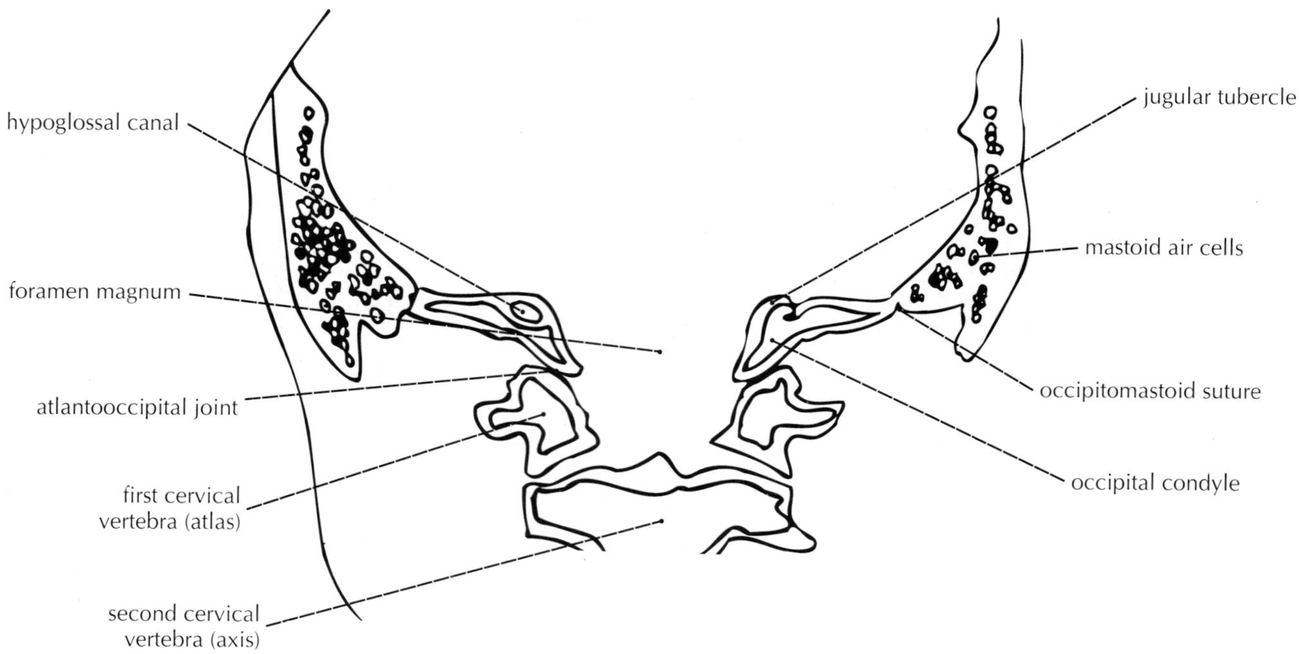

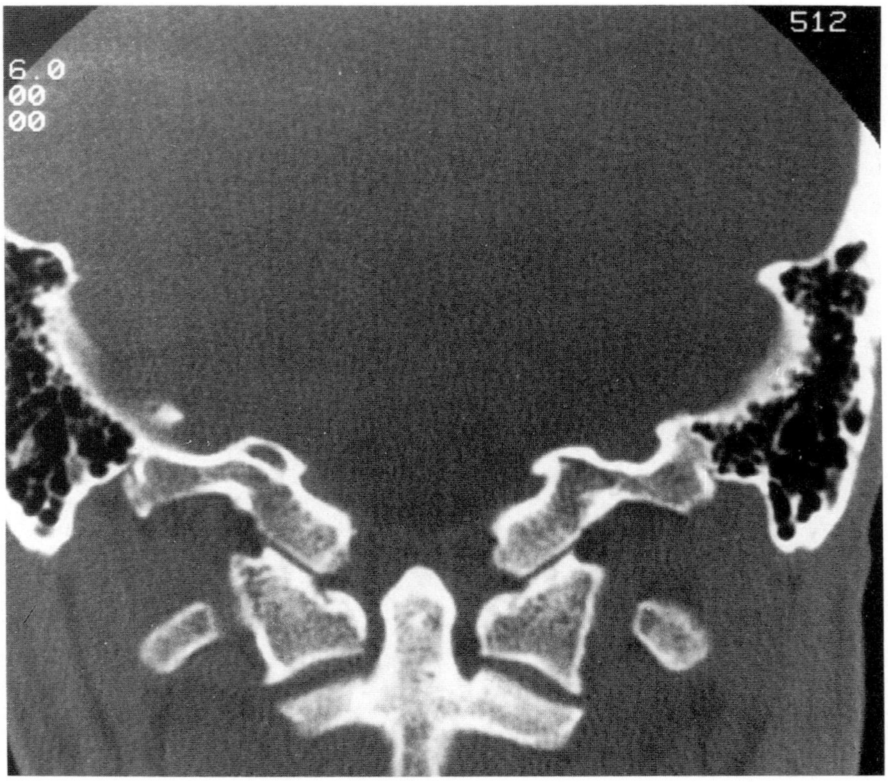

1-15 Coronal CT scan through skull base (section 19 in Fig. 1-11).

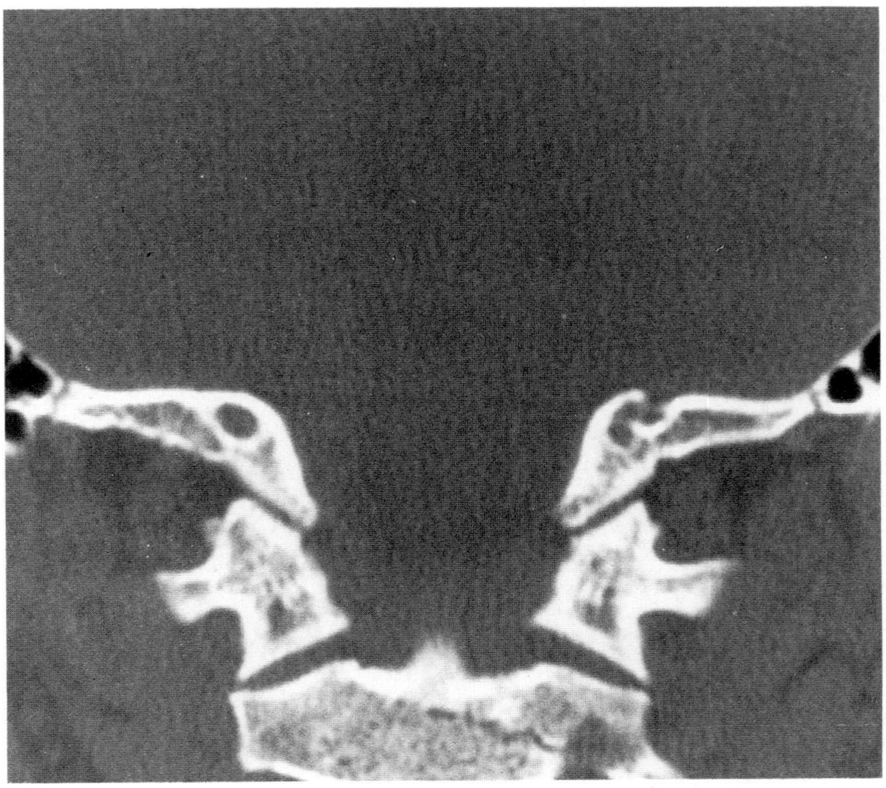

1-16 Coronal CT scan through skull base at foramen magnum (section 24 in Fig. 1-11).

1/Paranasal Sinuses and Facial Area, Scout and Axial CT

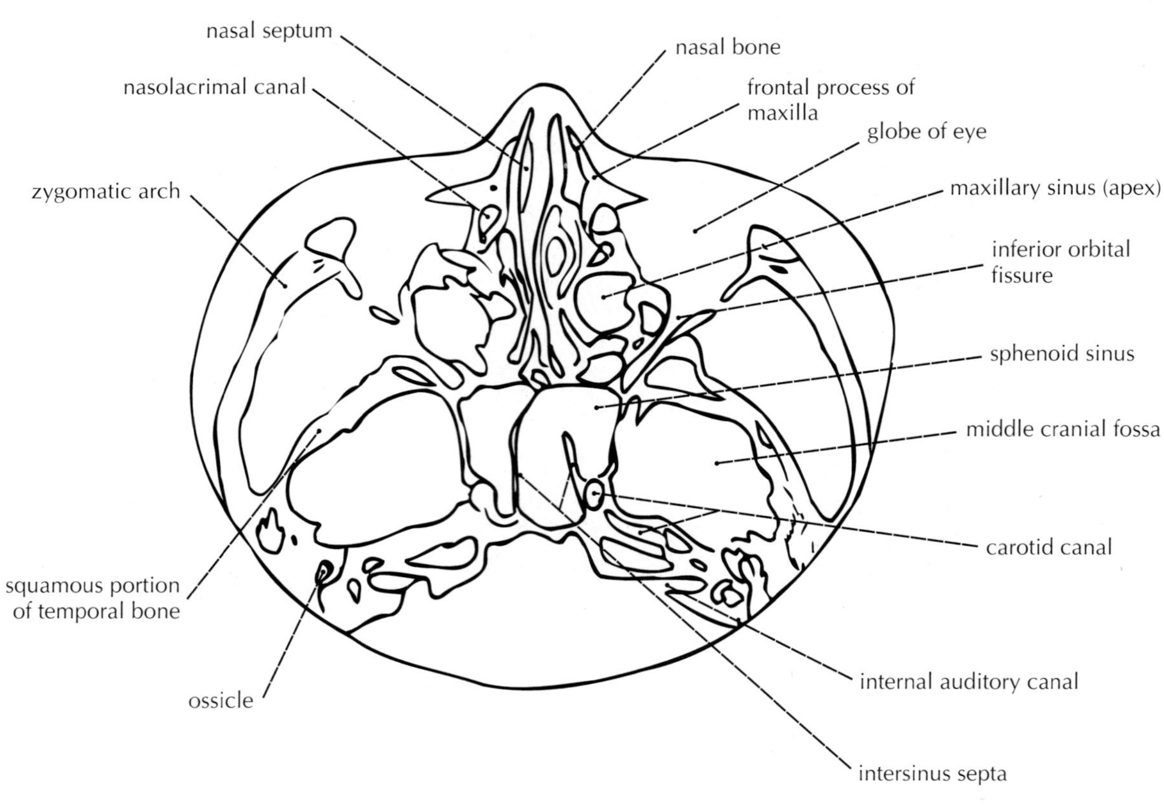

1/Paranasal Sinuses and Facial Area, Scout and Axial CT

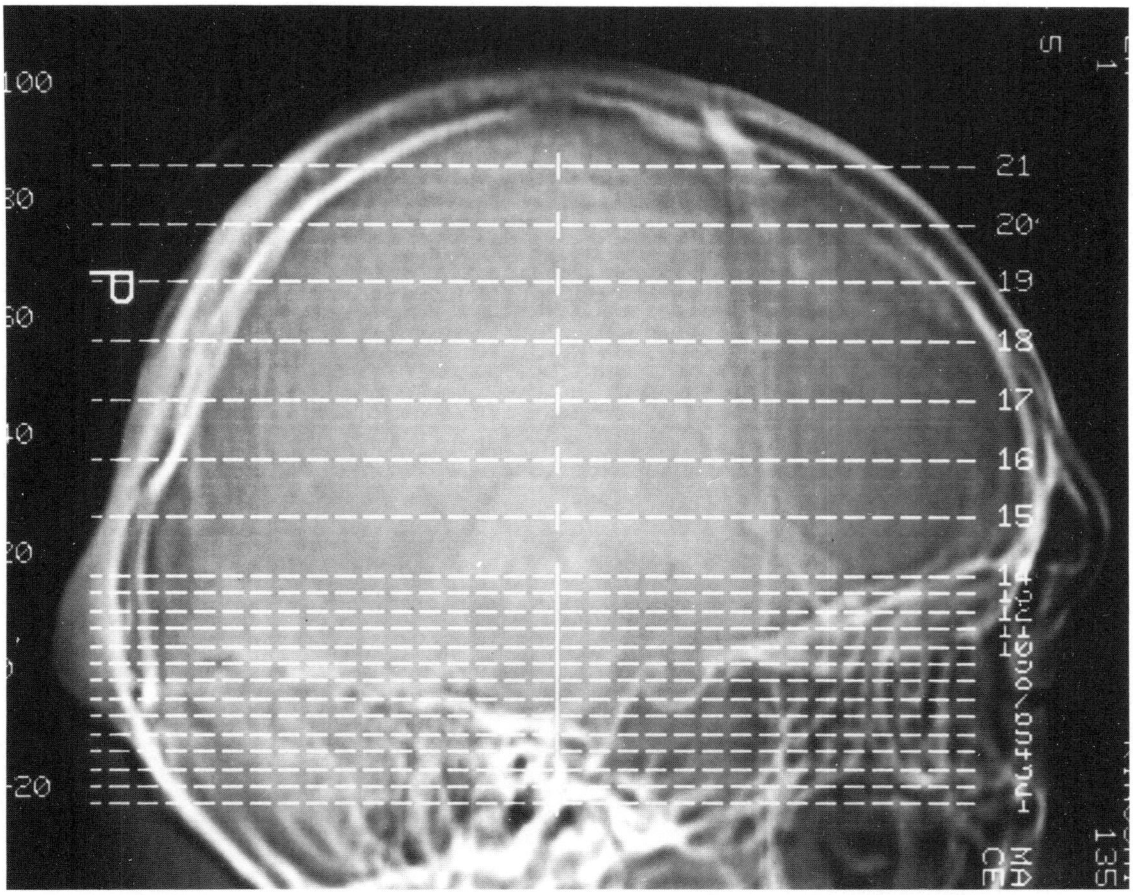

1-17 Sagittal scout CT scan of the head used to demonstrate the location of selected axial CT scans of the paranasal sinuses and facial area.

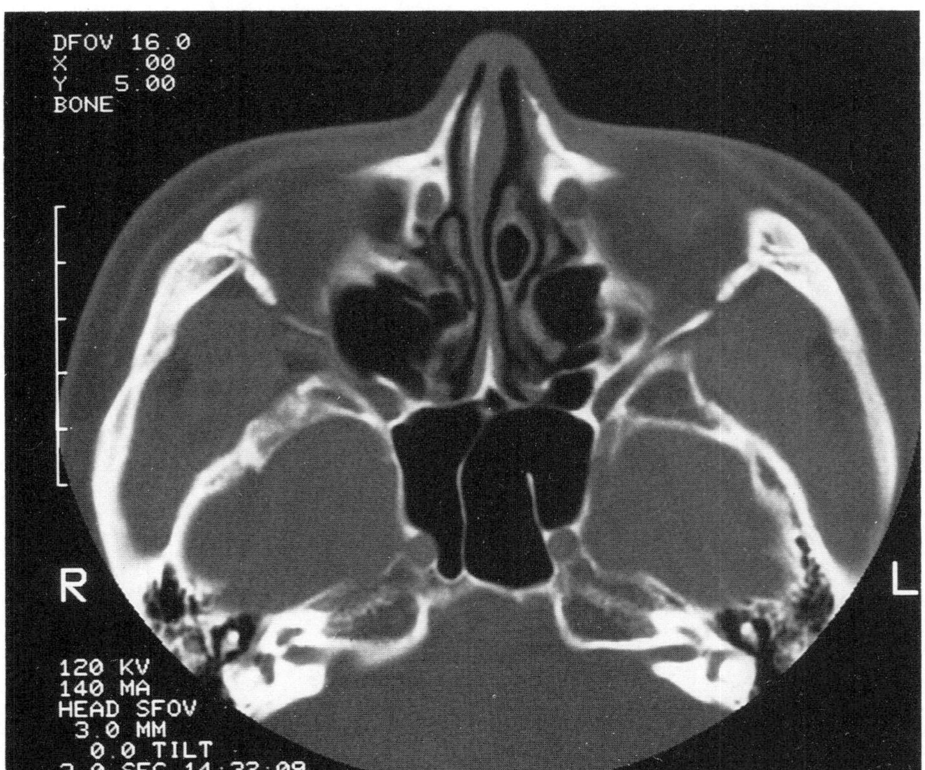

1-18 Axial facial CT scan (inferior orbit, bone window). Section 3 in Fig. 1-17.

1/Paranasal Sinuses and Facial Area, Axial CT

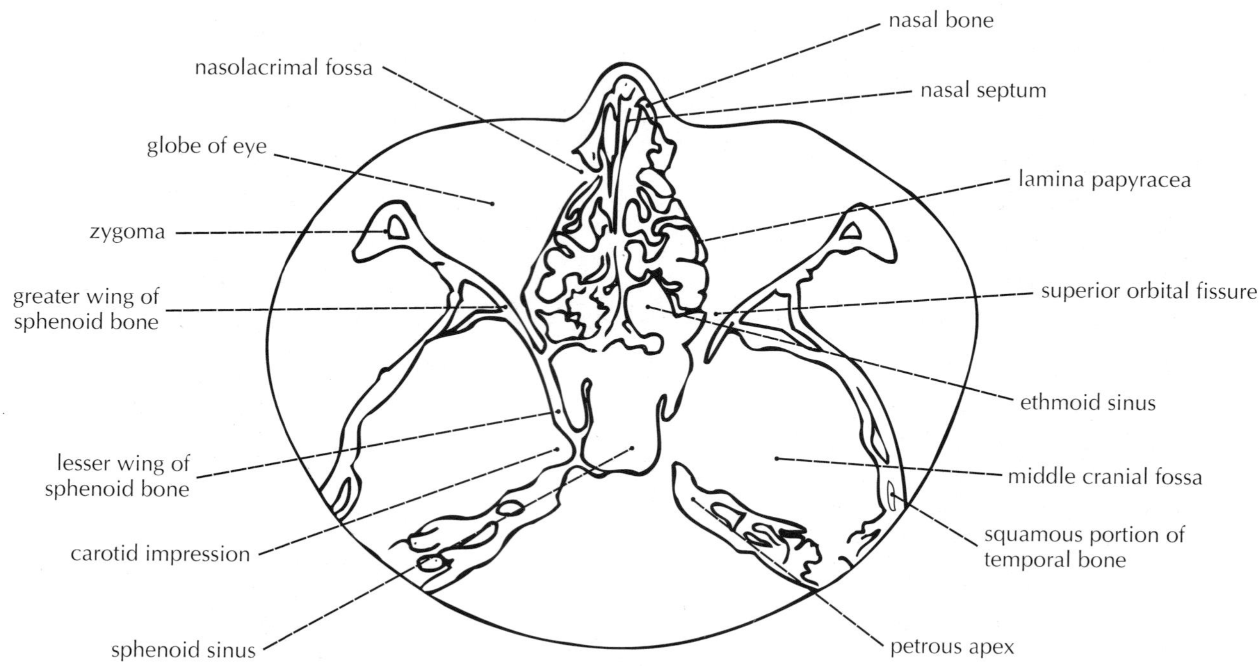

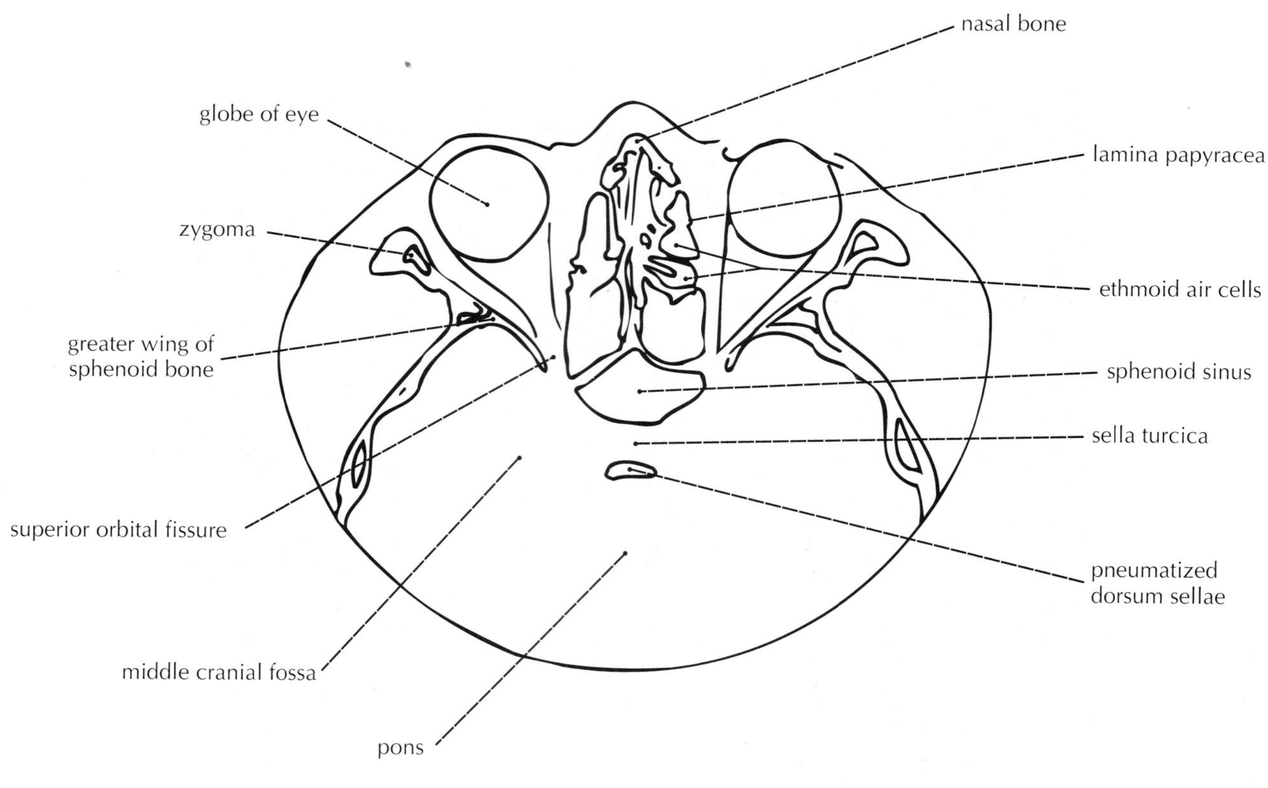

1/Paranasal Sinuses and Facial Area, Axial CT

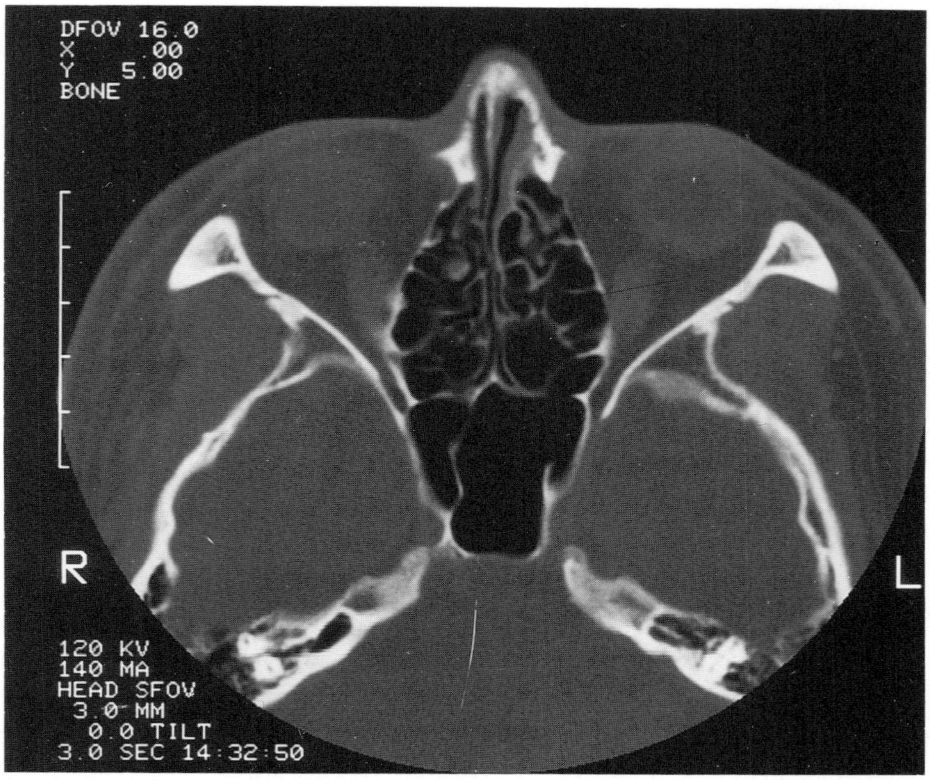

1-19 Axial facial CT scan (inferior orbit, bone window). Section 5 in Fig. 1-17.

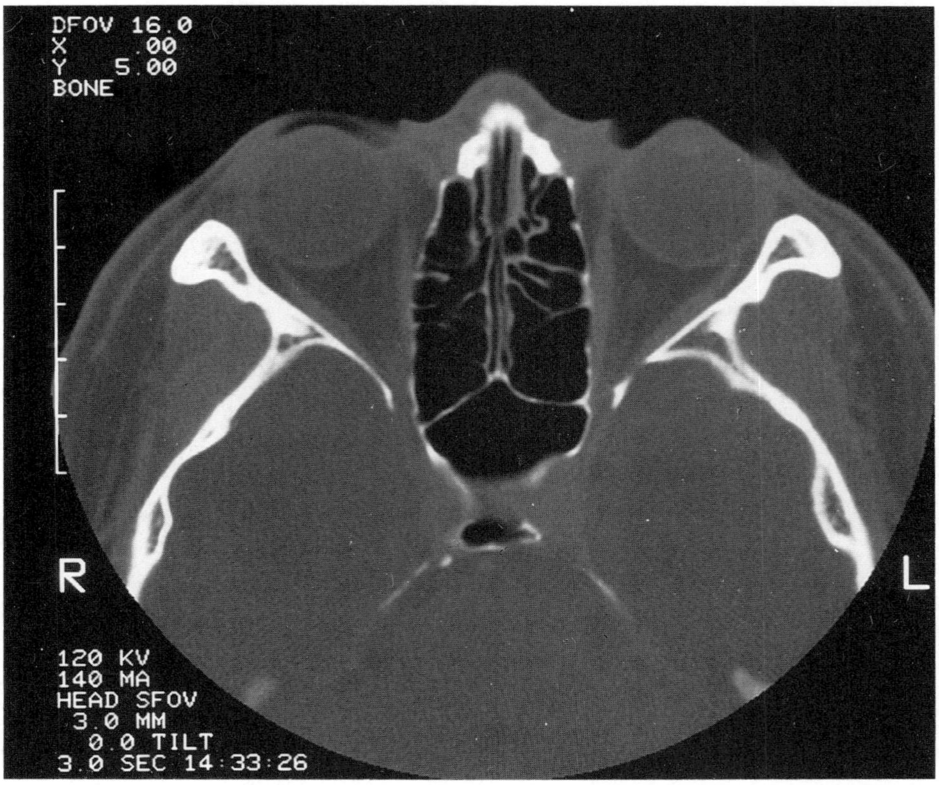

1-20 Axial facial CT scan (midorbit, bone window). Section 7 in Fig. 1-17.

1/Paranasal Sinuses and Facial Area, Axial CT

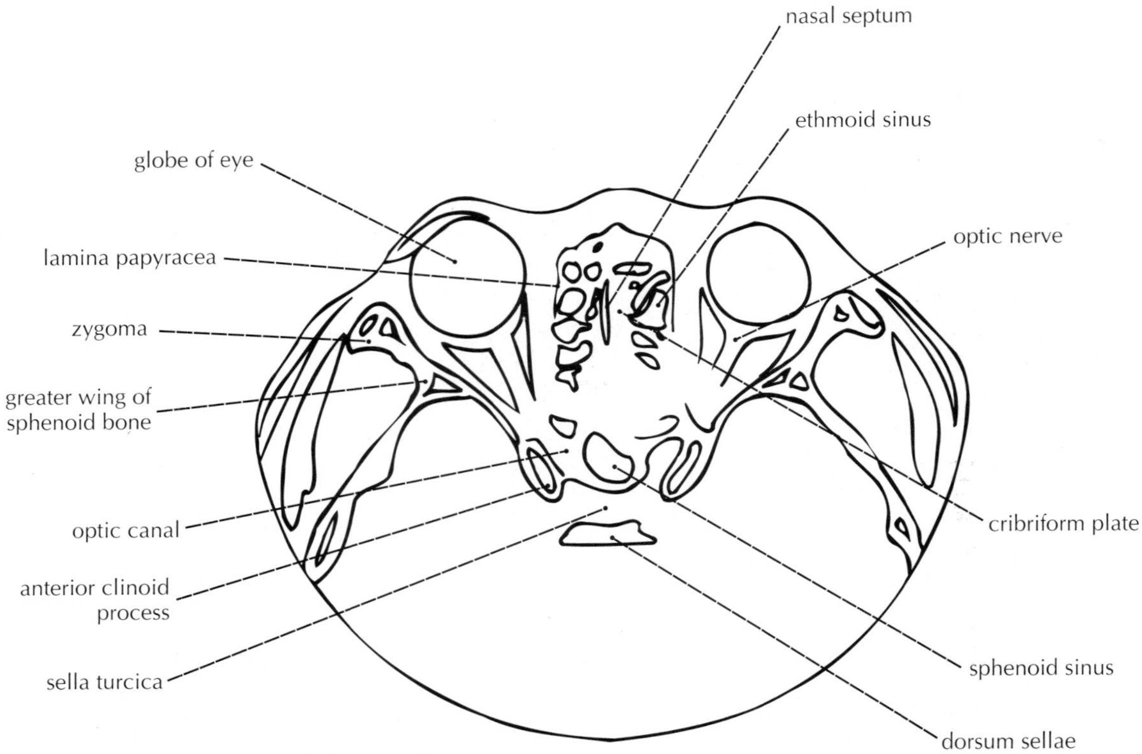

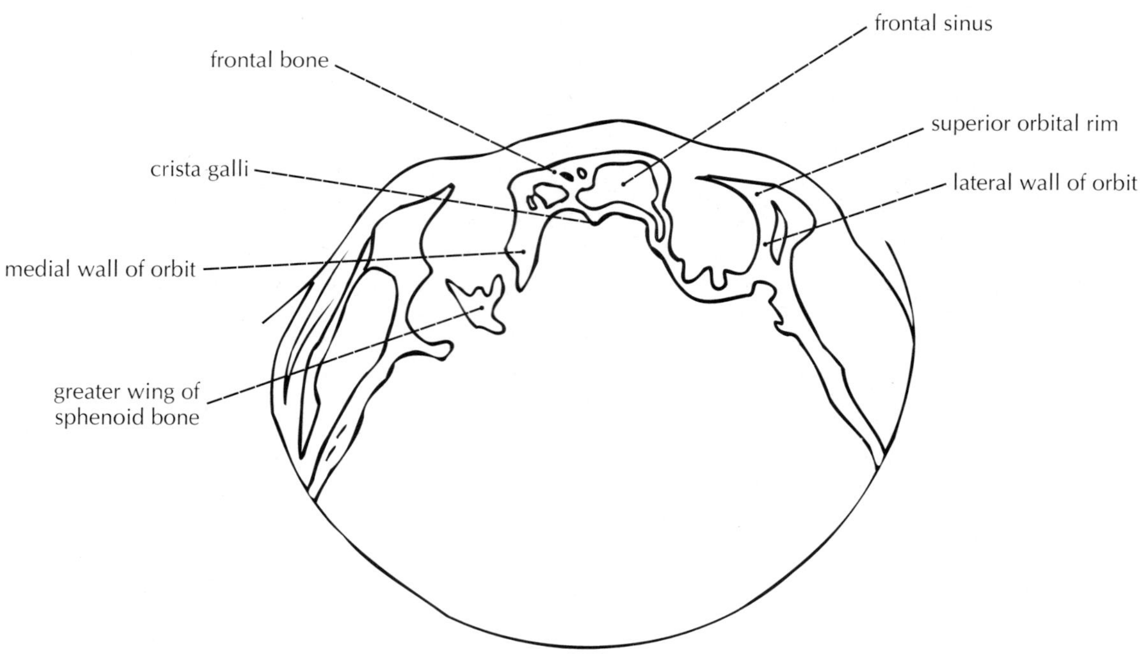

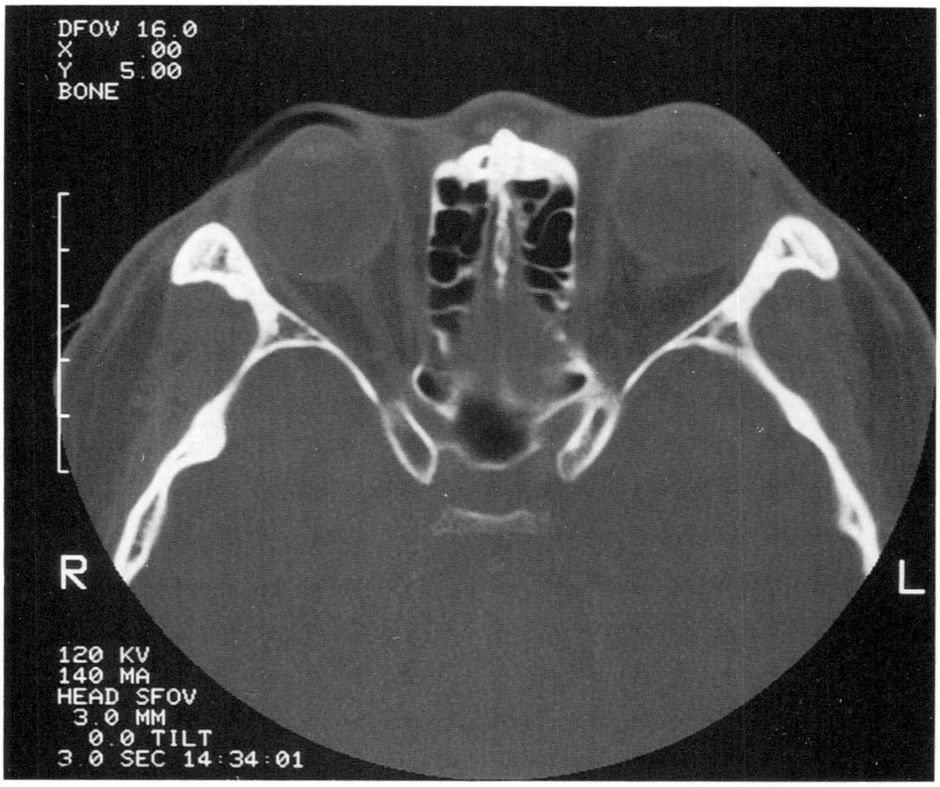

1-21 Axial facial CT scan (midorbit, bone window). Section 8 in Fig. 1-17.

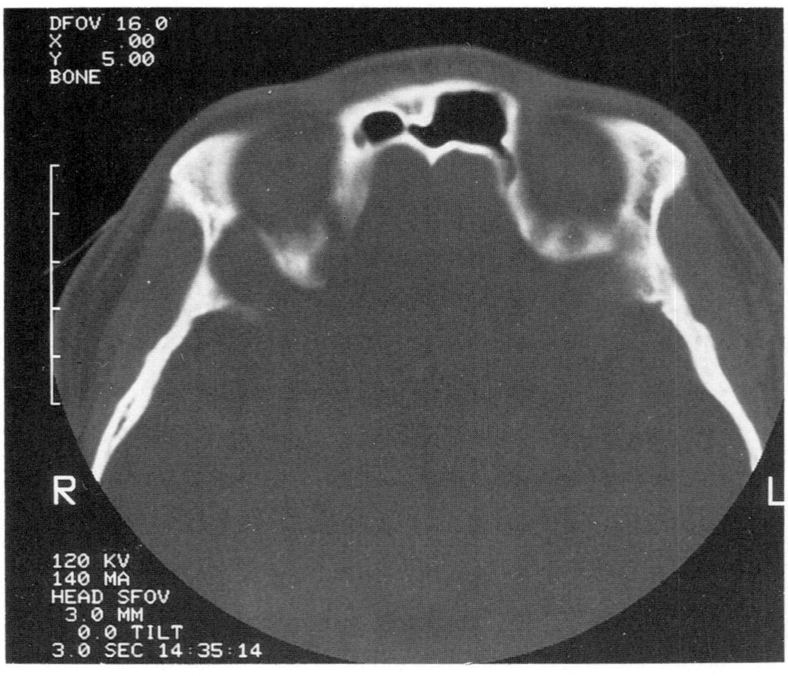

1-22 Axial facial CT scan (superior orbit, bone window). Section 12 in Fig. 1-17.

1/Facial Area, Sagittal Scout and Coronal CT

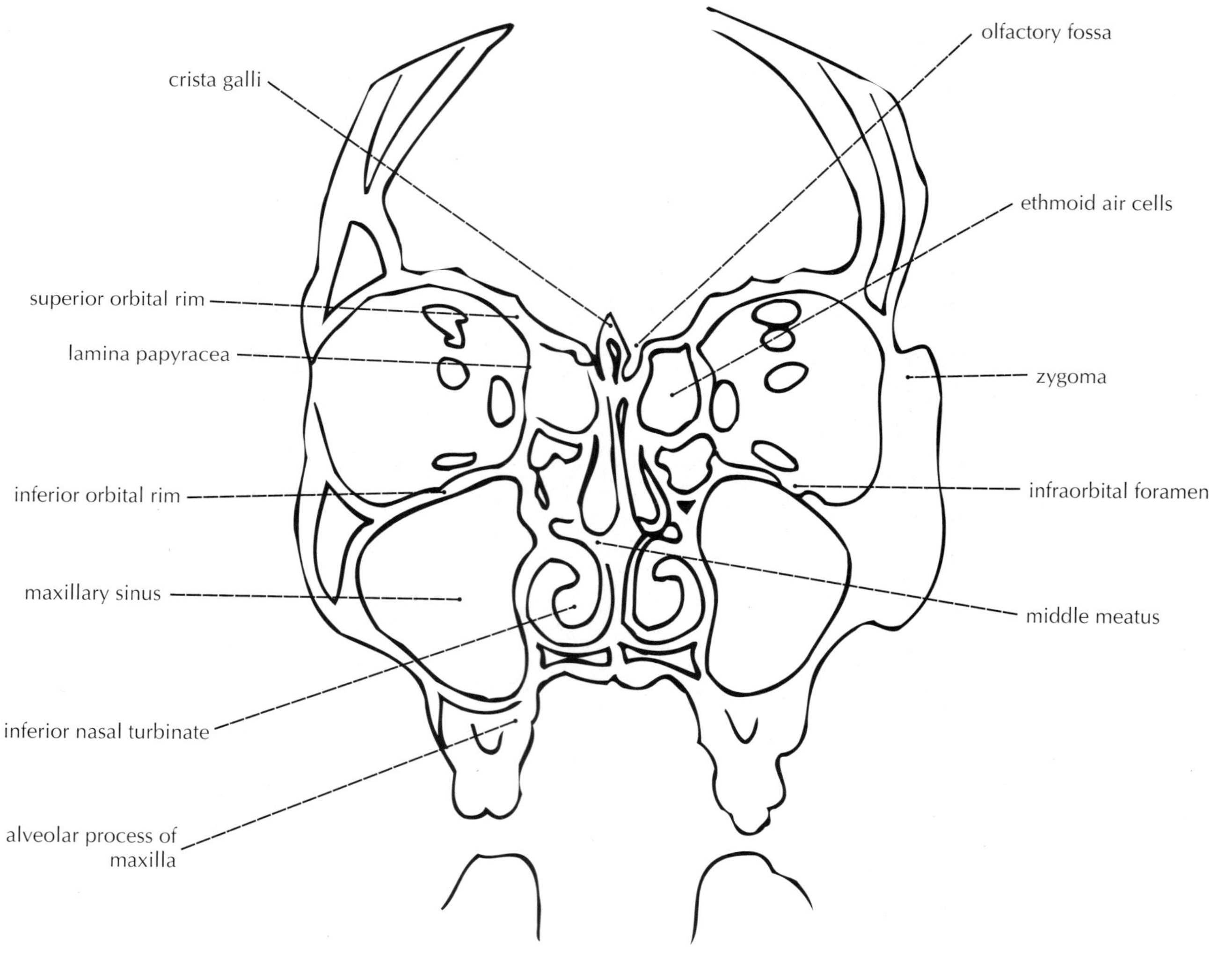

1/Facial Area, Sagittal Scout and Coronal CT

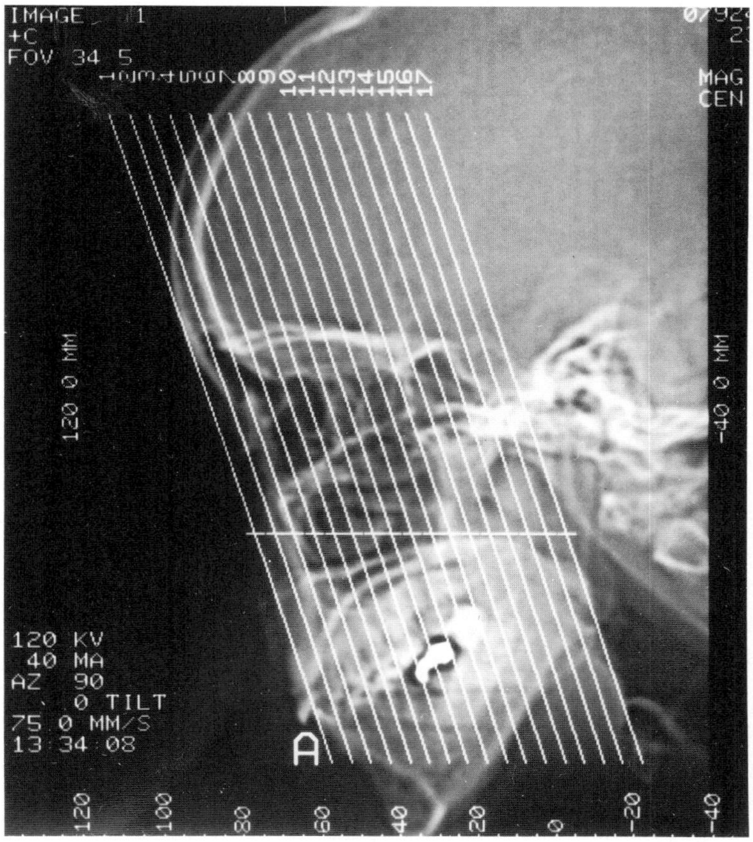

1-23 Sagittal CT scan used for demonstrating the orientation of selected coronal CT scans of the face and orbits.

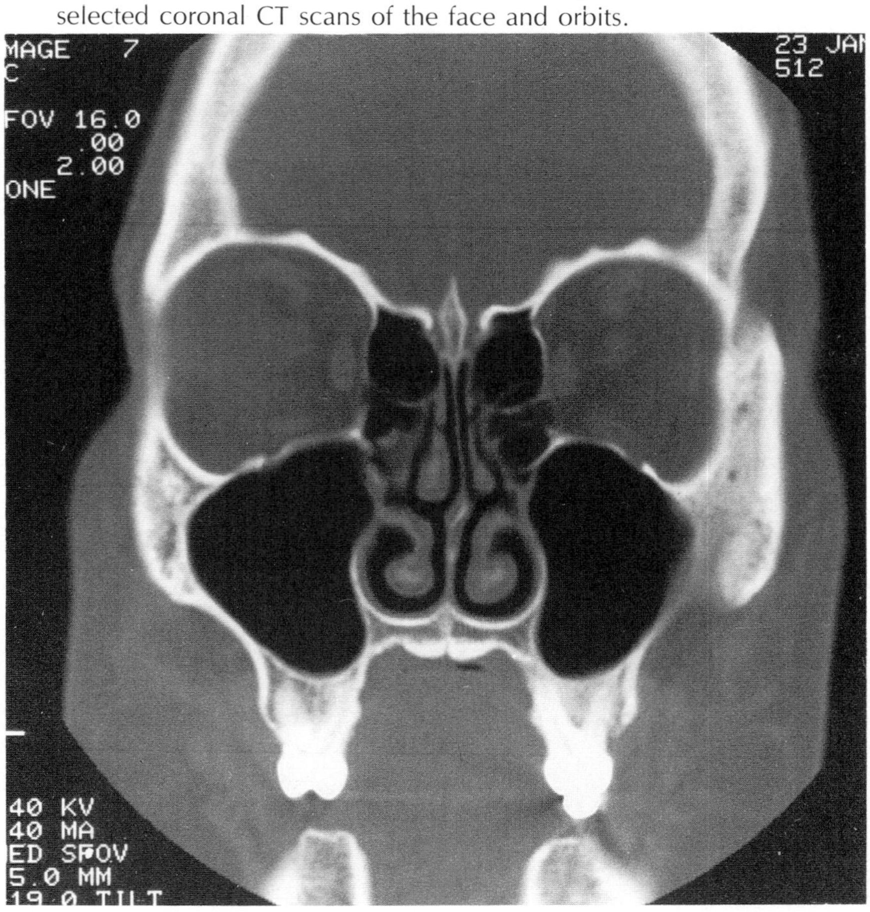

1-24 Coronal CT scan at level of orbits and central nasal cavity (section 7 in Fig. 1-23).

1/Facial Area, Coronal CT and Axial MRI

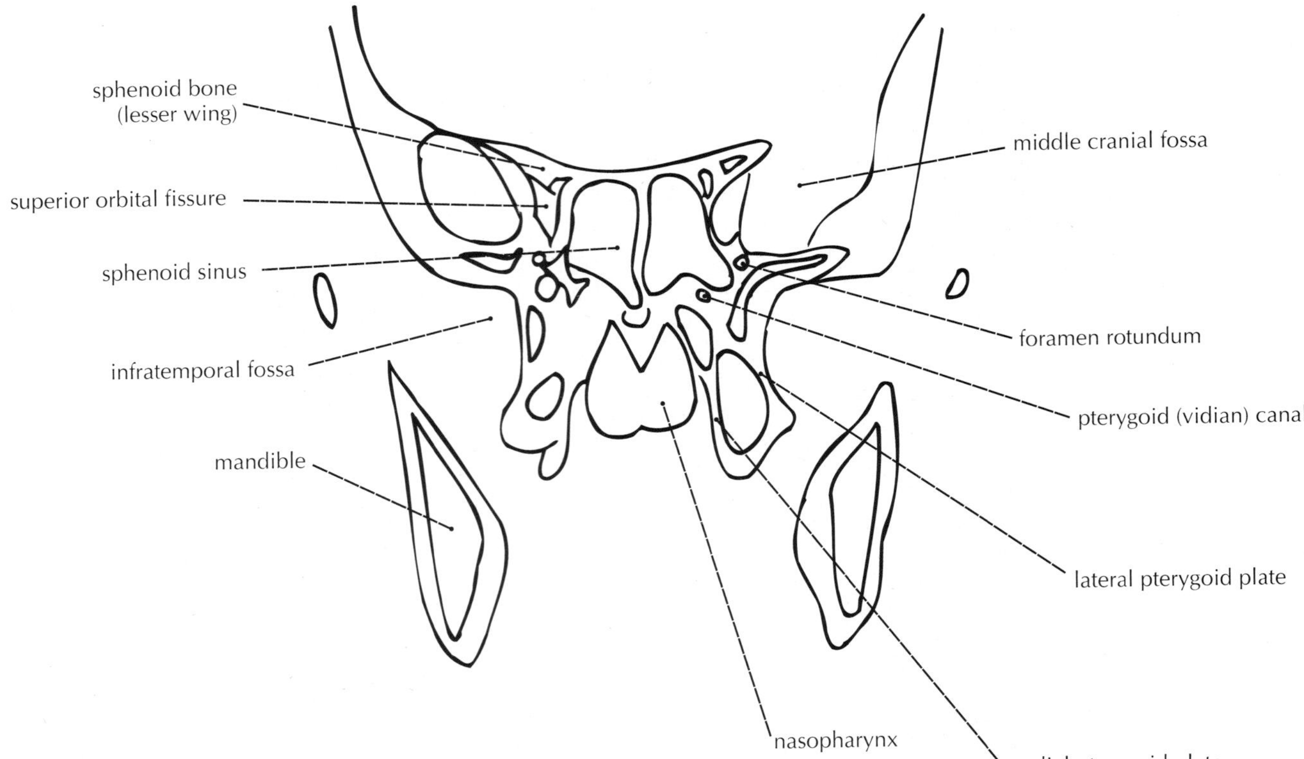

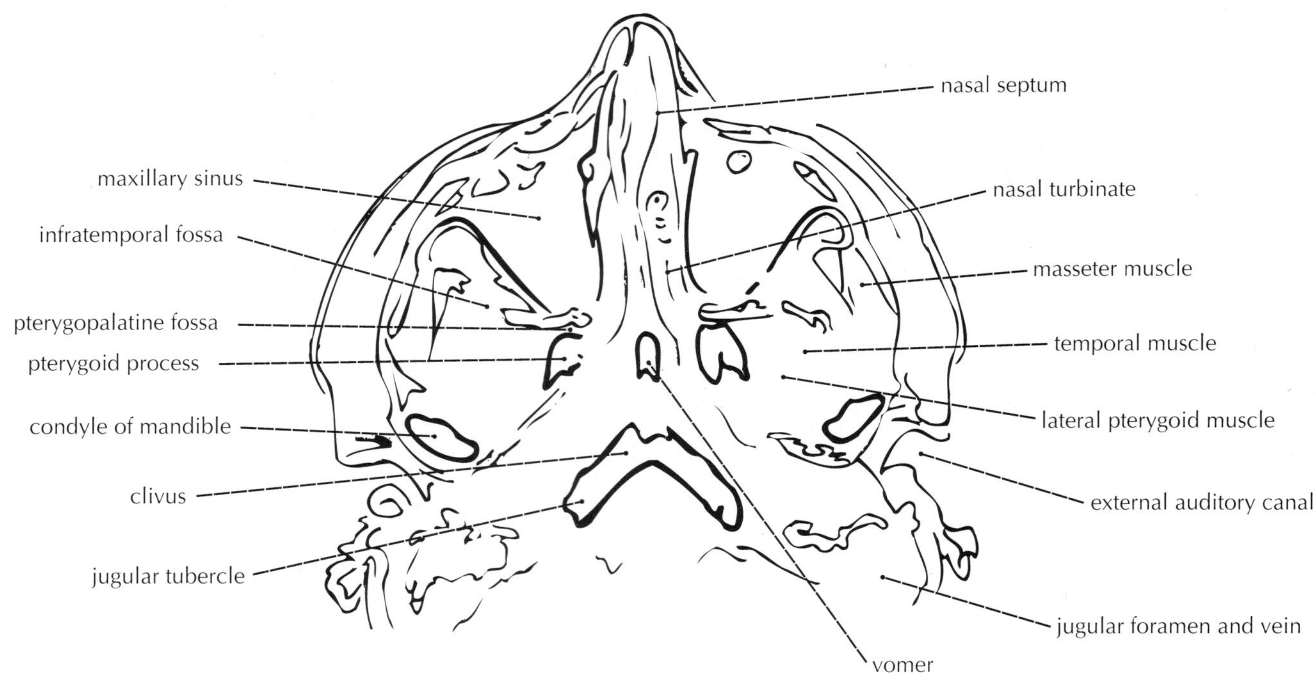

1/Facial Area, Coronal CT and Axial MRI

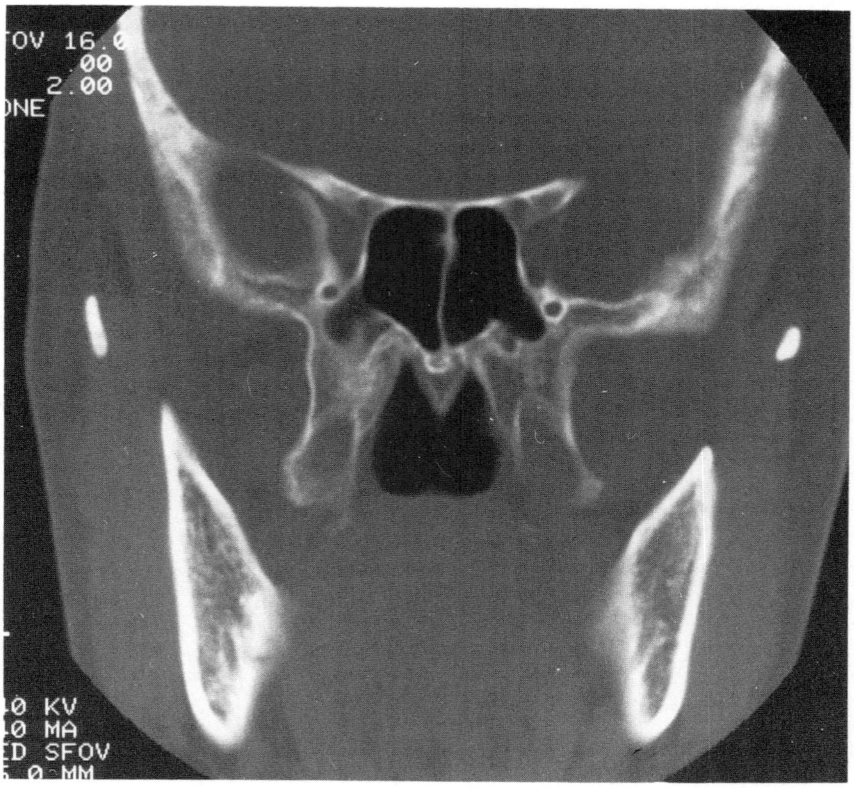

1-25 Coronal CT scan at level of lesser wing of sphenoid (section 13 in Fig. 1-23).

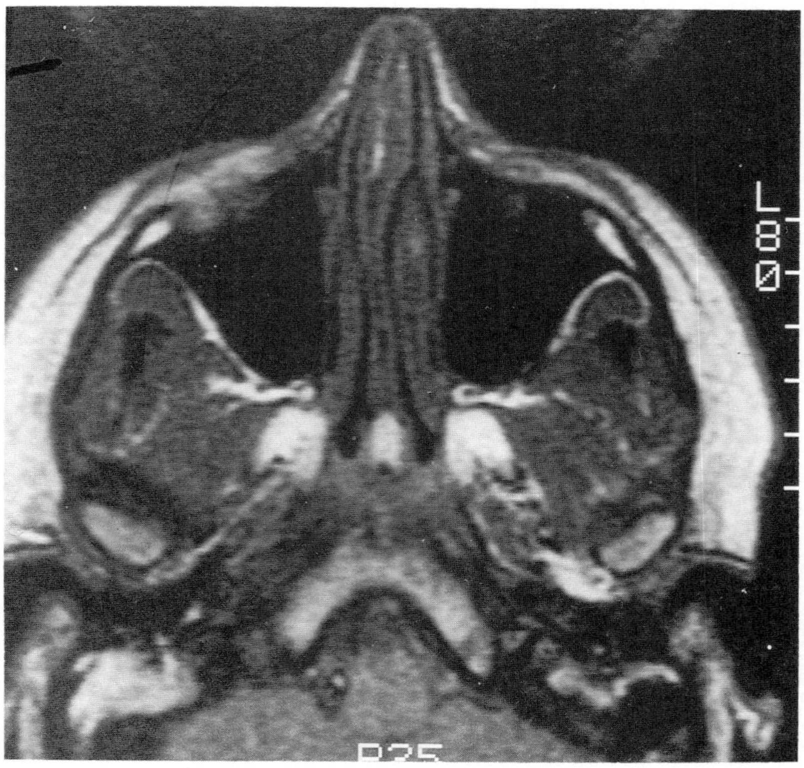

1-26 Axial MR scan through maxillary sinus and infratemporal fossa (600/20).

1/Optic Foramen, X-Ray; Orbit, Axial CT

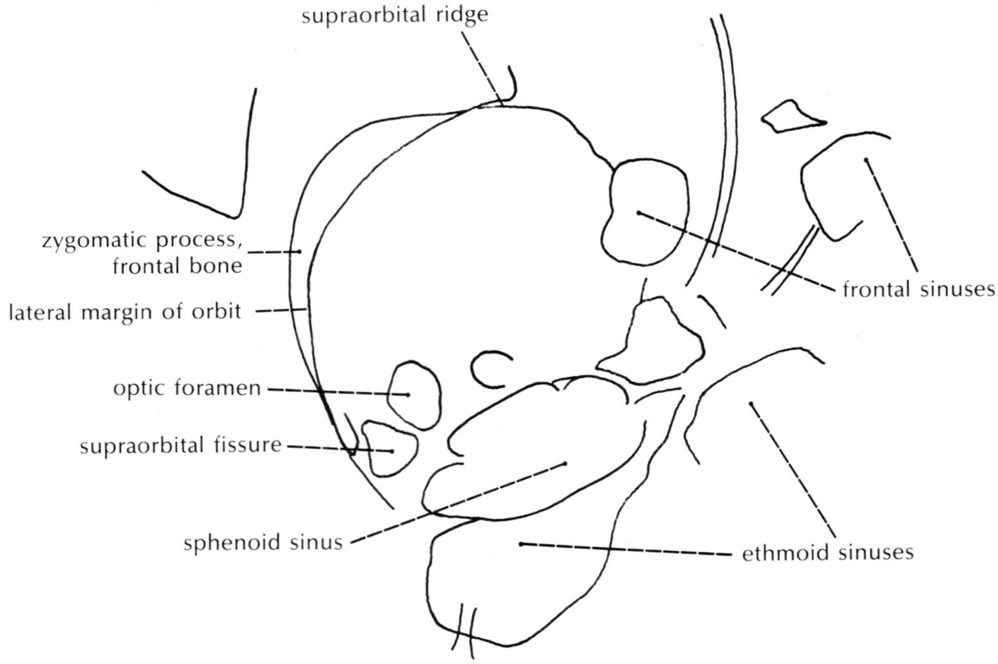

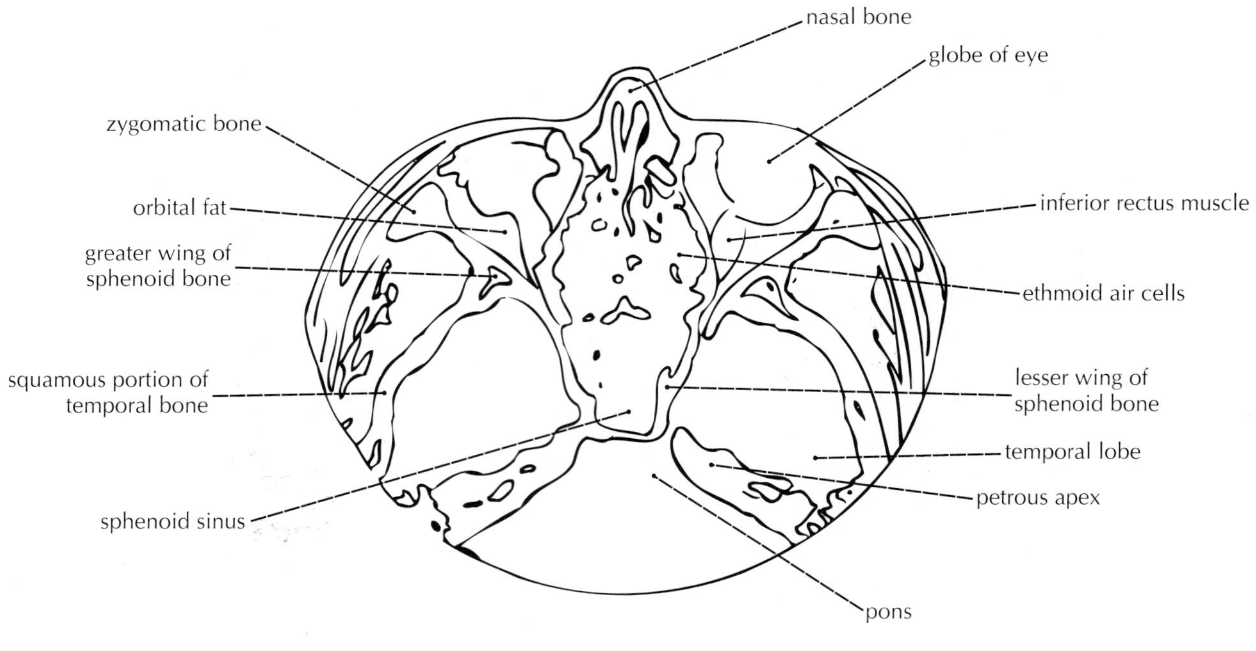

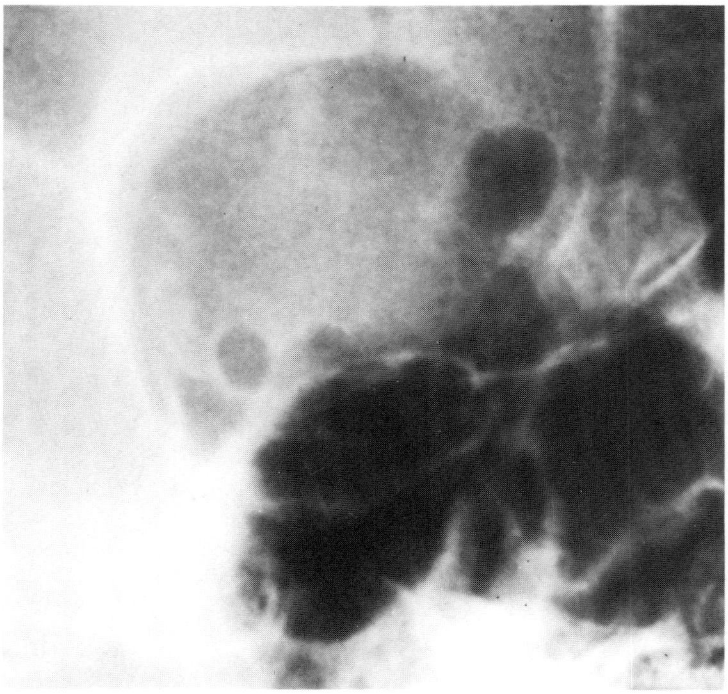

1-27 Optic foramen, oblique view.

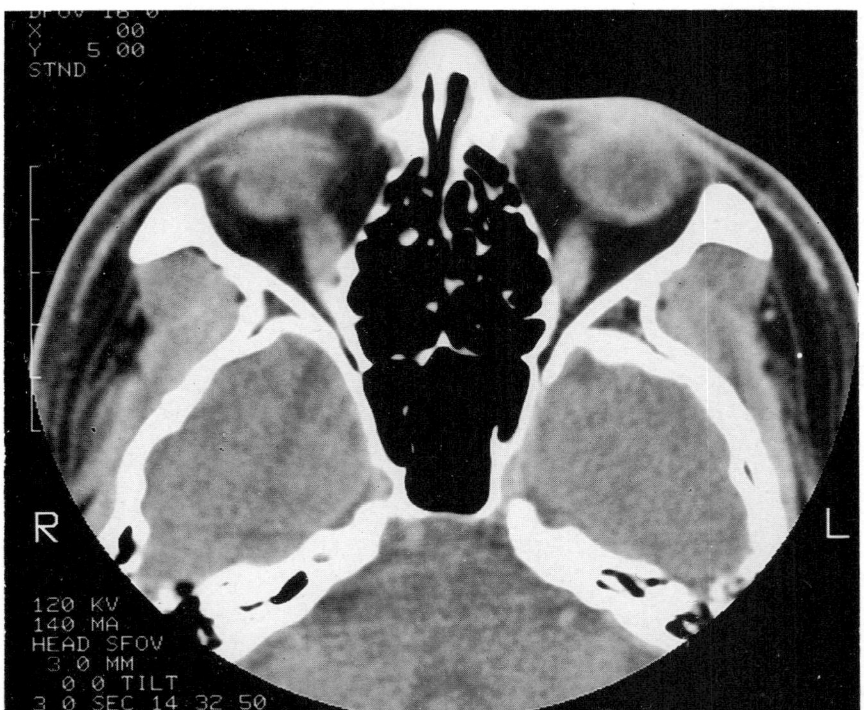

1-28 Axial orbital CT scan (section 4 in Fig. 1-17).

1/Orbit, Axial CT

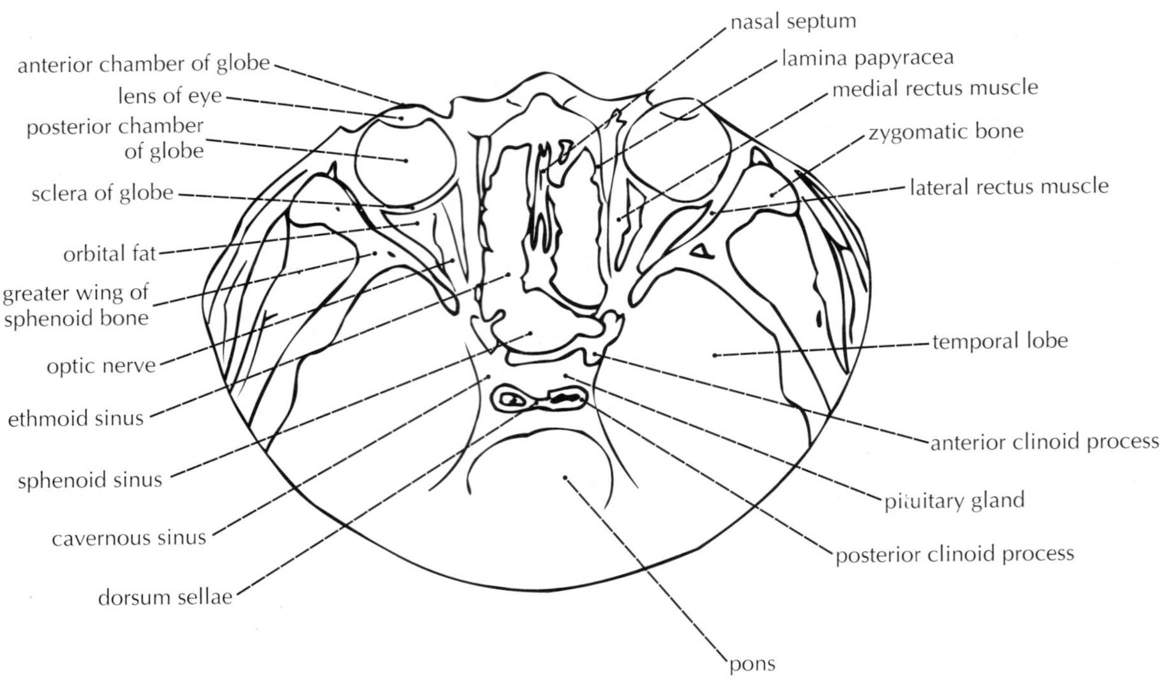

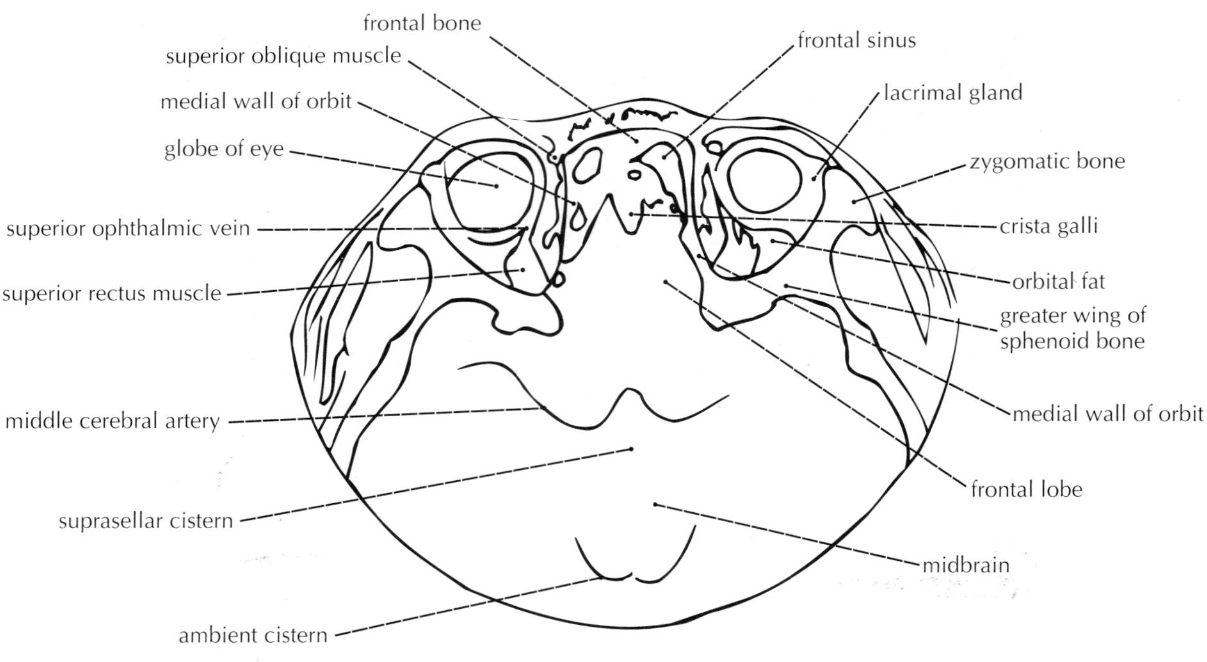

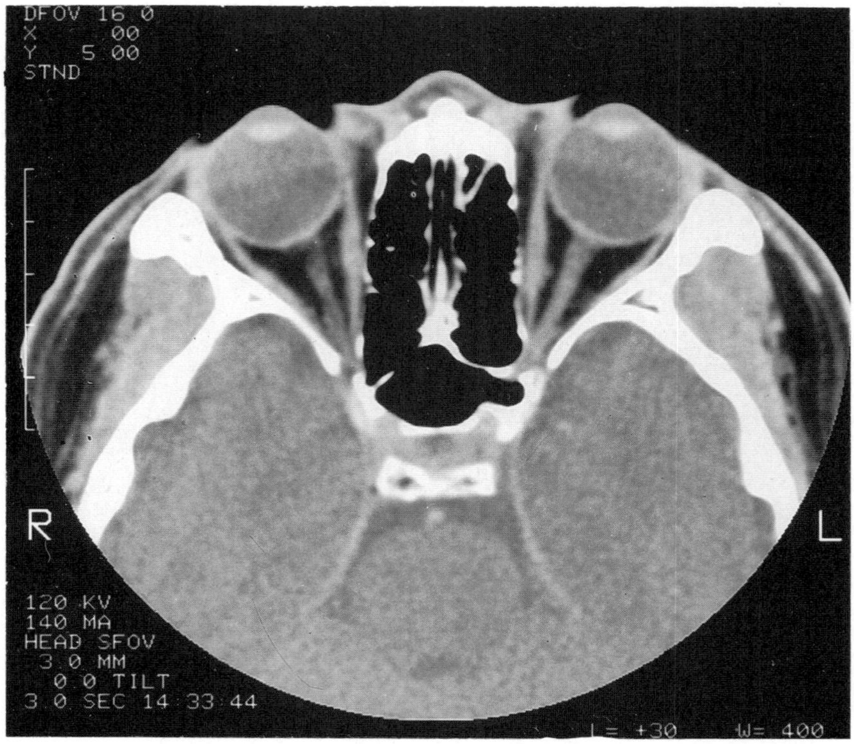

1-29 Axial orbital CT scan (section 7 in Fig. 1-17).

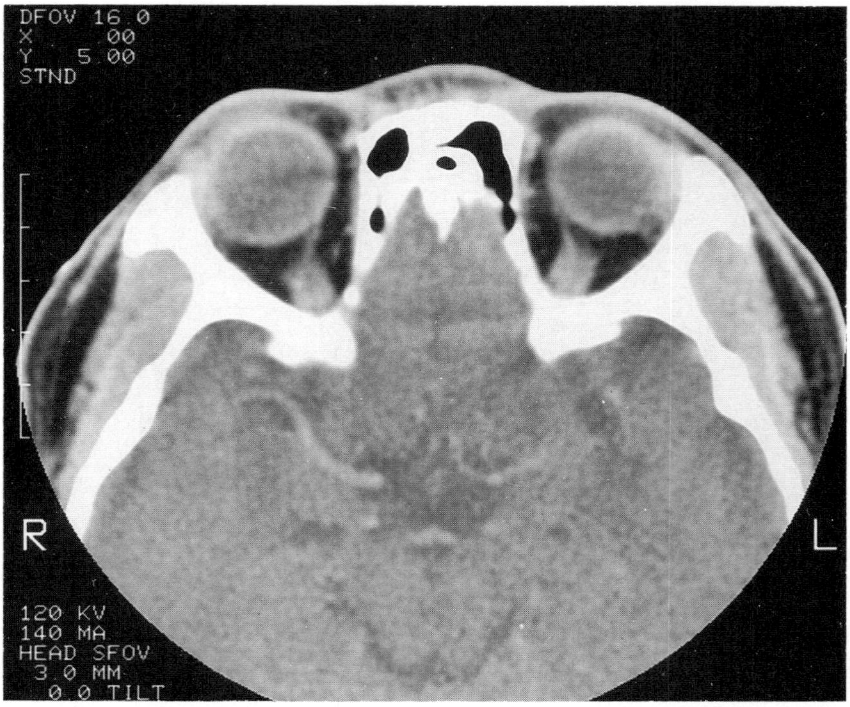

1-30 Axial orbital CT scan (section 10 in Fig. 1-17).

1/Orbit, Coronal CT

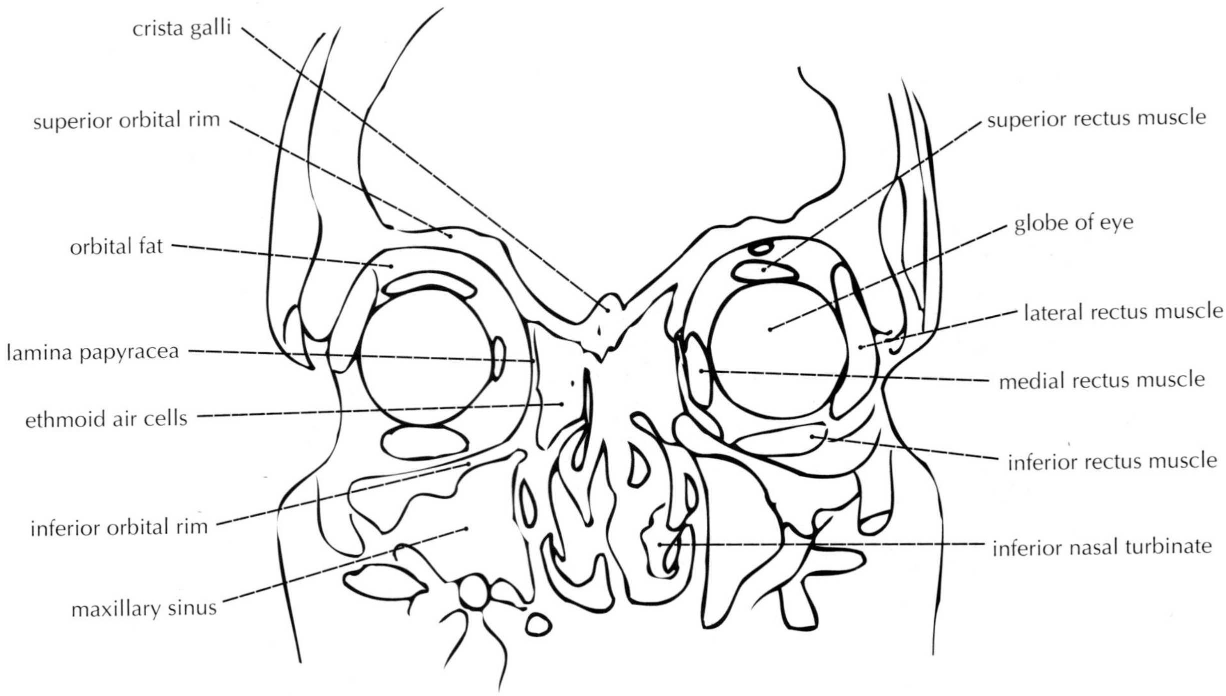

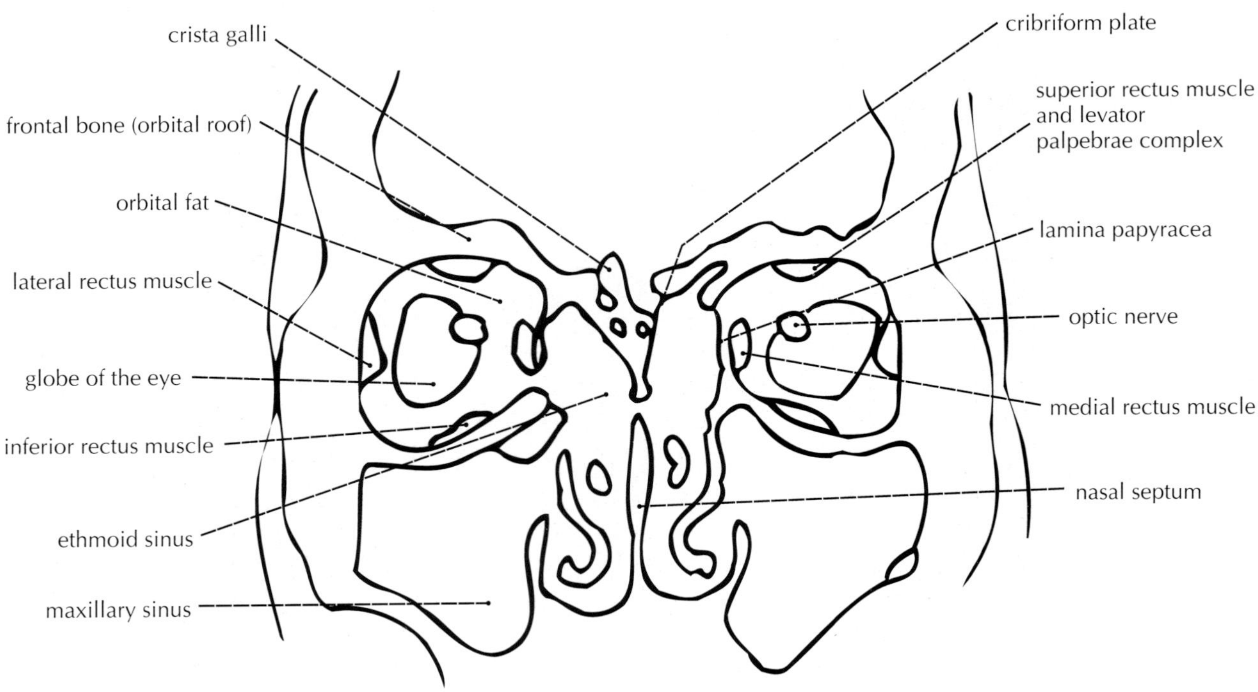

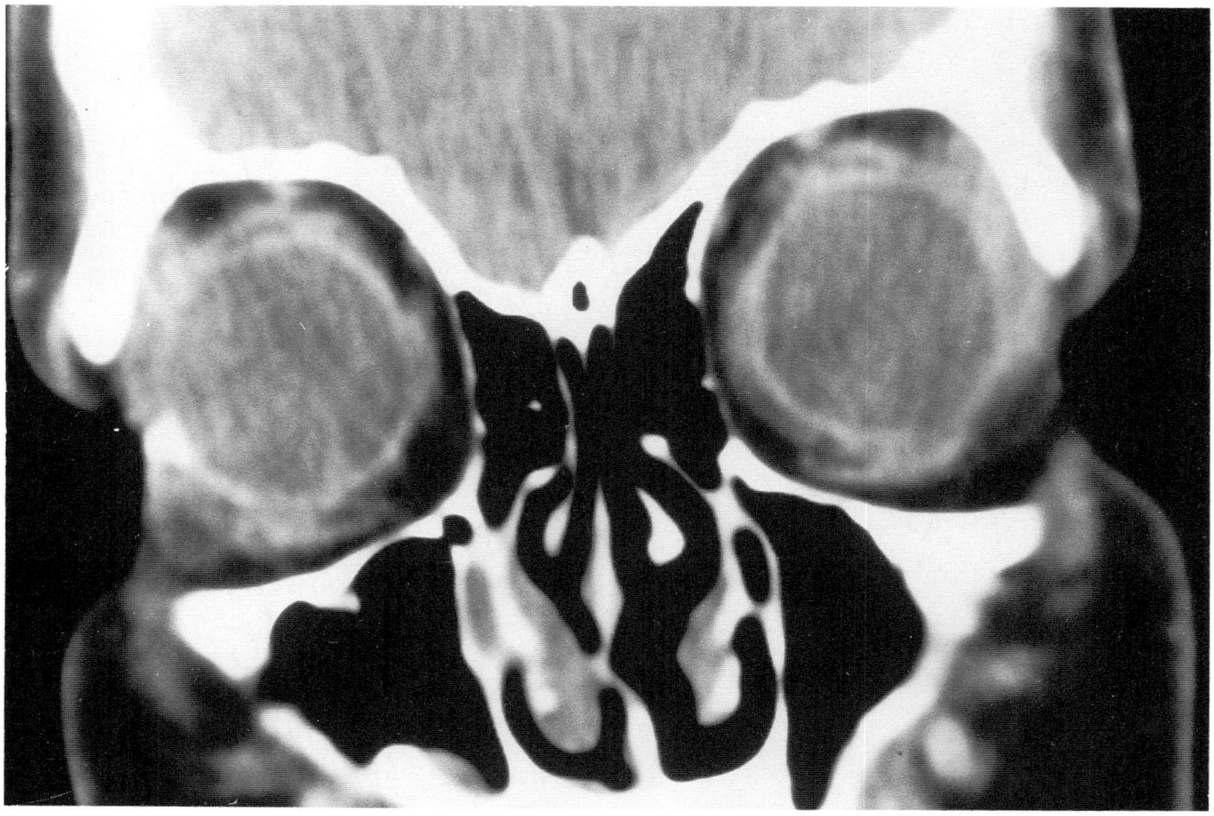

1-31 Coronal CT scan through anterior orbit (section 4 in Fig. 1-23).

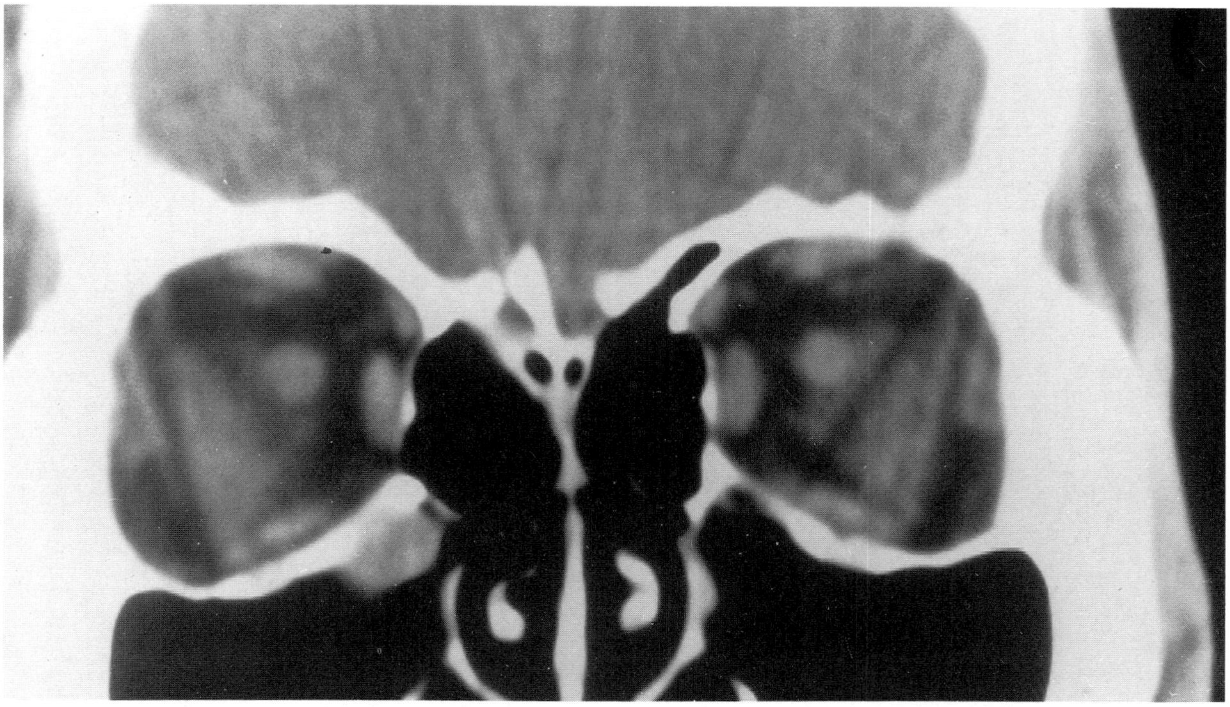

1-32 Coronal CT scan through the orbit (section 6 in Fig. 1-23).

1/Orbit, Coronal CT

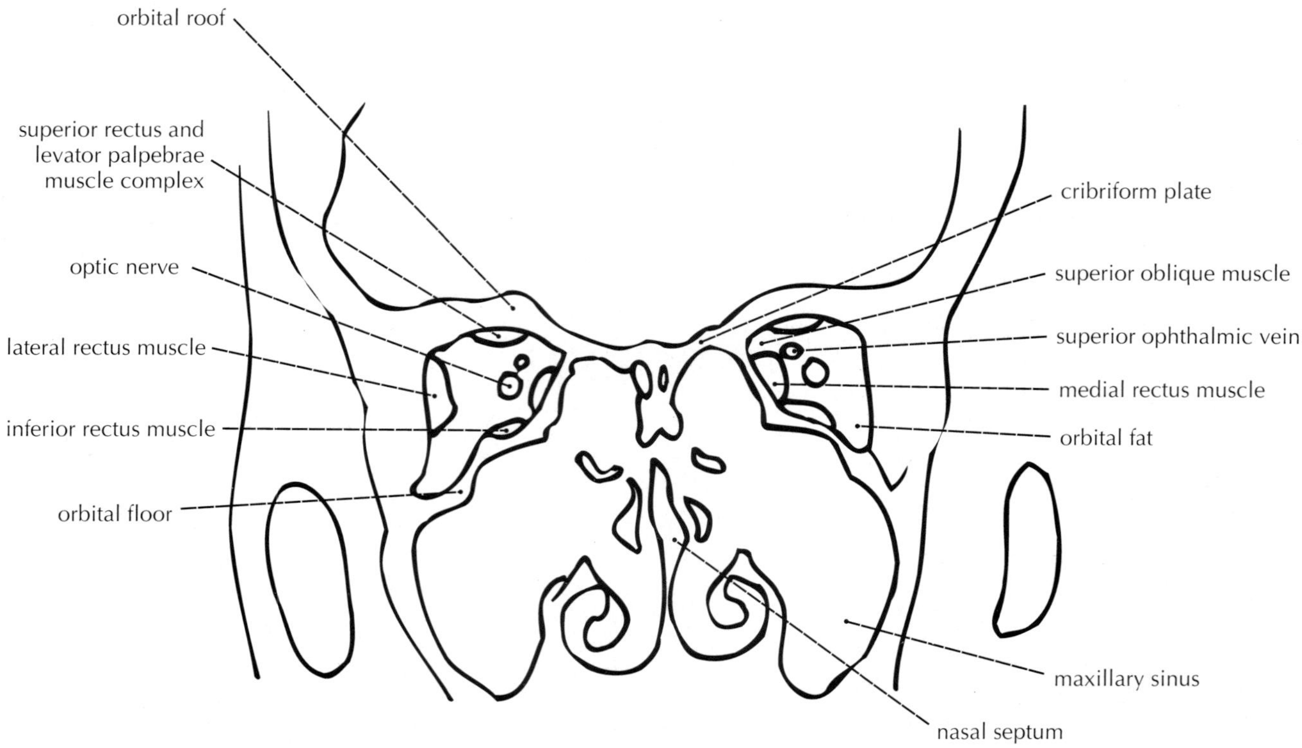

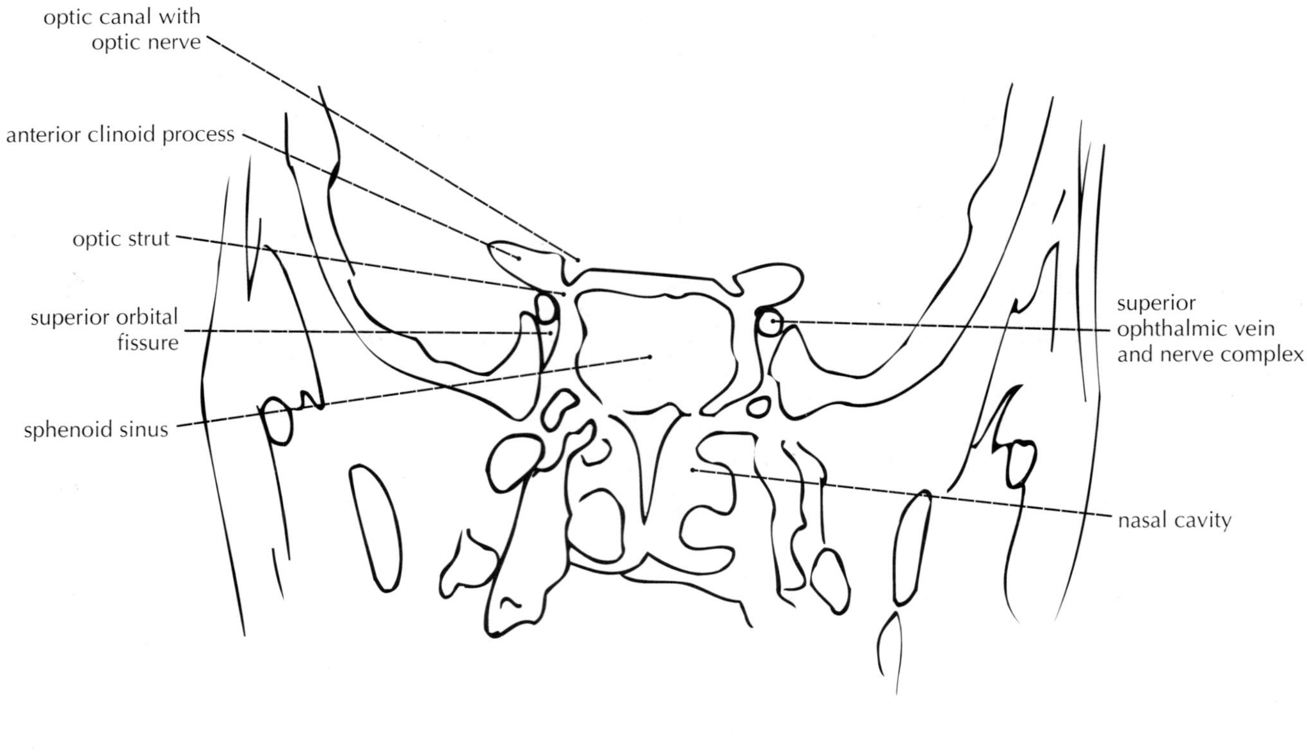

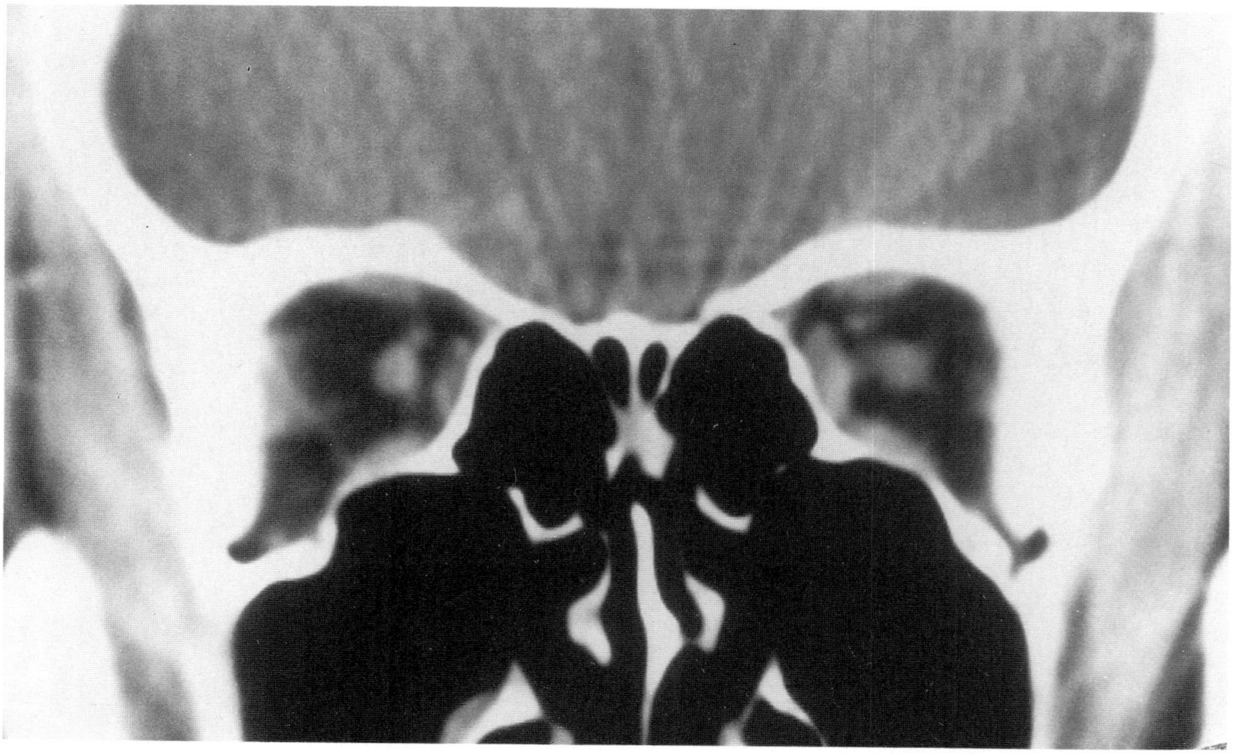

1-33 Coronal CT scan through the orbit (section 10 in Fig. 1-23).

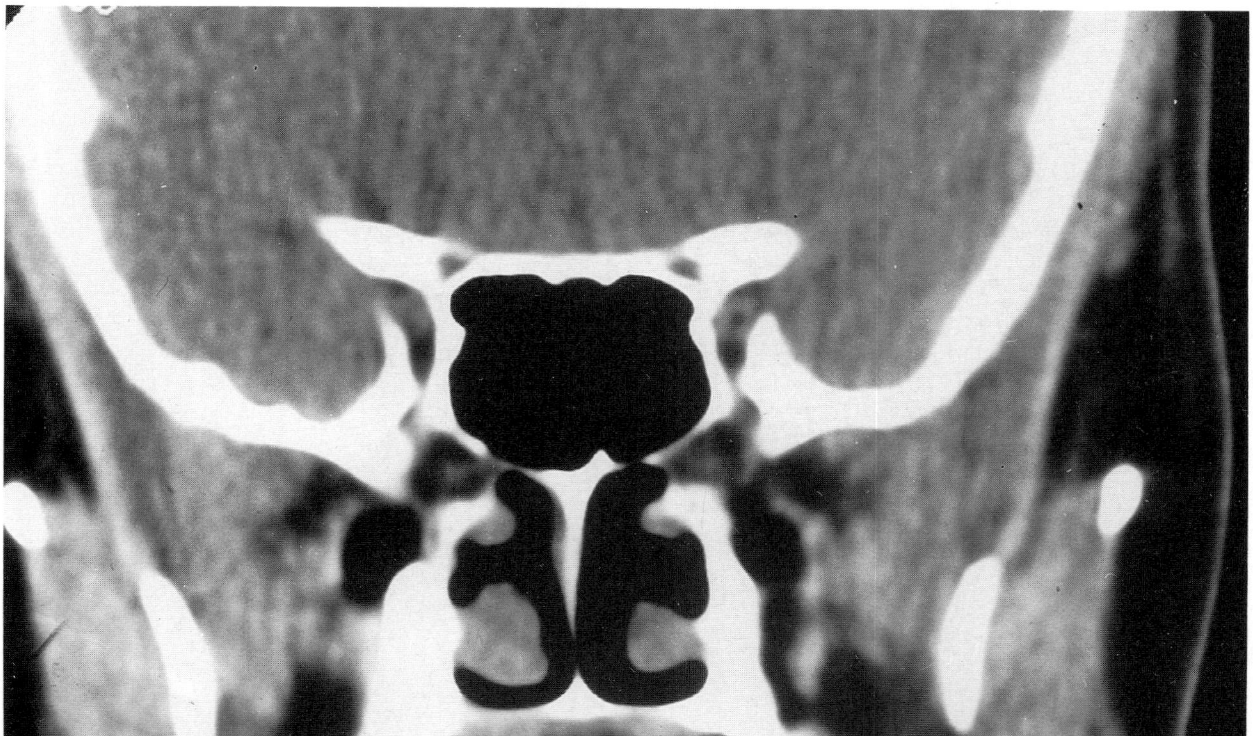

1-34 Coronal CT scan through orbital apex (section 14 in Fig. 1-23).

1/Orbit, Coronal Scout and Axial MR

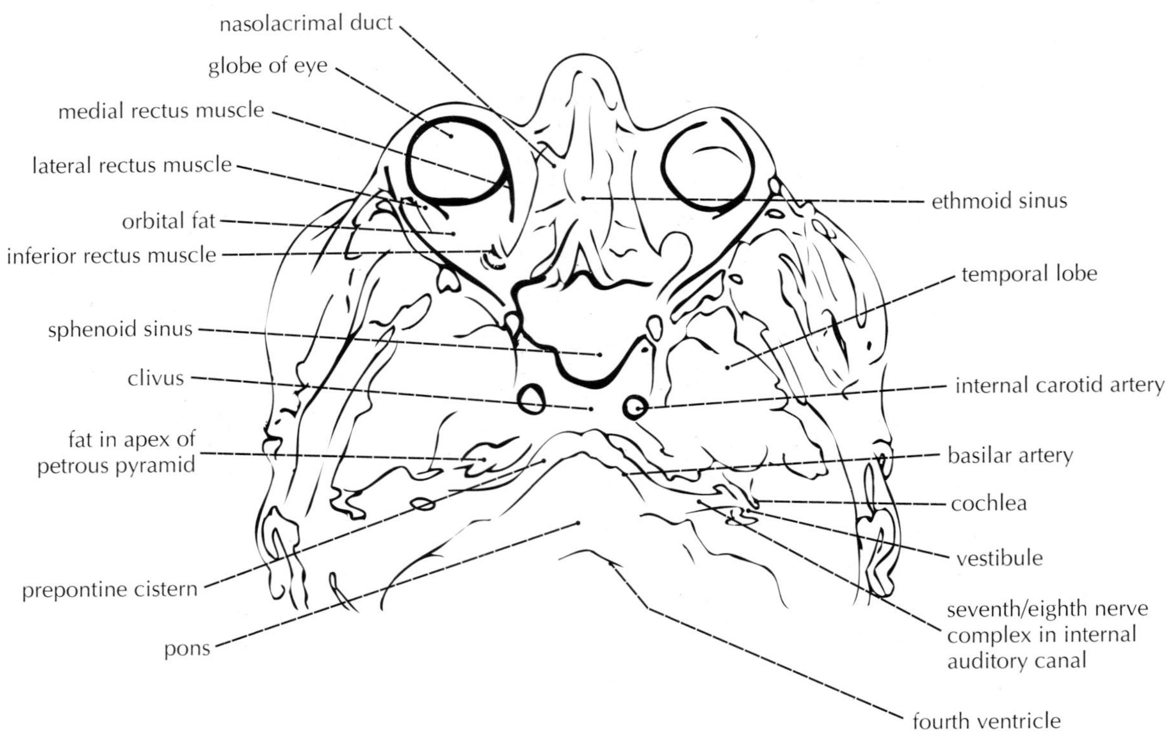

1/Orbit, Coronal Scout and Axial MR

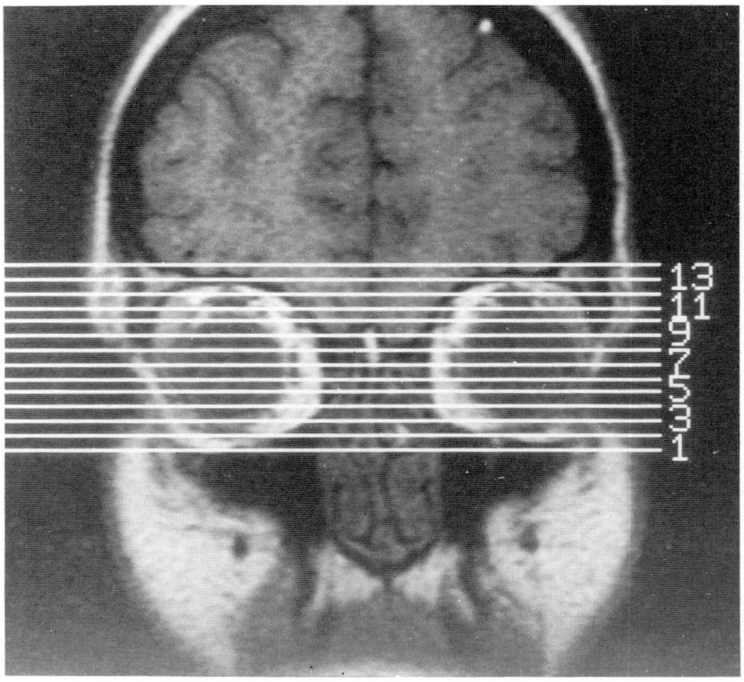

1-35 Coronal MR scout image to demonstrate selected axial orbital MR sections.

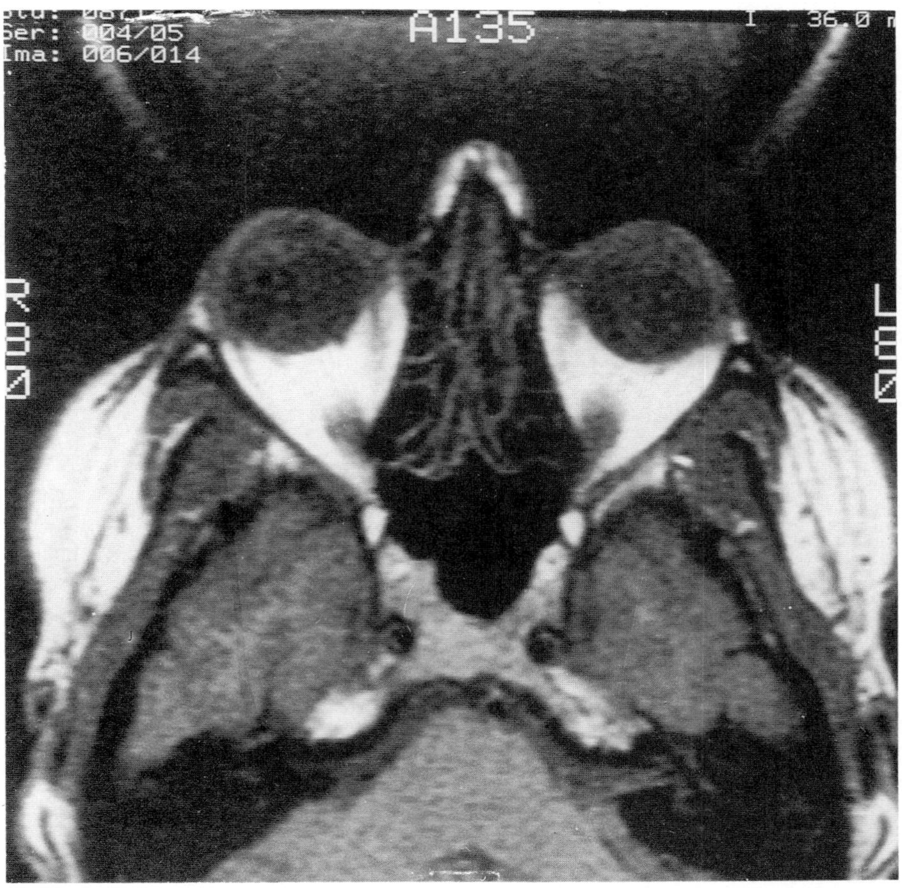

1-36 Axial MR scan through lower orbit (600/20) (section 6 in Fig. 1-35).

1/Orbit, Axial MR

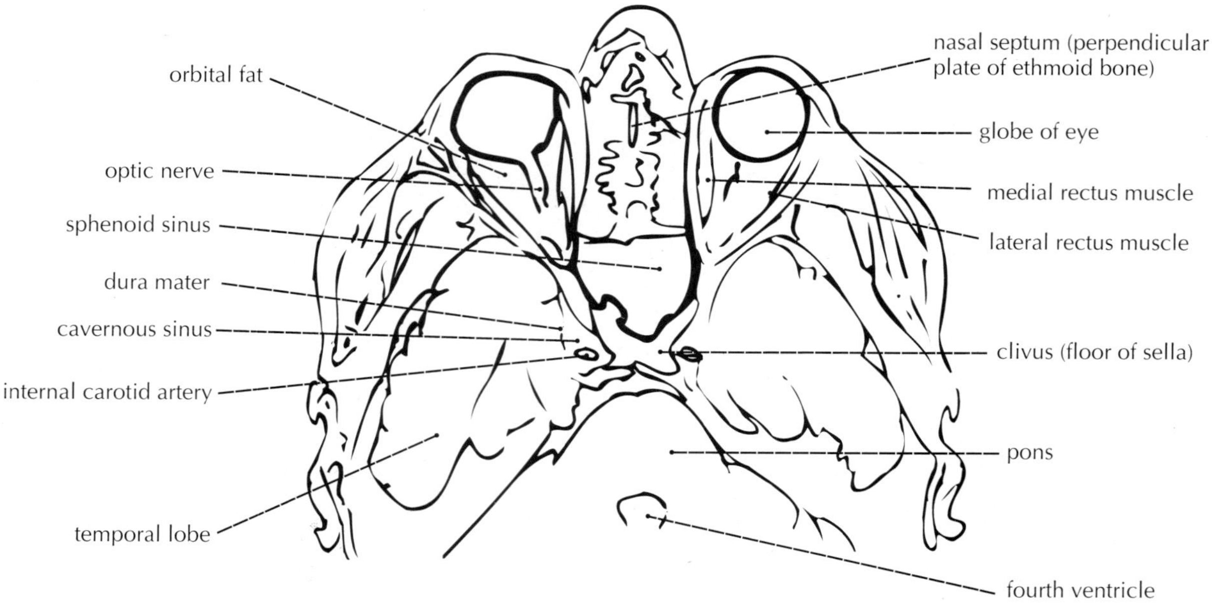

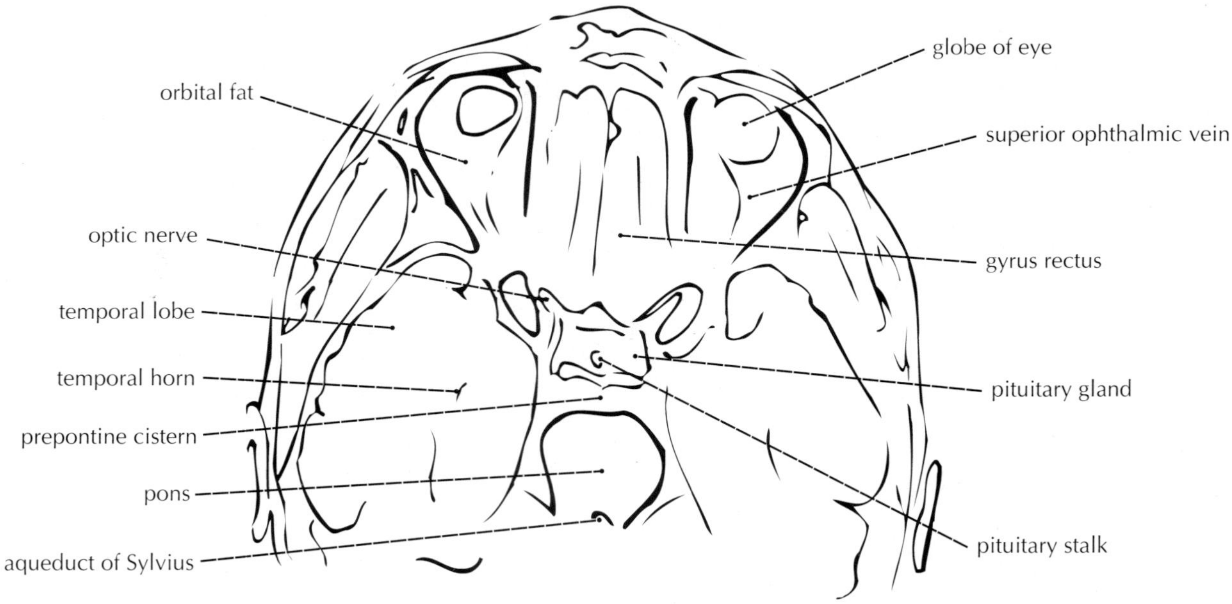

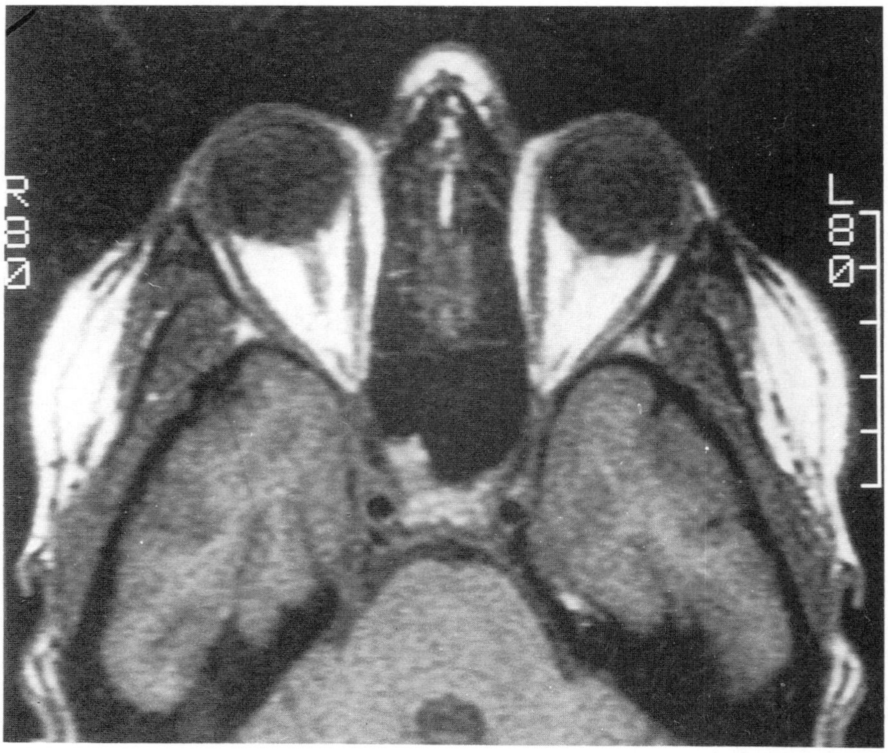

1-37 Axial MR scan through midorbit (600/20) (section 8 in Fig. 1-35).

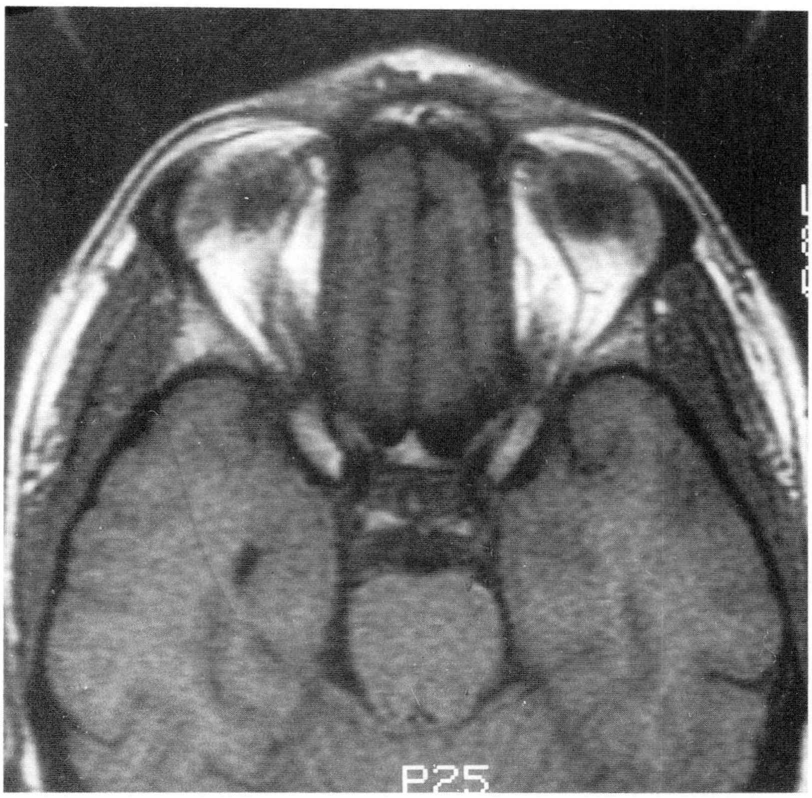

1-38 Axial orbital MR scan (600/20) (section 11 in Fig. 1-35).

1/Orbit, Axial MR

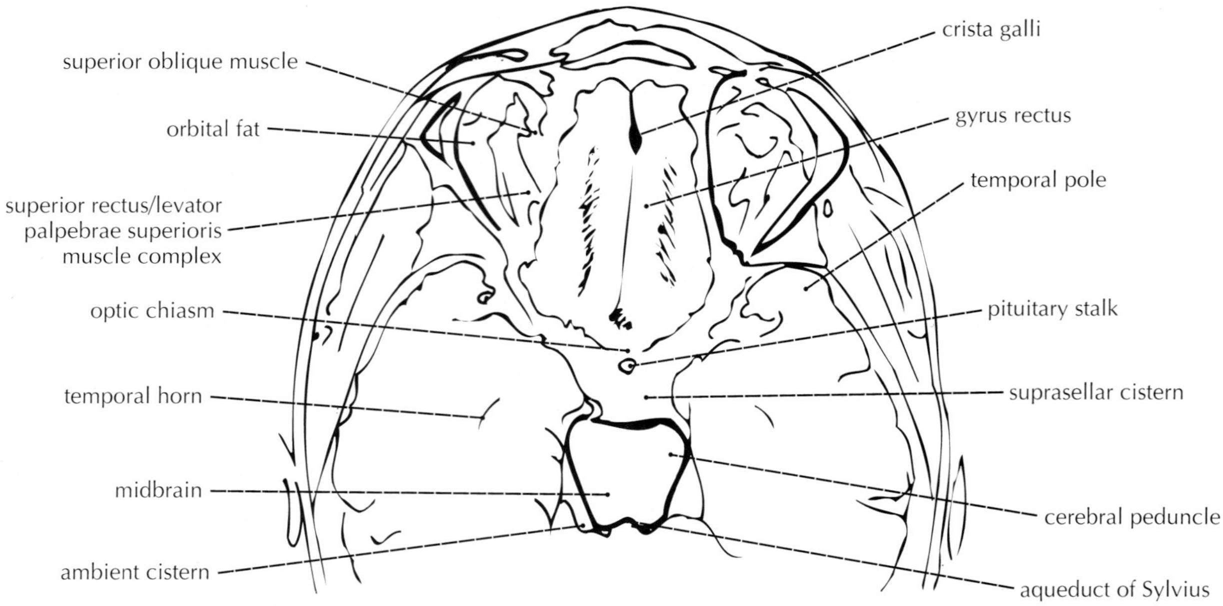

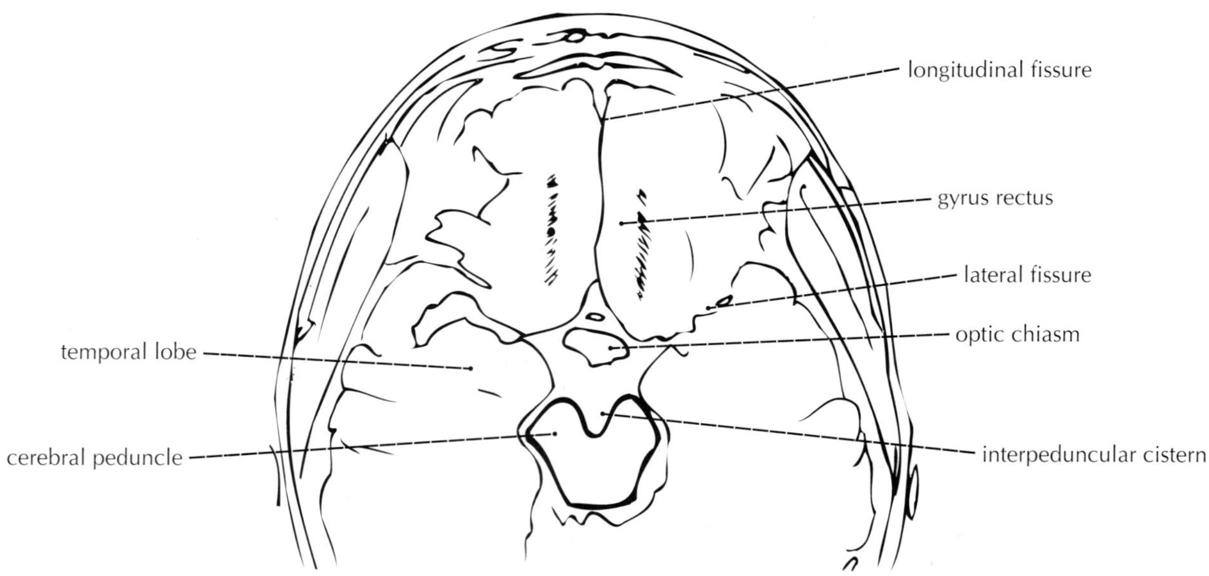

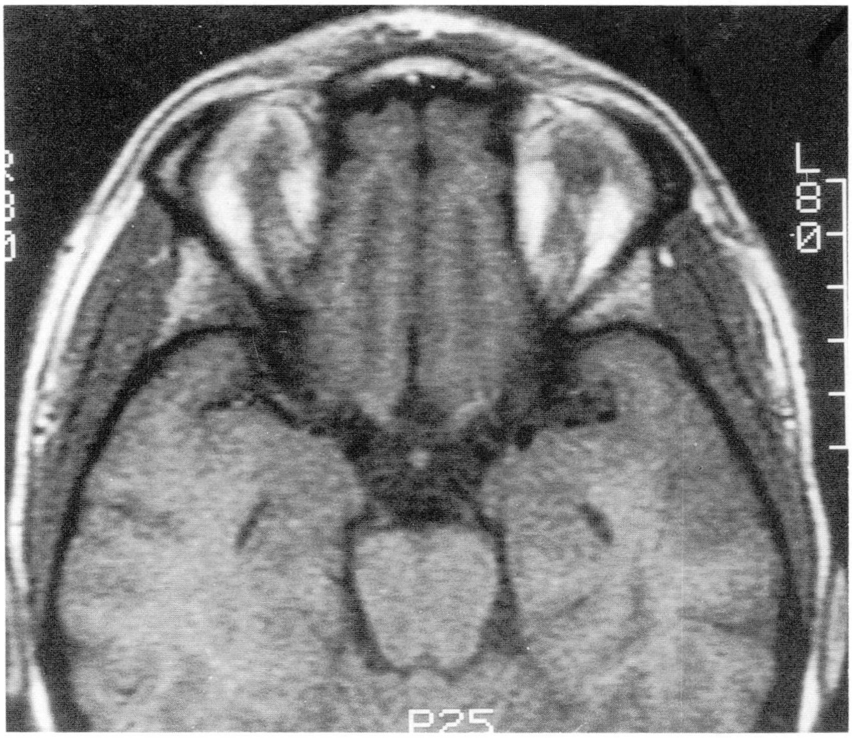

1-39 Axial orbital MR scan (600/20) (section 12 in Fig. 1-35).

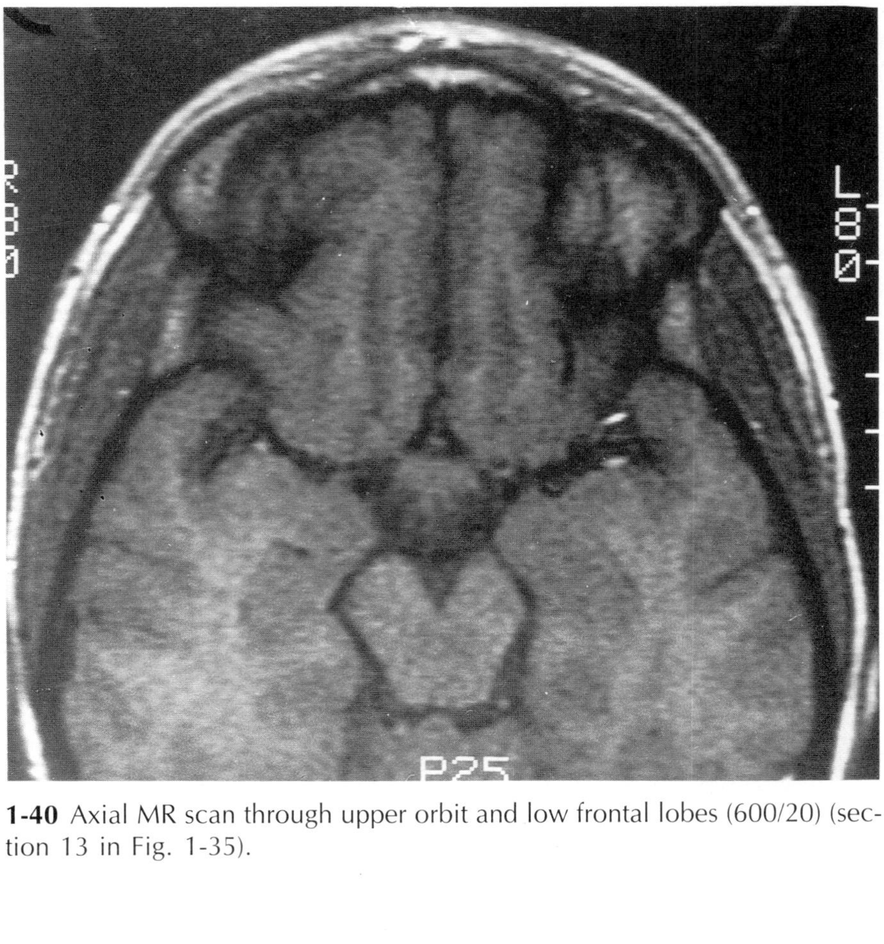

1-40 Axial MR scan through upper orbit and low frontal lobes (600/20) (section 13 in Fig. 1-35).

1/Orbit, Sagittal Scout and Coronal MR

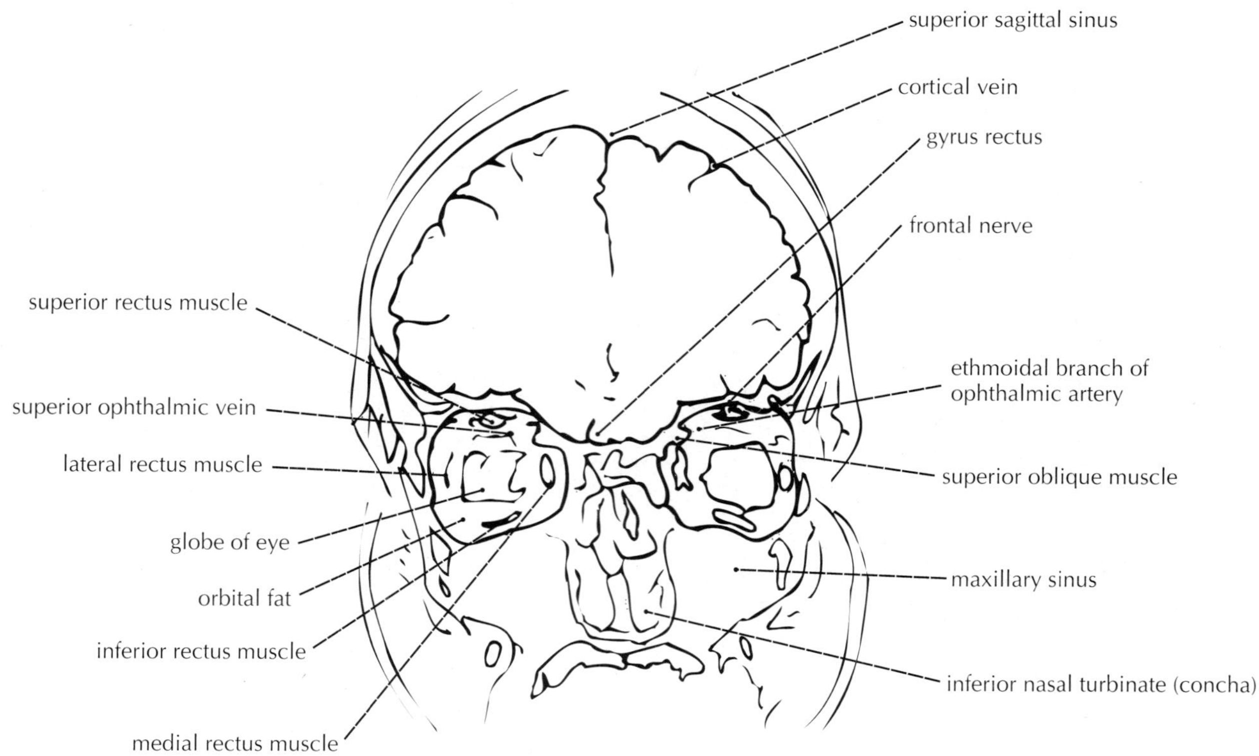

1/Orbit, Sagittal Scout and Coronal MR

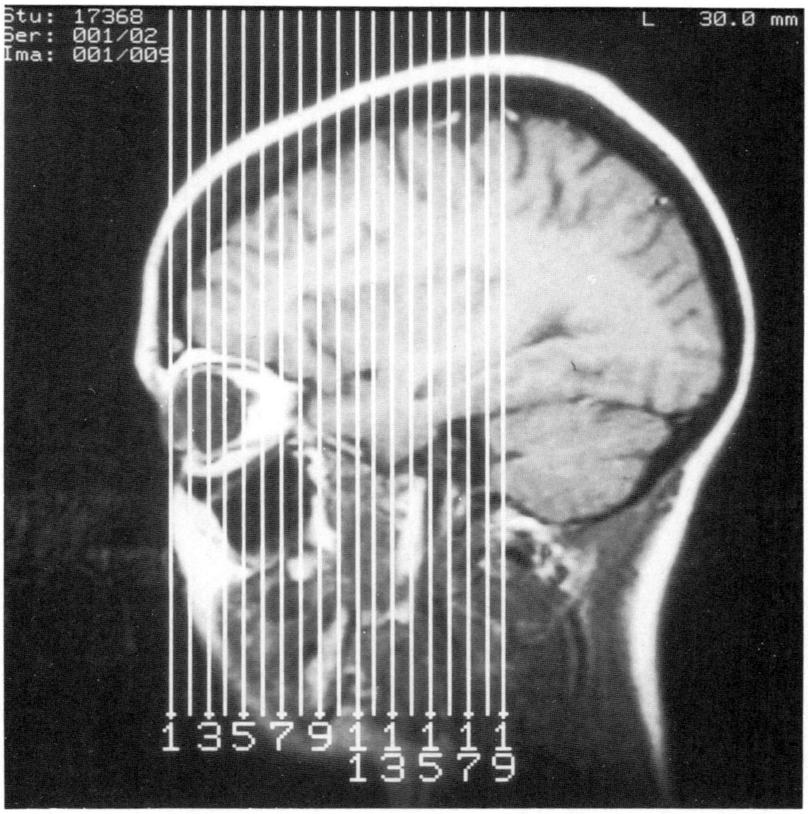

1-41 Sagittal scout MR scan used to demonstrate the location of selected coronal MR scans of the orbit.

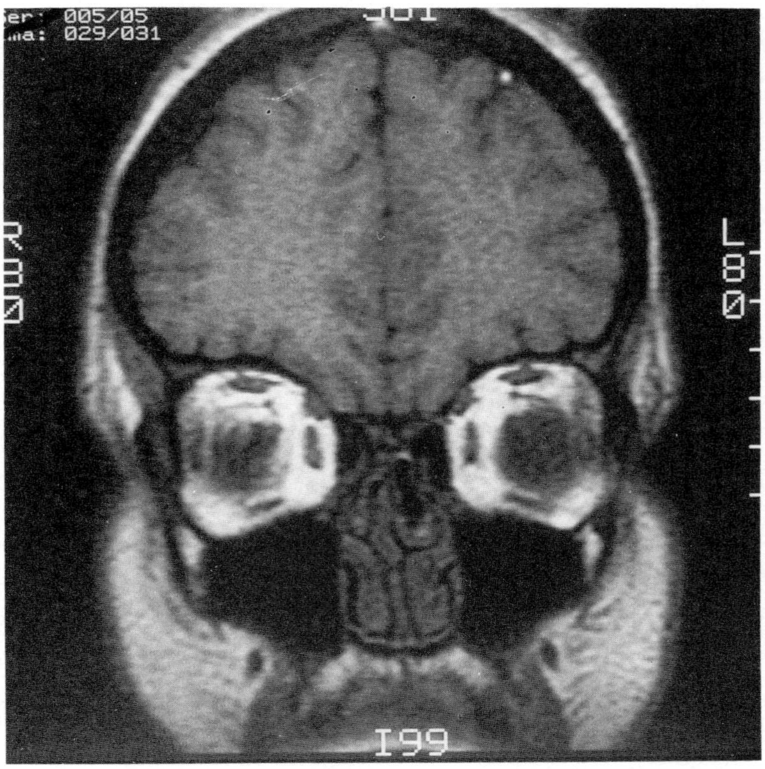

1-42 Coronal MR scan through orbits (600/20) (section 4 in Fig. 1-41).

1/Orbit, Coronal MR

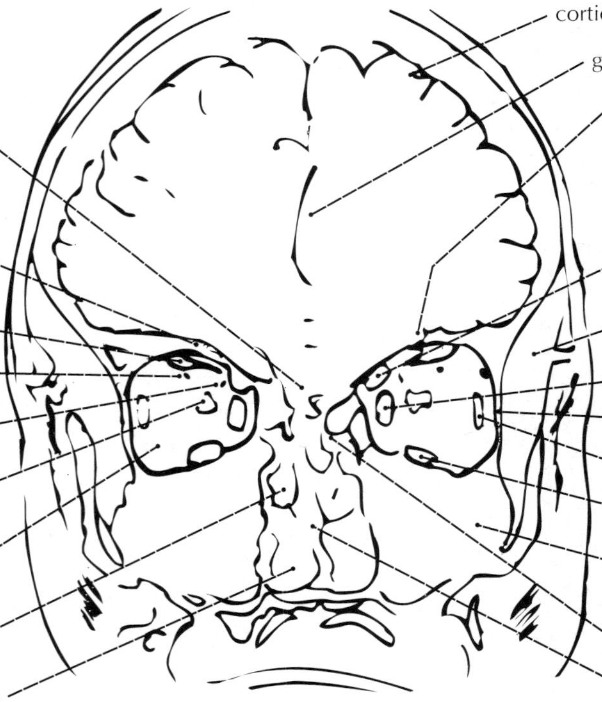

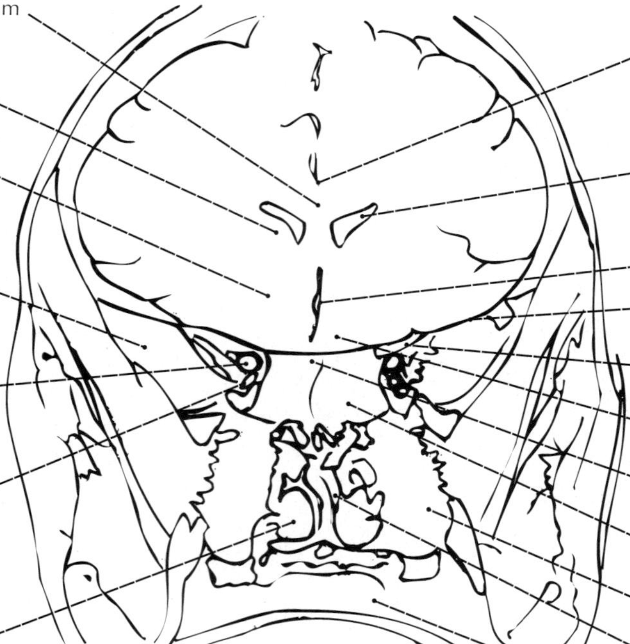

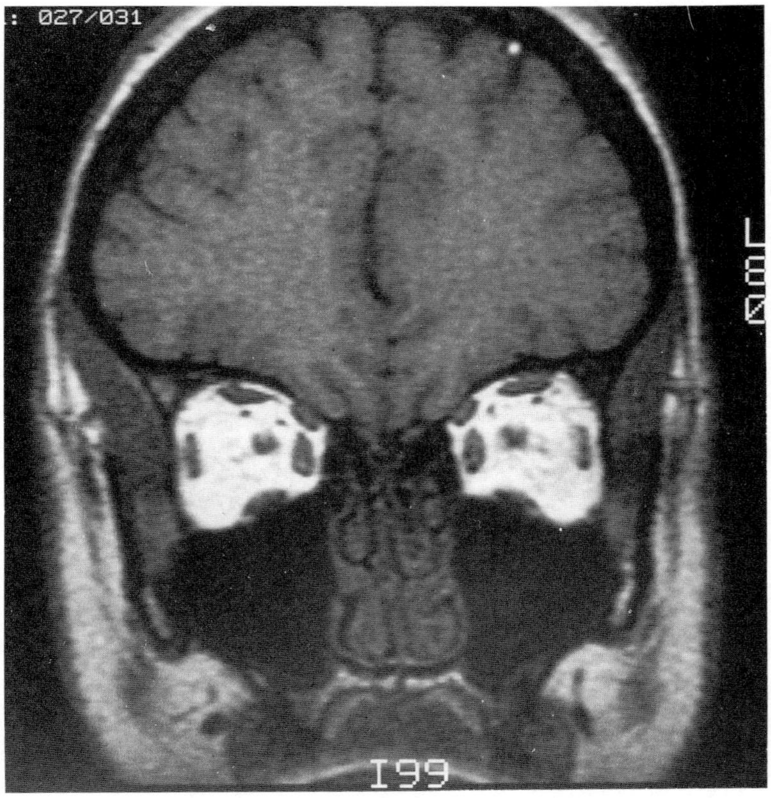

1-43 Coronal MR scan through orbit (posterior to globe) (600/20). Section 7 in Fig. 1-41.

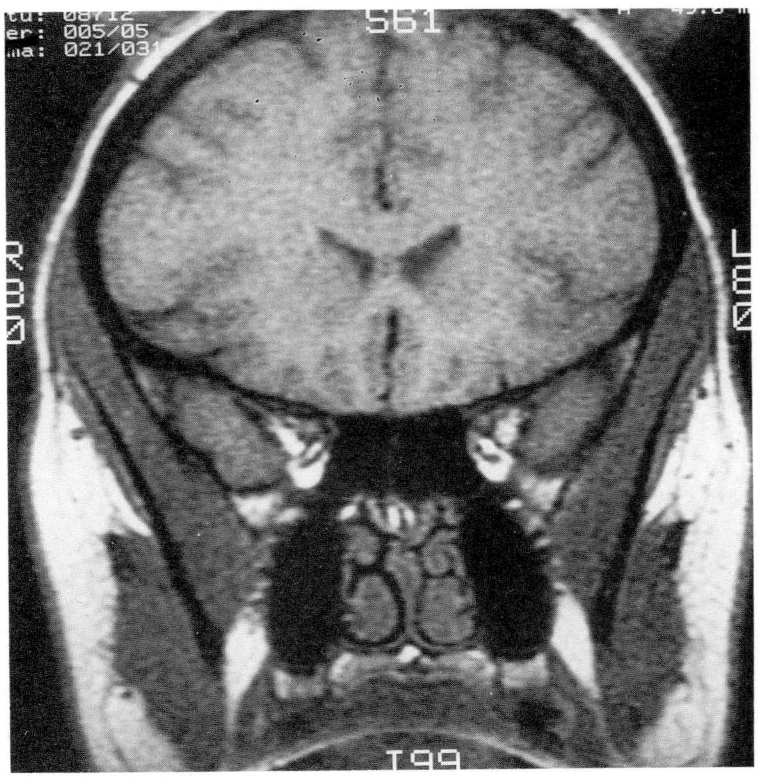

1-44 Coronal MR scan through posterior orbit (600/20). Section 9 in Fig. 1-41.

1/Optic Chiasm and Pituitary Gland, Coronal MR

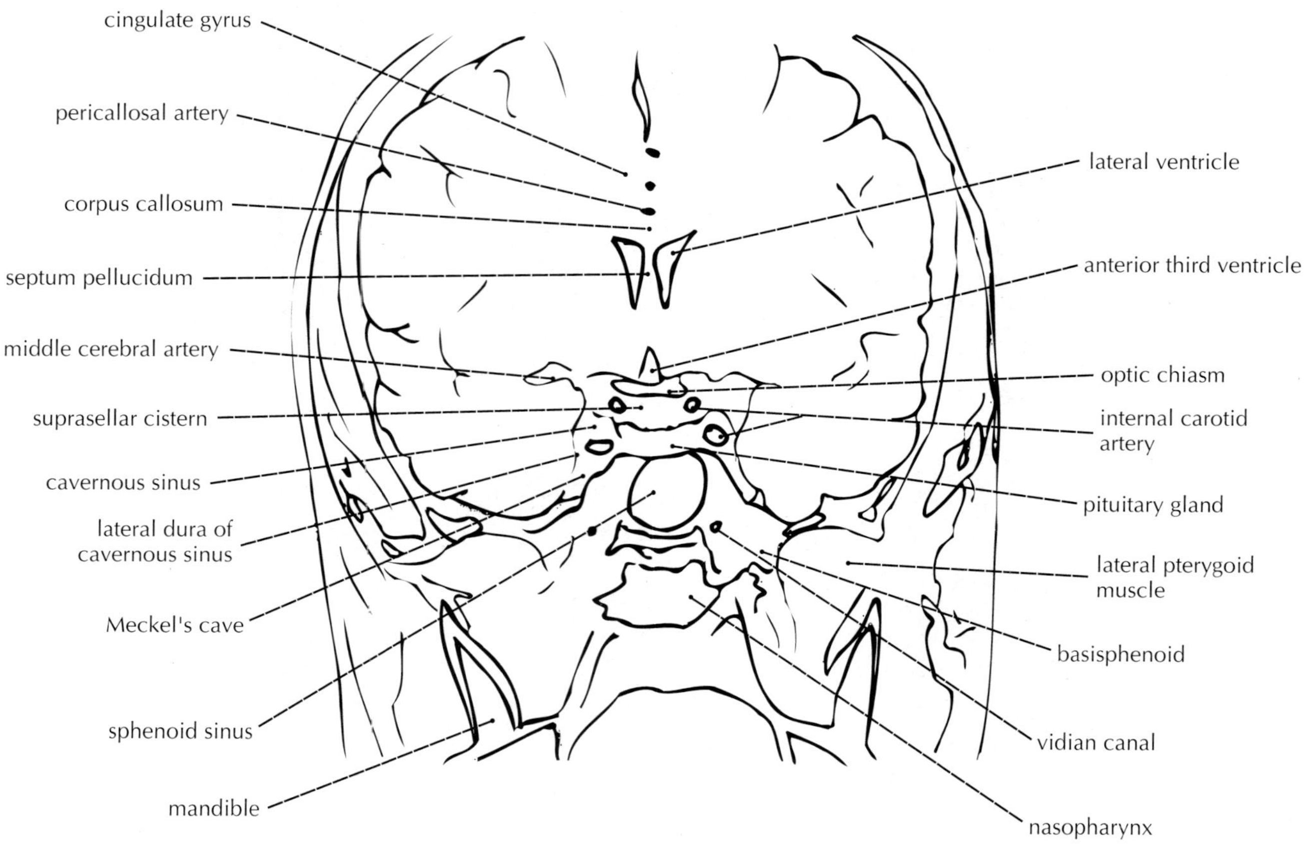

1/Optic Chiasm and Pituitary Gland, Coronal MR

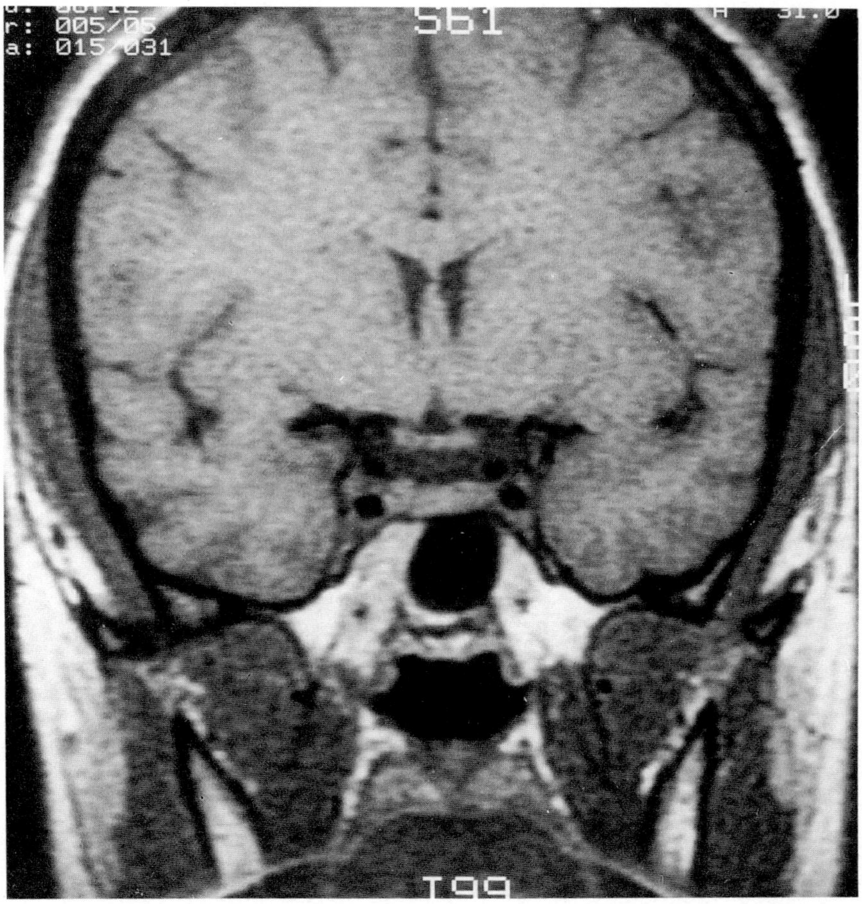

1-45 Coronal MR scan through optic chiasm and pituitary gland (600/20). Section 12 in Fig. 1-41.

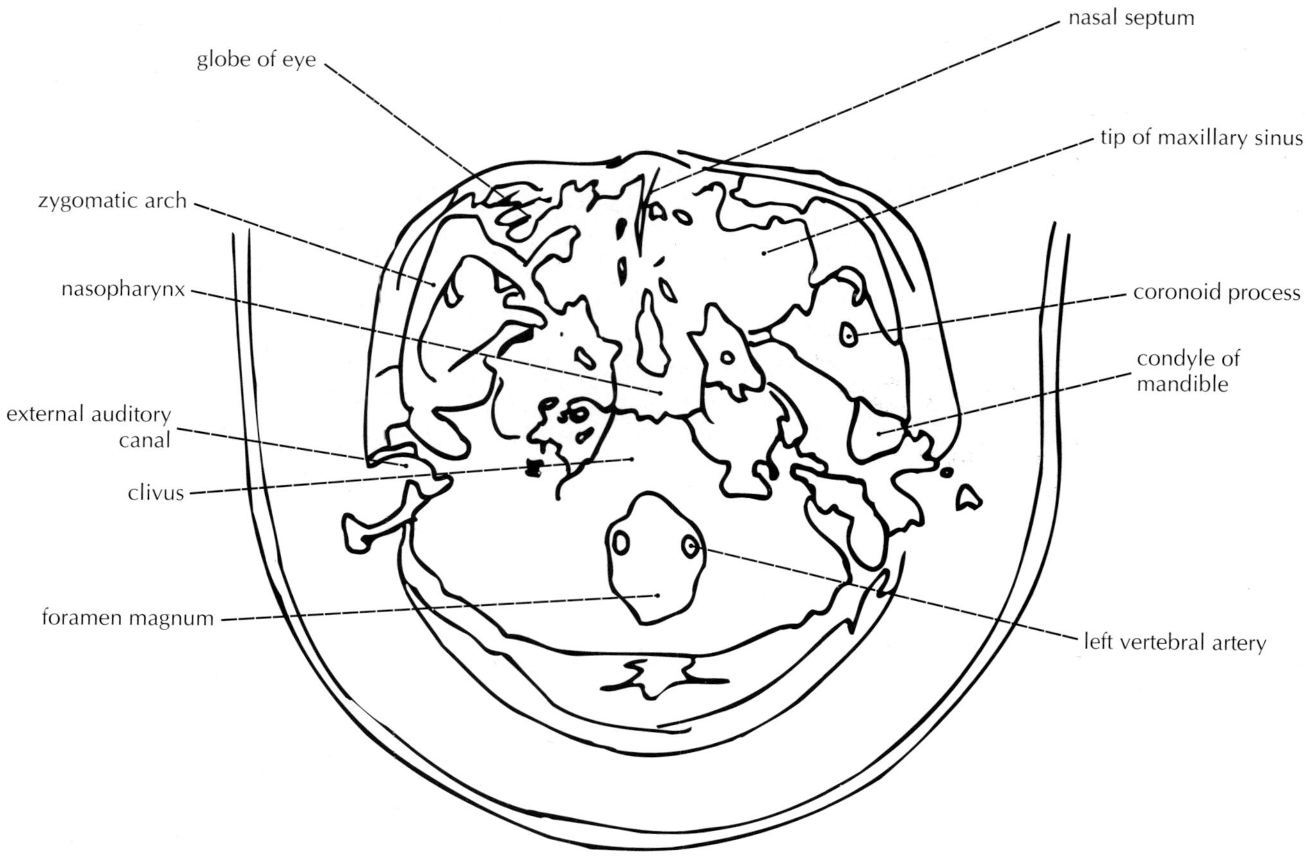
nasal septum
globe of eye
tip of maxillary sinus
zygomatic arch
nasopharynx
coronoid process
condyle of mandible
external auditory canal
clivus
foramen magnum
left vertebral artery

2/Brain, Sagittal Scout CT and Axial CT

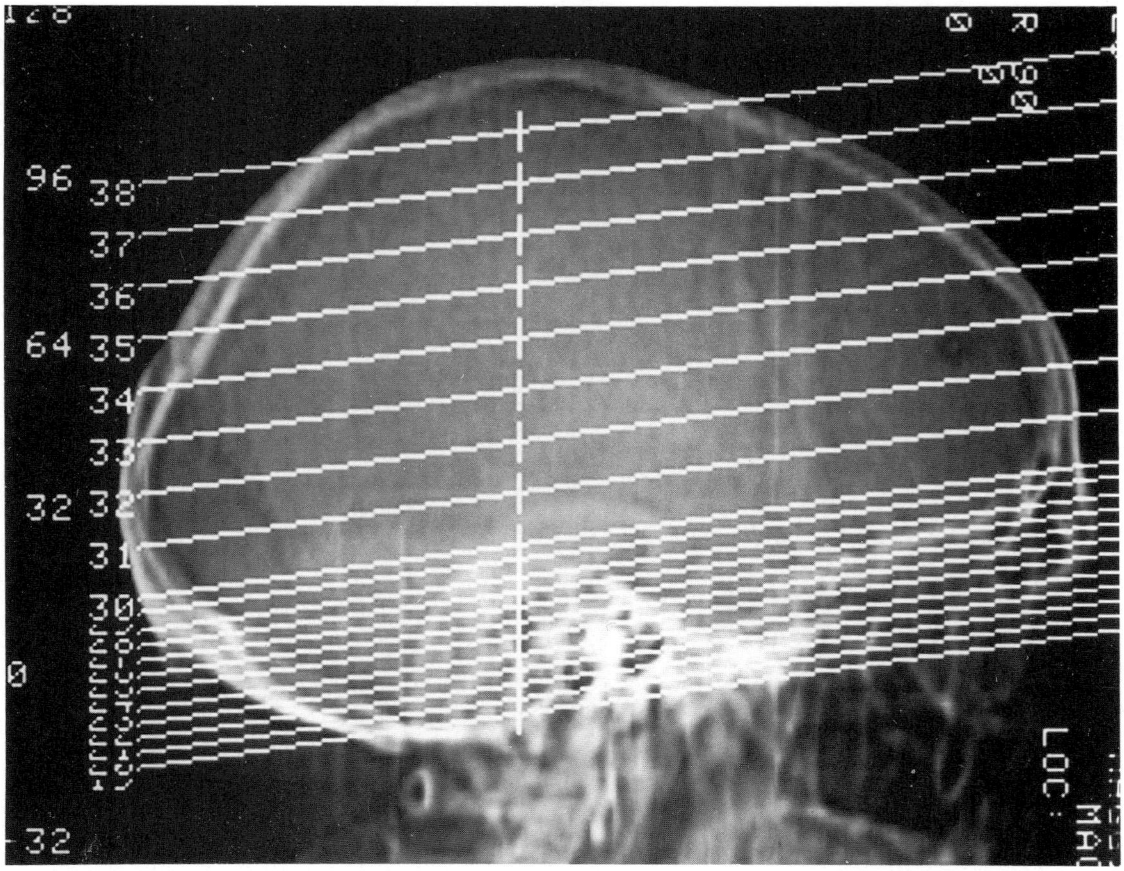

2-1 Sagittal CT scout of the head used for demonstration of axial CT sections (Figs. 2-2 through 2-11).

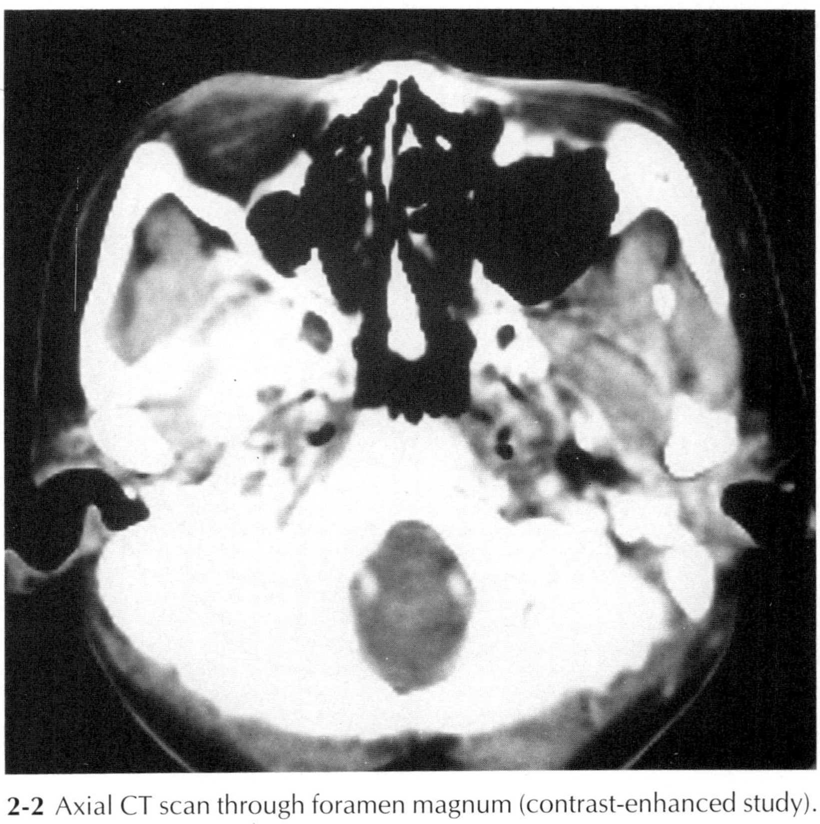

2-2 Axial CT scan through foramen magnum (contrast-enhanced study). Section 19 in Fig. 2-1.

2/Brain, Axial CT

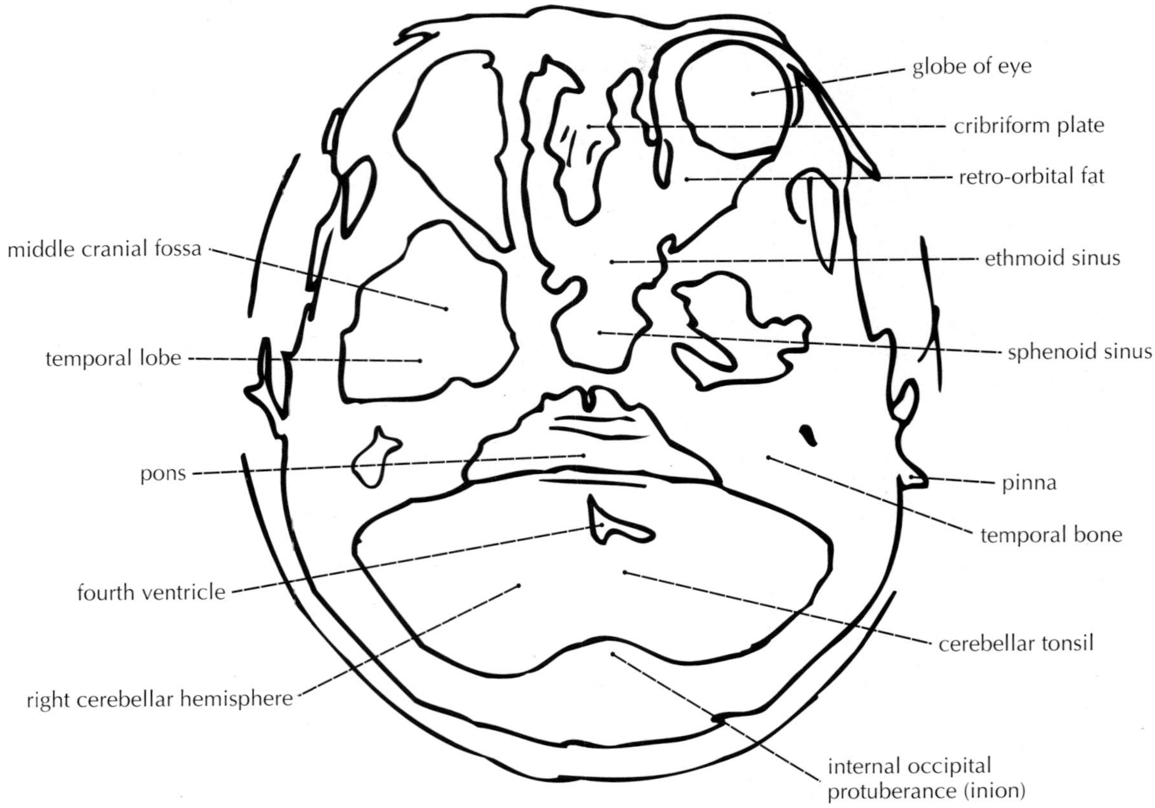

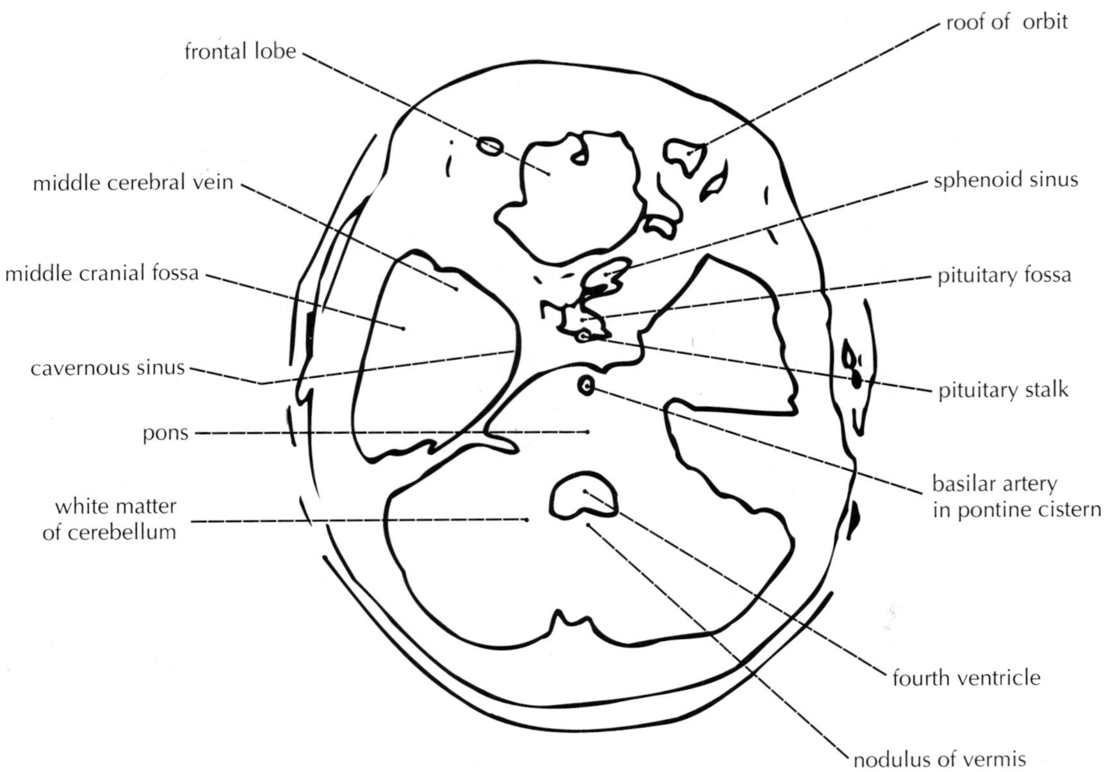

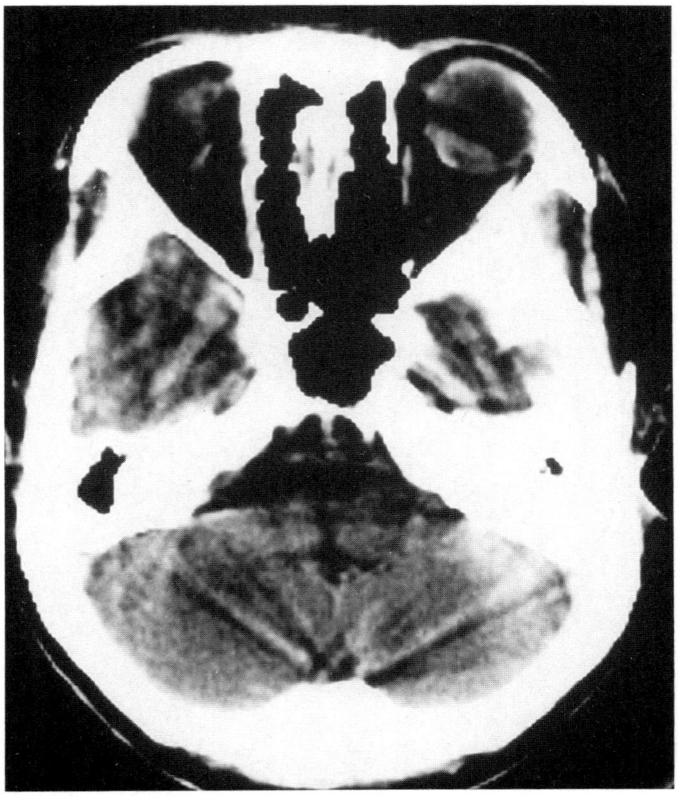

2-3 Axial CT scan through lower posterior fossa (contrast-enhanced study). Section 25 in Fig. 2-1.

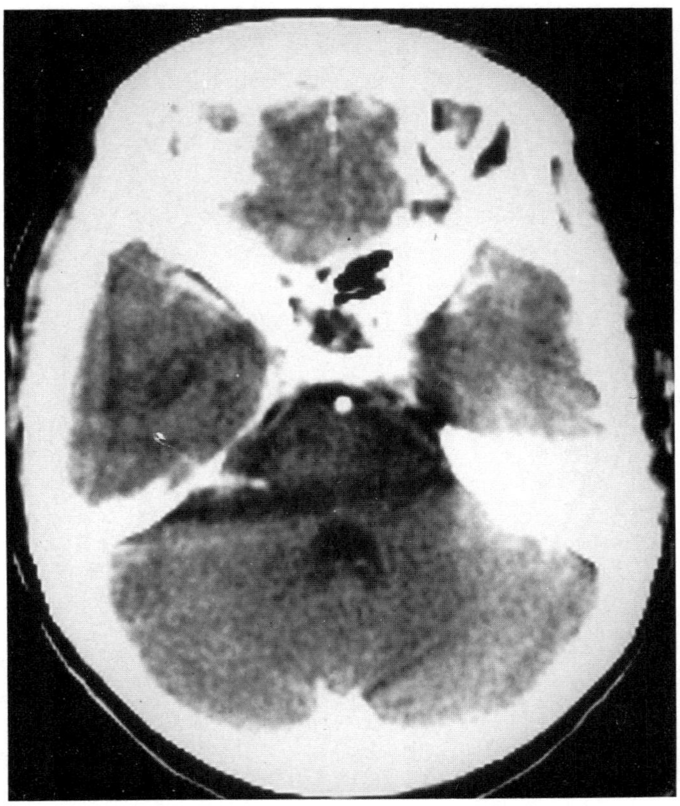

2-4 Axial CT scan through fourth ventricle (contrast-enhanced study). Section 27 in Fig. 2-1.

2/Brain, Axial CT

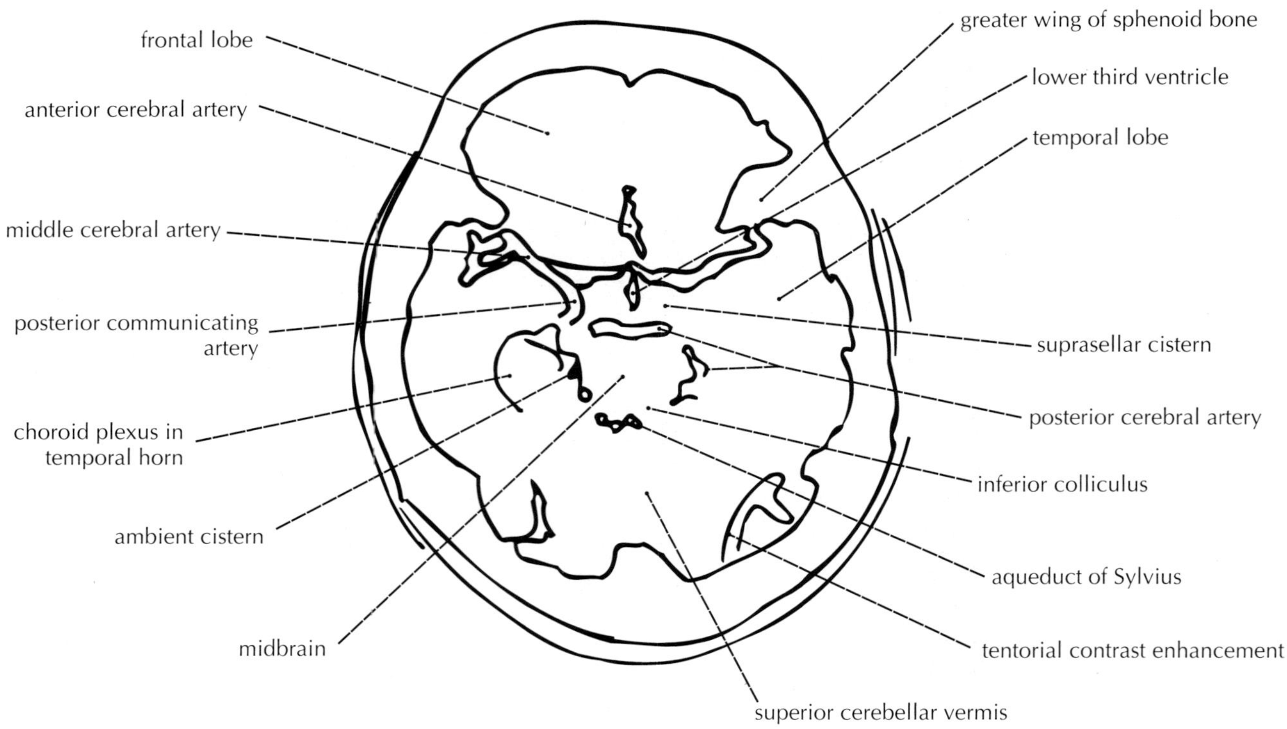

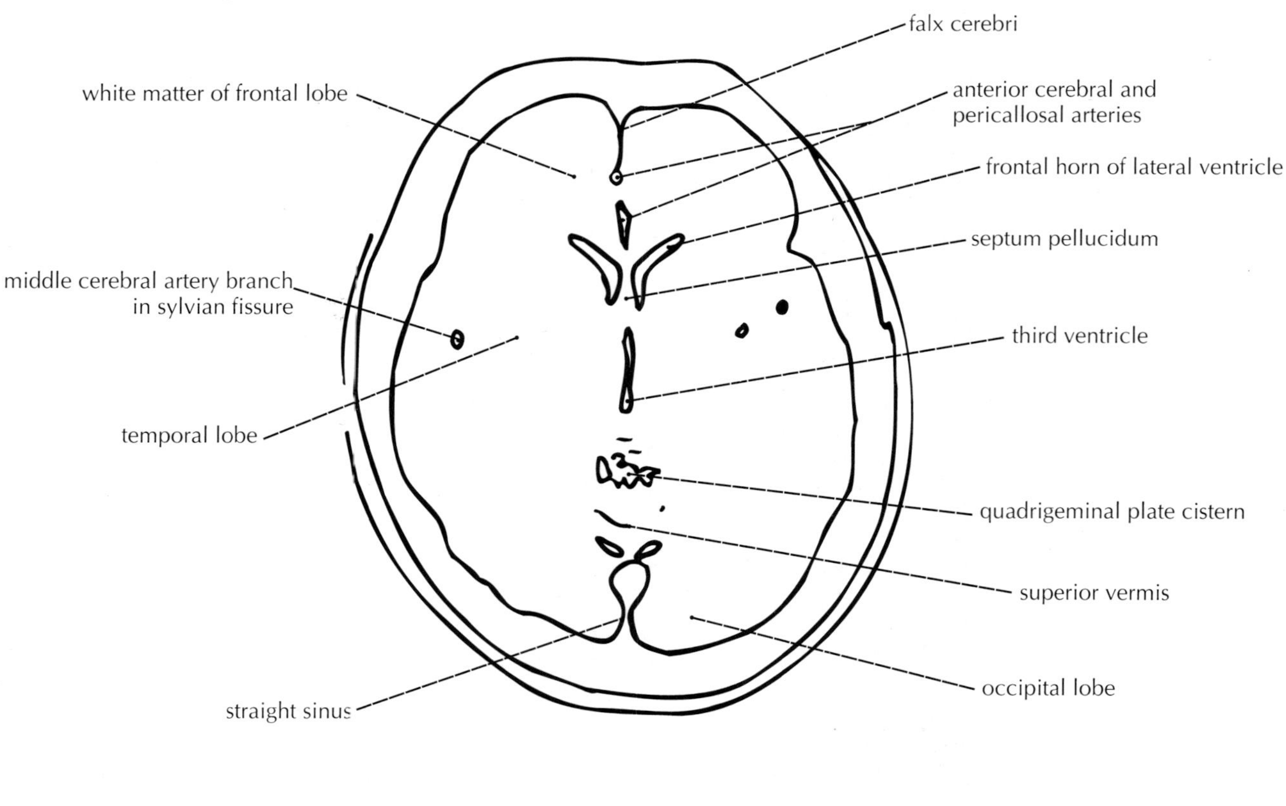

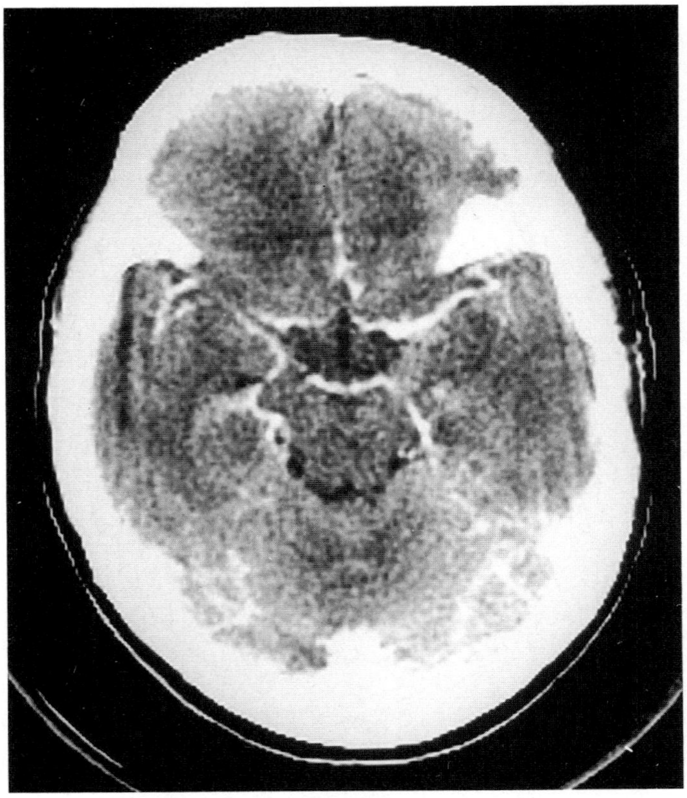

2-5 Axial CT scan through midbrain (contrast-enhanced study). Section 30 in Fig. 2-1.

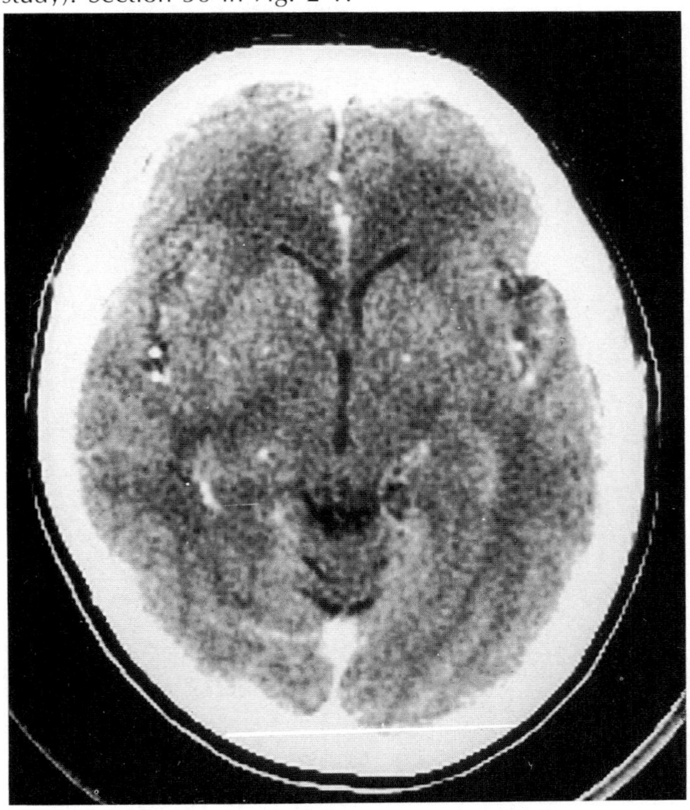

2-6 Axial CT scan through third ventricle (contrast-enhanced study). Section 32 in Fig. 2-1.

2/Brain, Axial CT

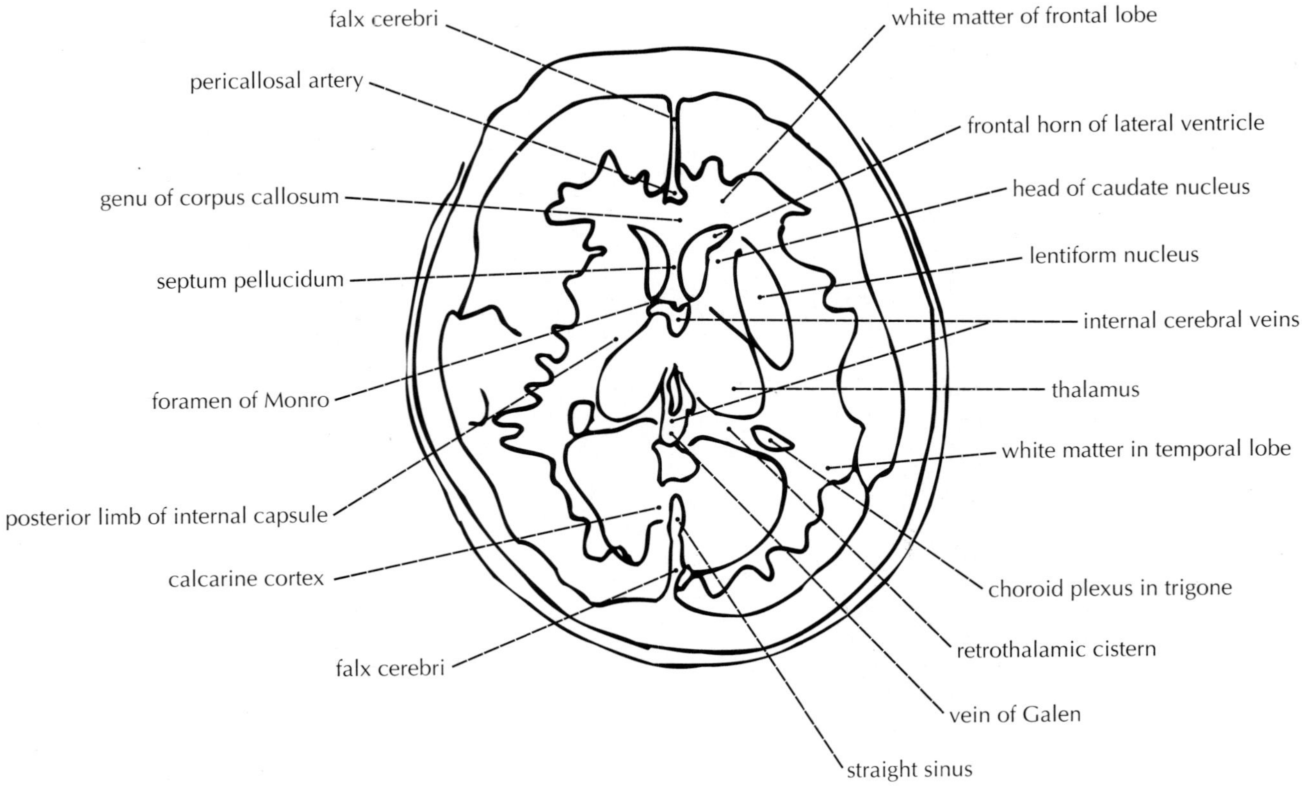

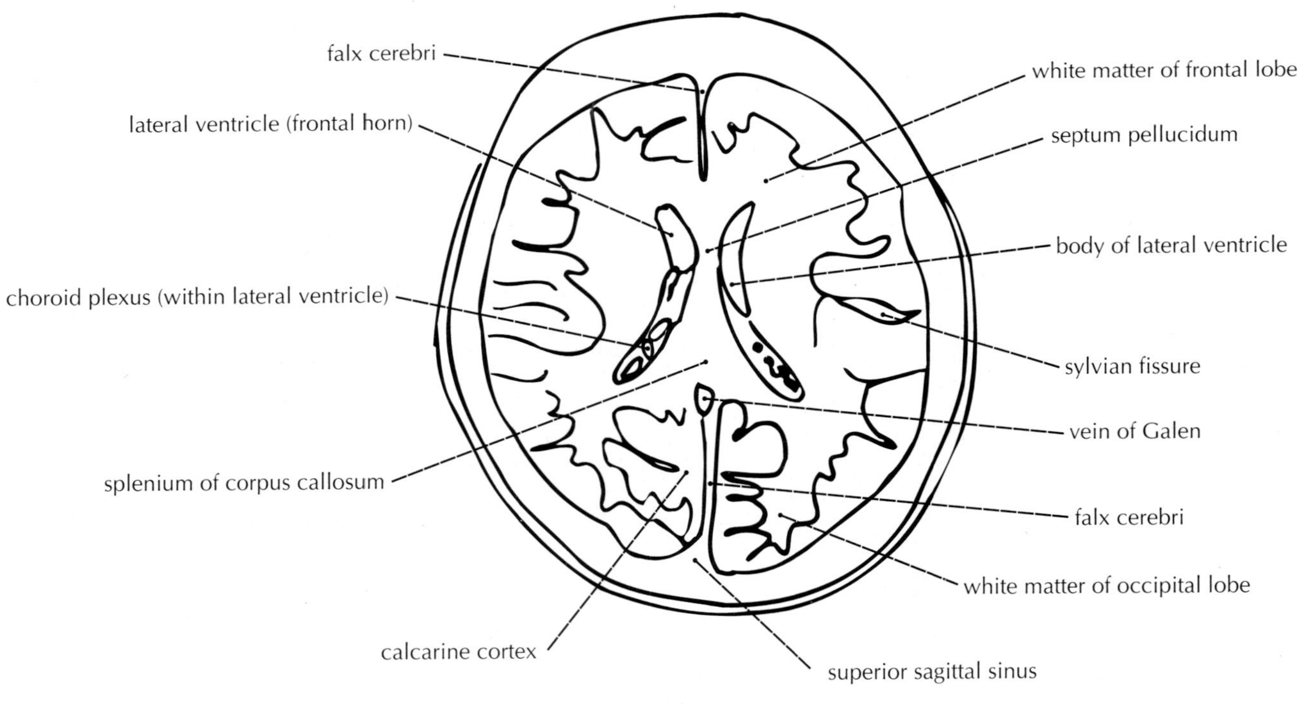

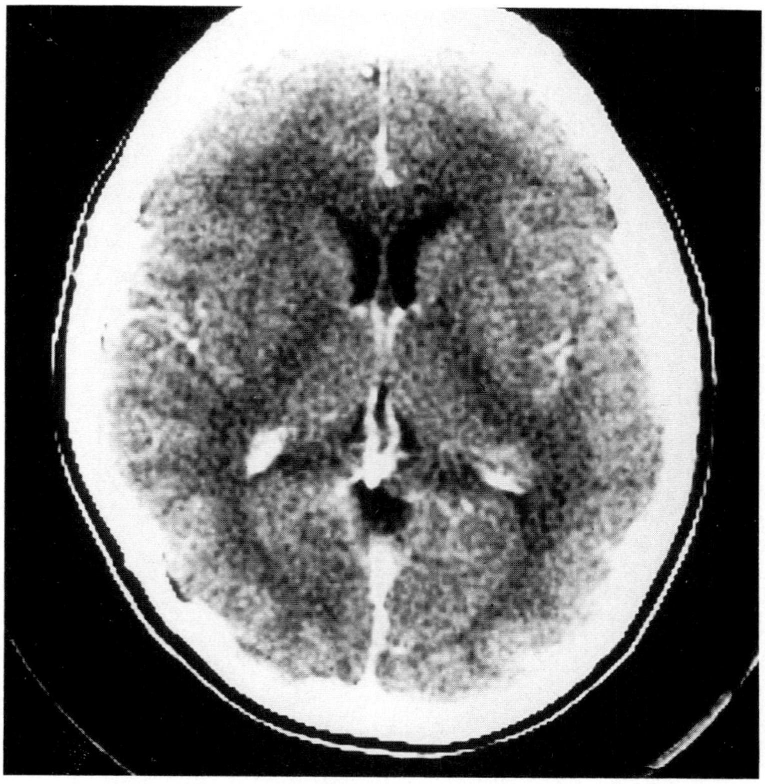

2-7 Axial CT scan through third ventricle and basal ganglia (contrast-enhanced study). Section 33 in Fig. 2-1.

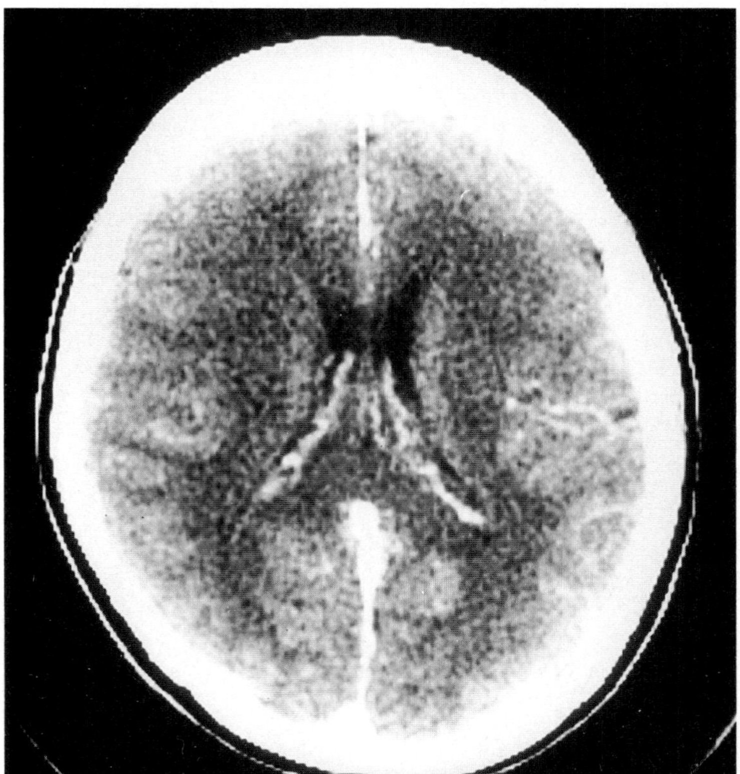

2-8 Axial CT scan through bodies of lateral ventricles (contrast-enhanced study). Section 34 in Fig. 2-1.

2/Brain, Axial CT

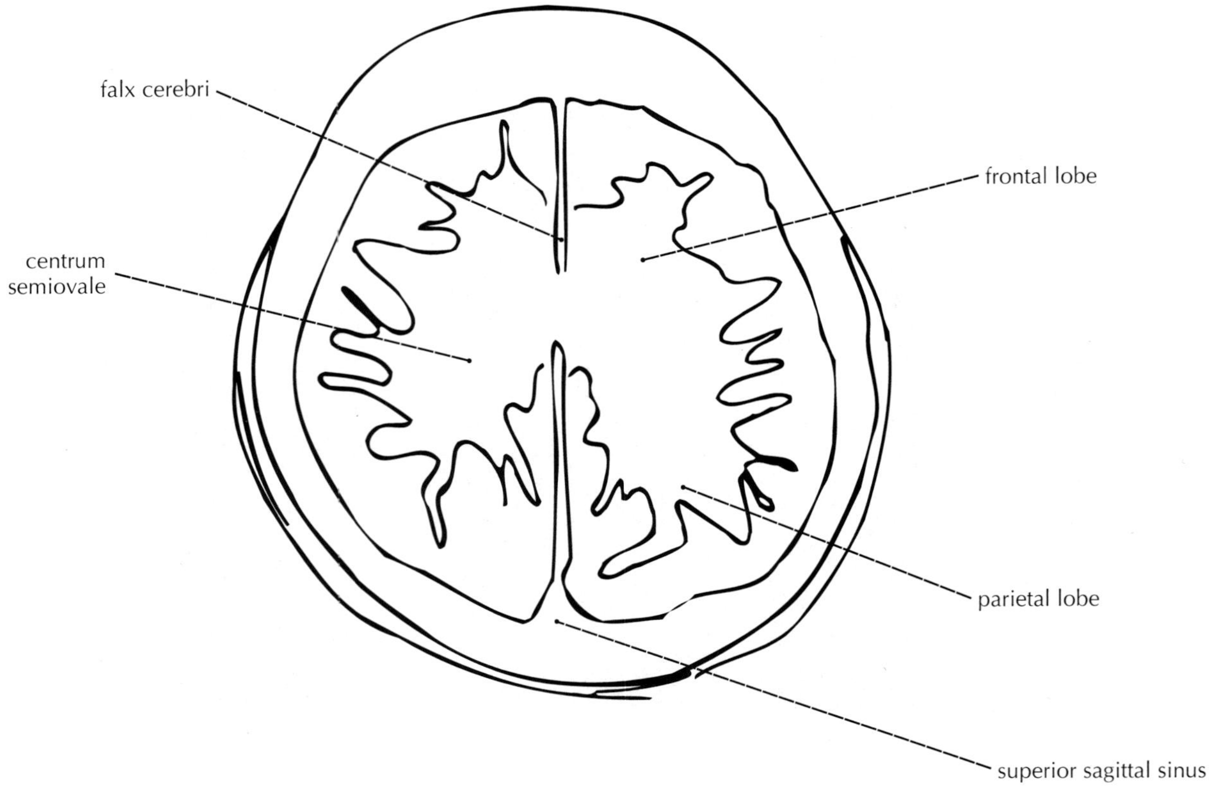

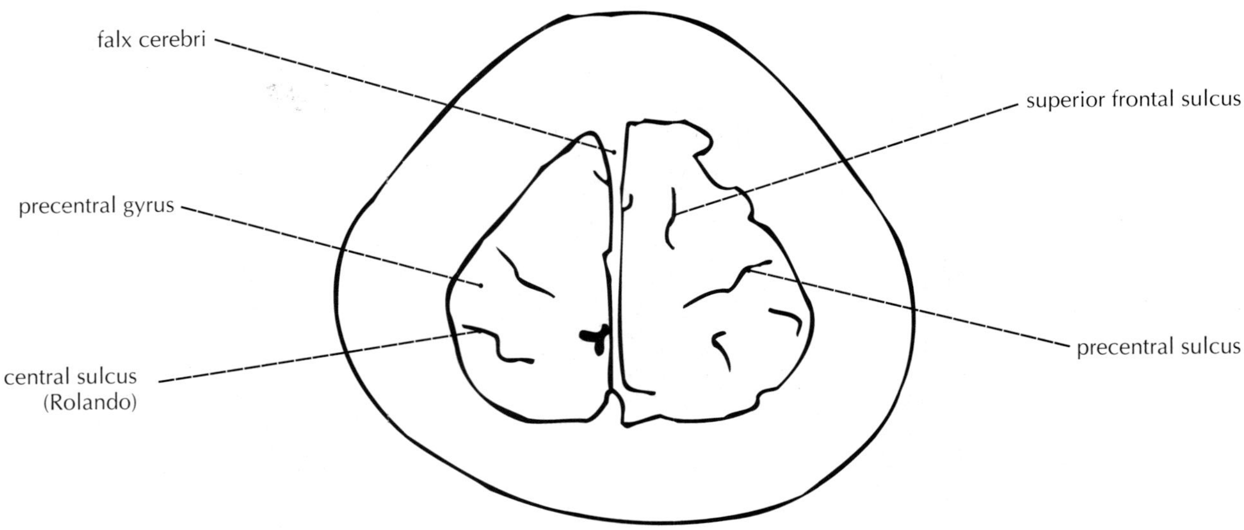

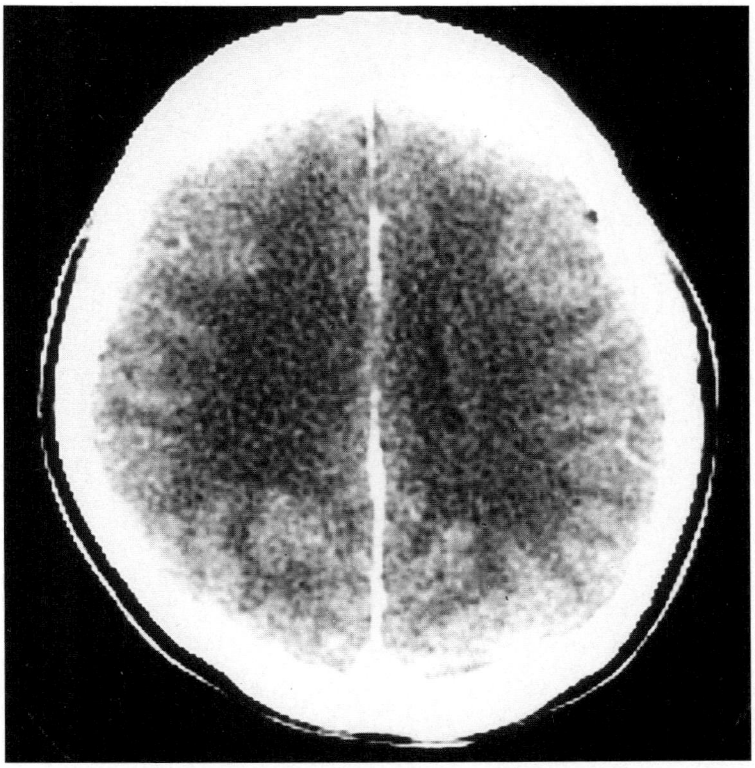

2-9 Axial CT scan through centrum semiovale (contrast-enhanced study). Section 36 in Fig. 2-1.

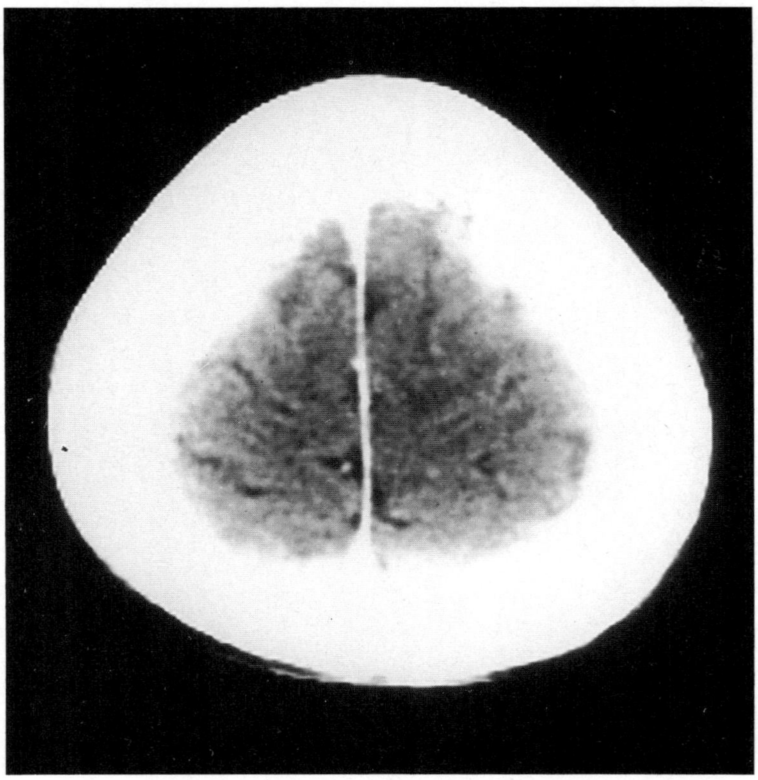

2-10 Axial CT scan through vertex (contrast-enhanced study). Section 38 in Fig. 2-1.

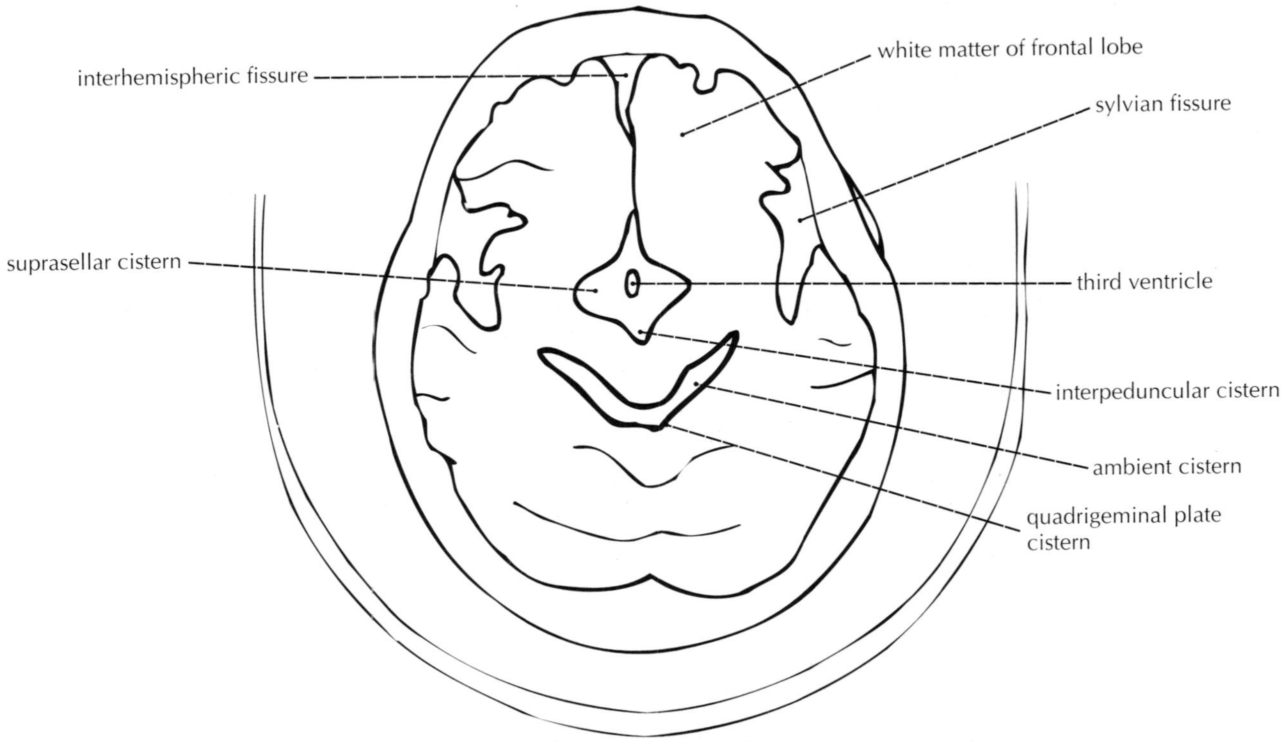

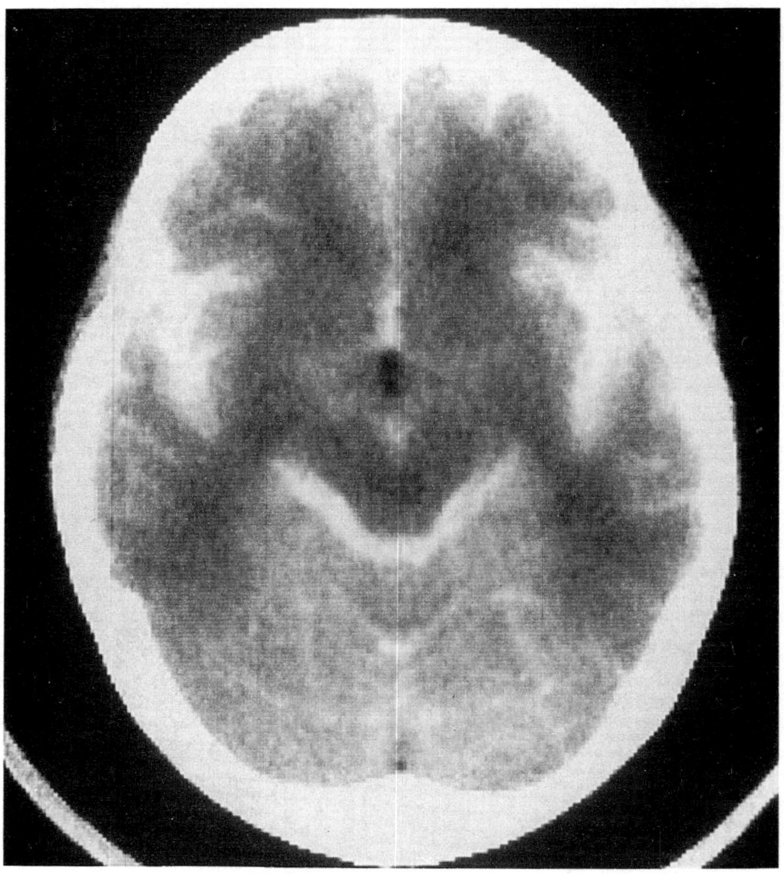

2-11 Contrast cisternogram through suprasellar area. Section 31 in Fig. 2-1.

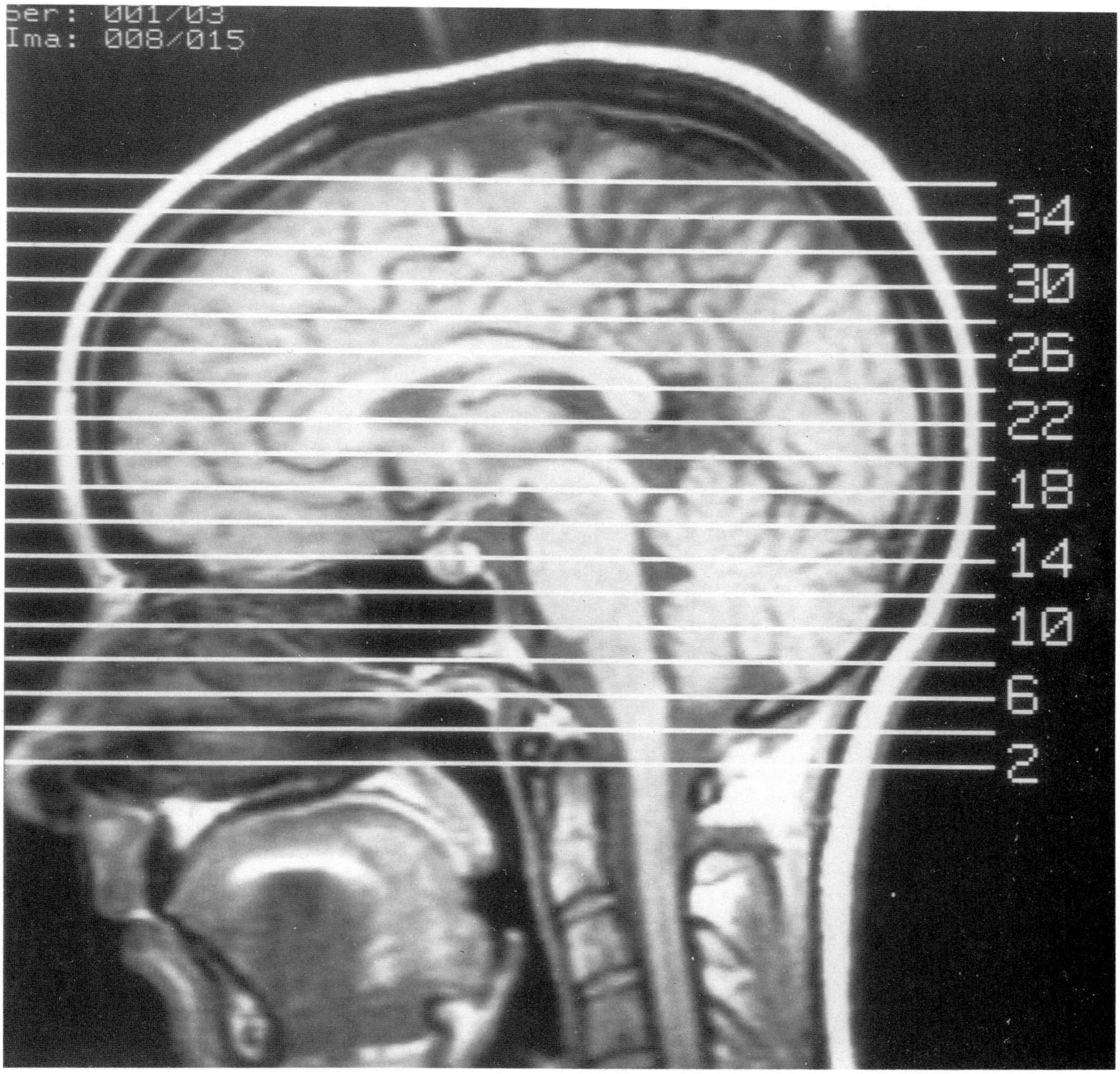

2-12 This sagittal scout MR scan is used to illustrate the locations of selected axial MR sections obtained with various techniques.

2/Brain, Axial MRI

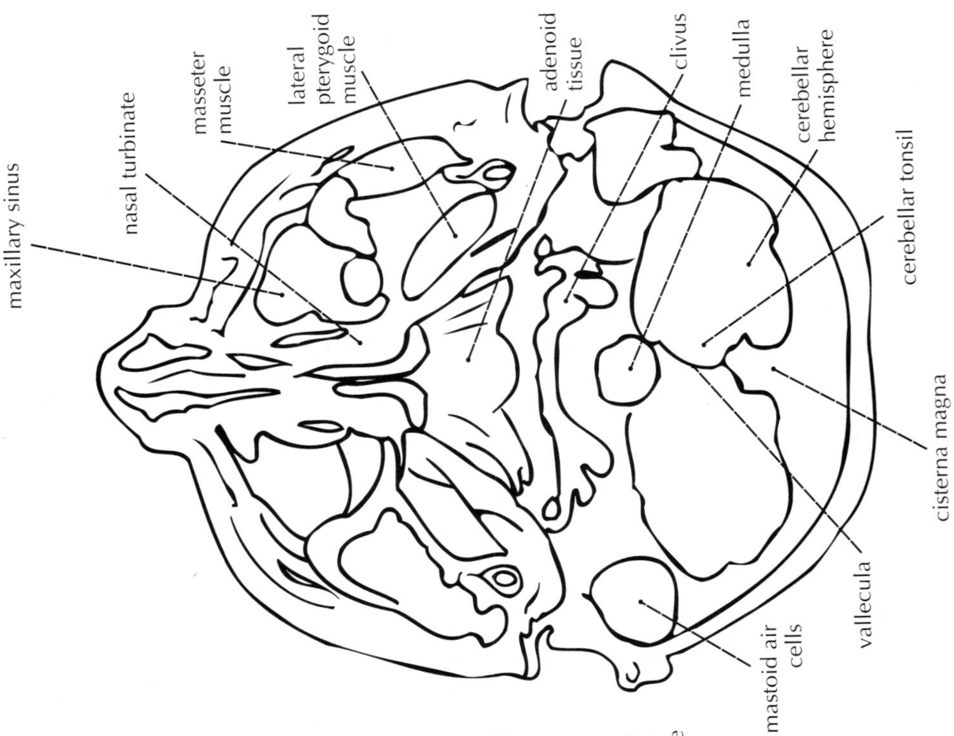

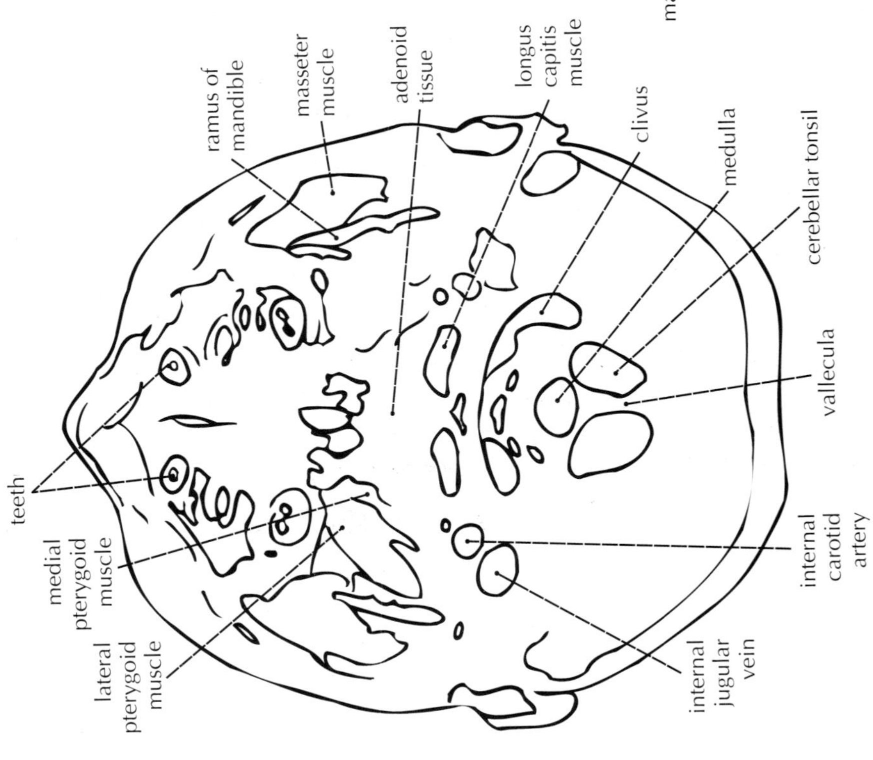

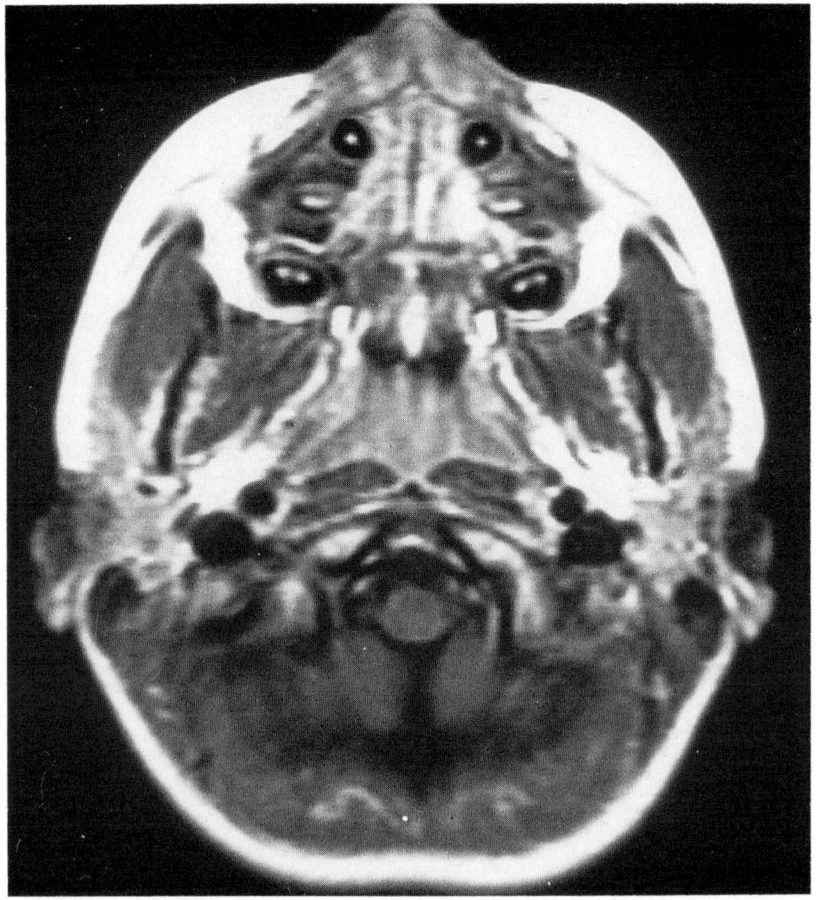

2-13 Axial MR scan of the head (600/15). Contrast-enhanced study. Image between sections 4 and 6 in Fig. 2-12.

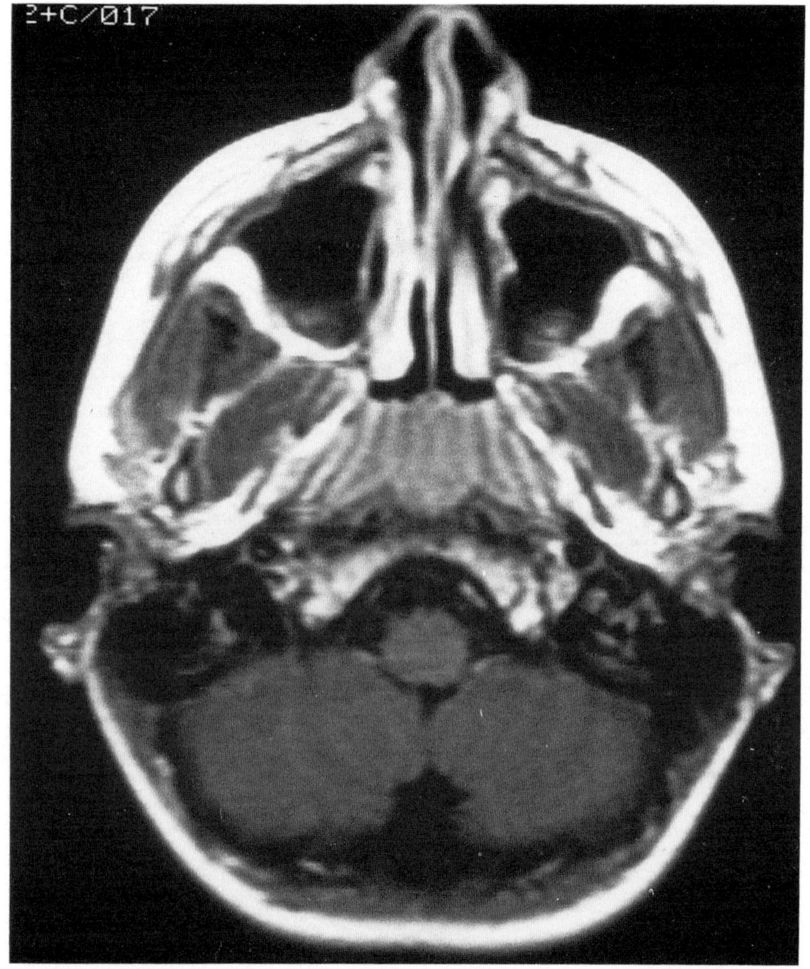

2-14 Axial MR scan through posterior fossa (600/15). Contrast-enhanced study. Section 6 in Fig. 2-12.

2/Brain, Axial MRI

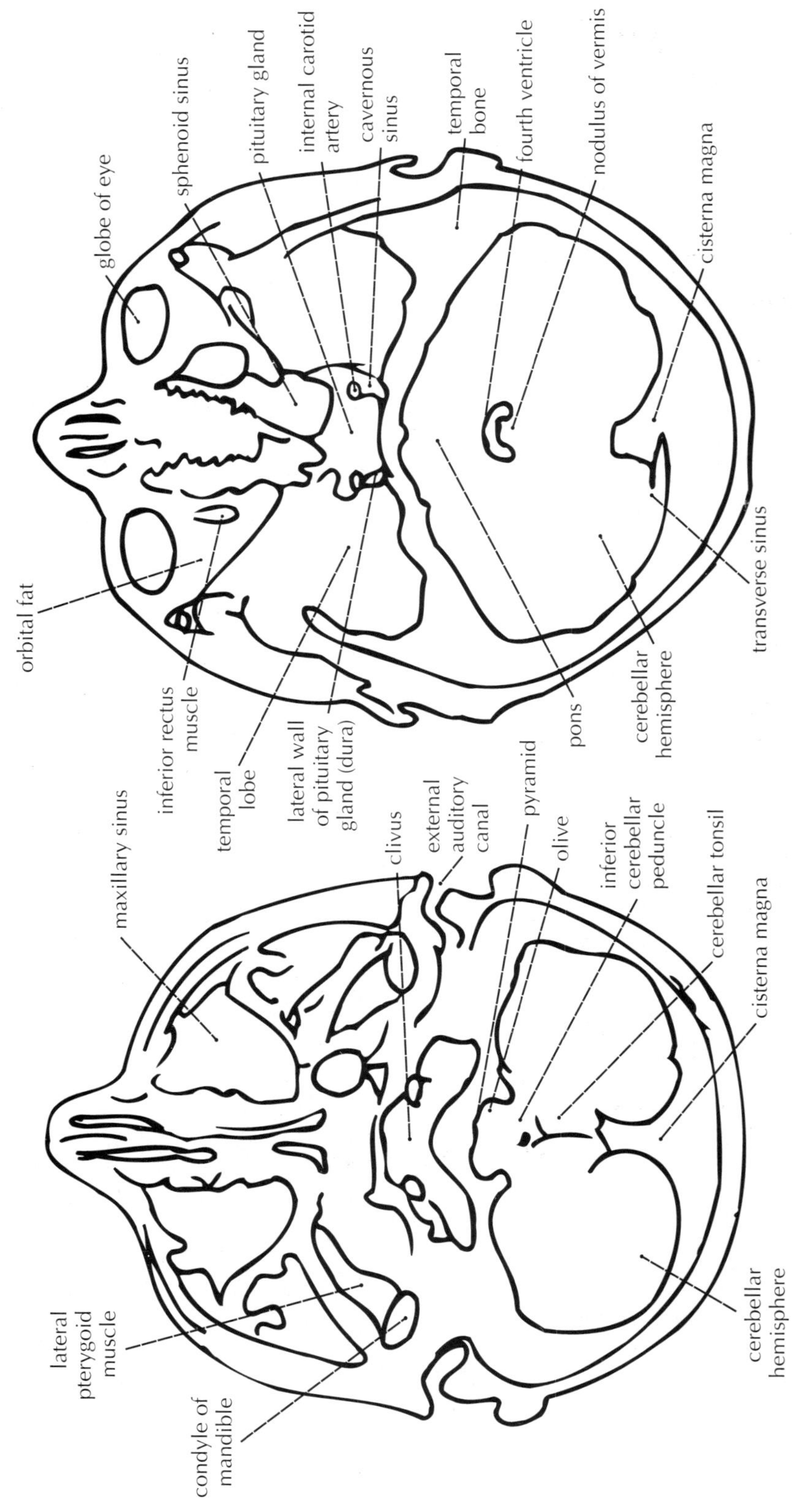

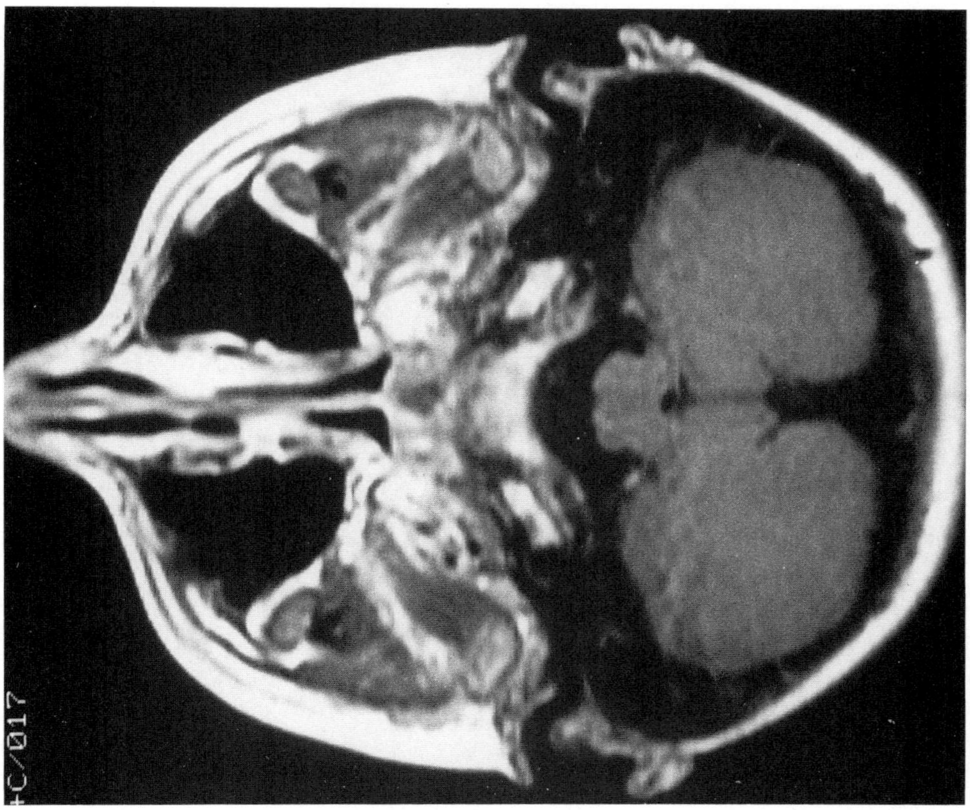

2-15 Axial MR scan through posterior fossa and tonsils (600/15). Contrast-enhanced study. Section 8 in Fig. 2-12.

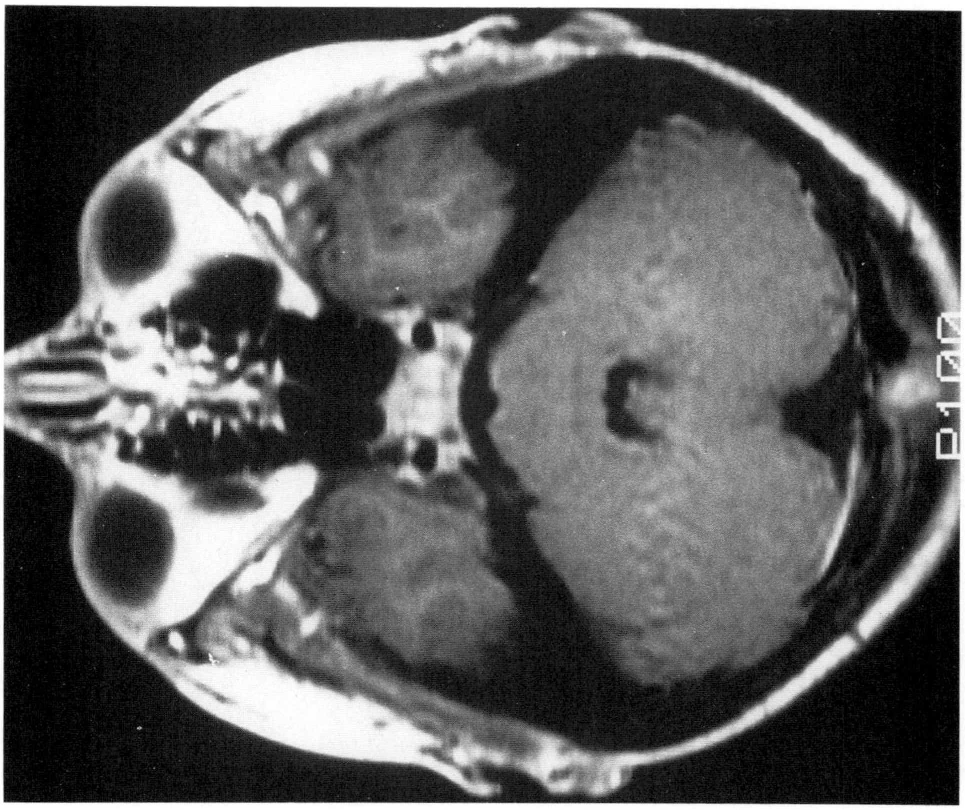

2-16 Axial MR scan through fourth ventricle (600/15). Contrast-enhanced study. Section 12 in Fig. 2-12.

2/Brain, Axial MRI

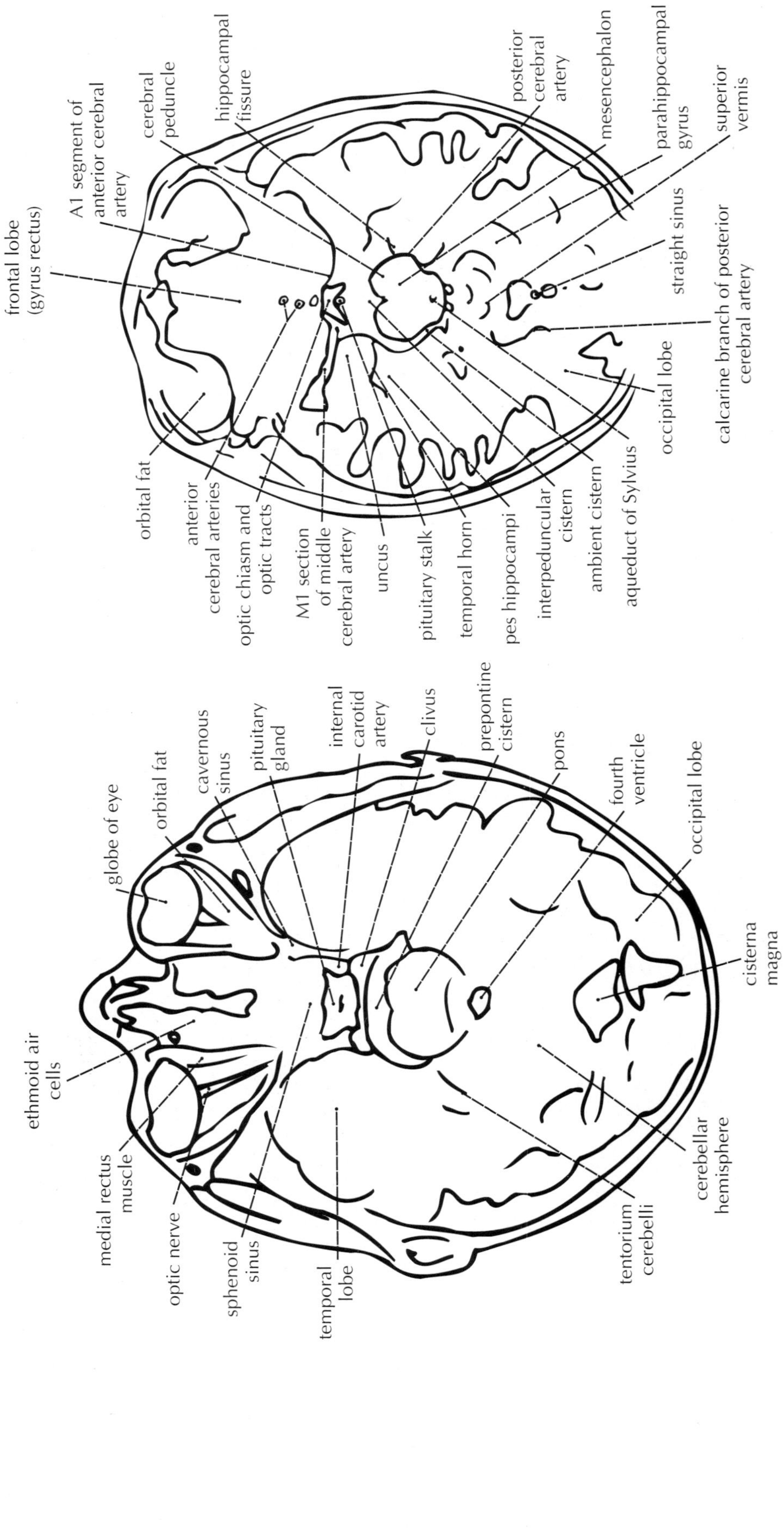

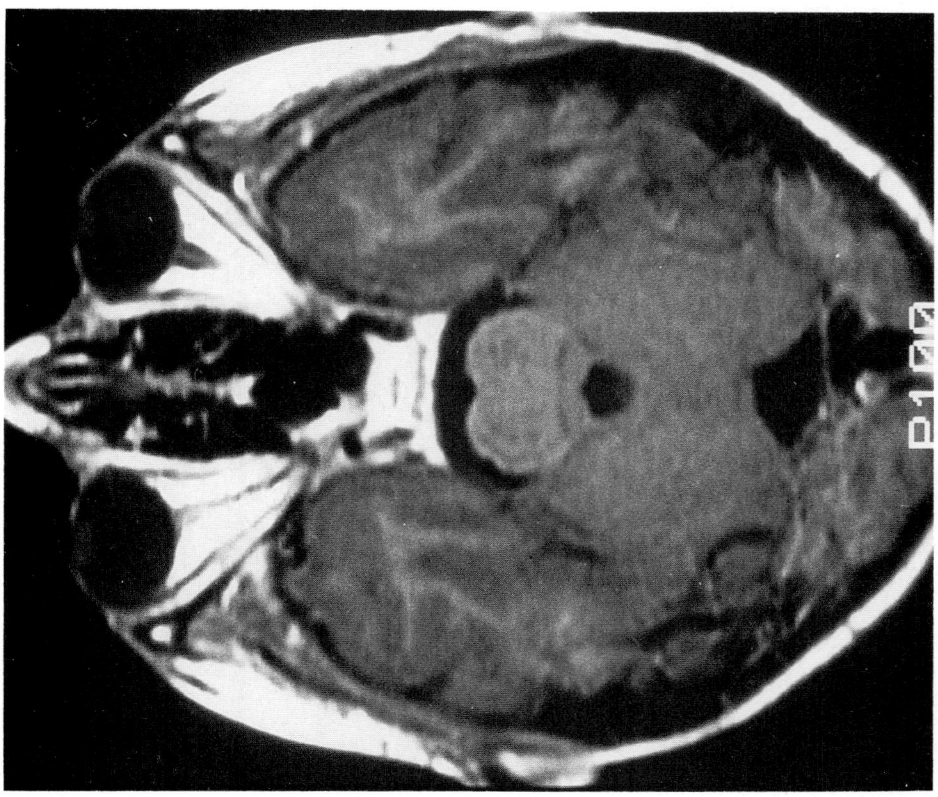

2-17 Axial MR scan through pons (600/15). Contrast-enhanced study. Section 14 in Fig. 2-12.

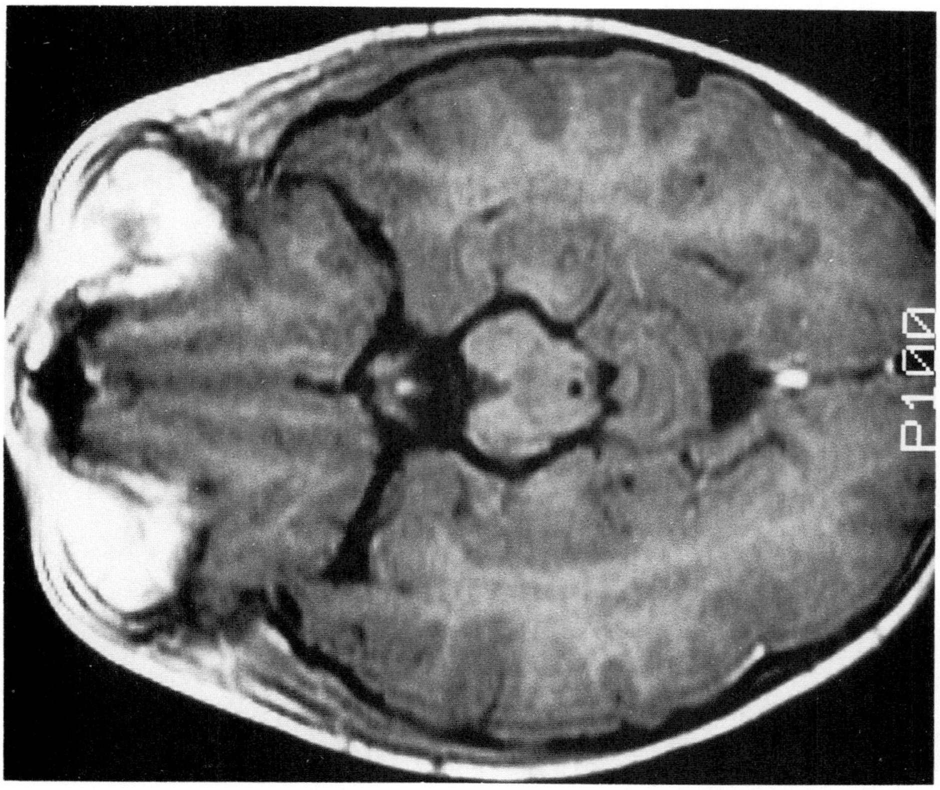

2-18 Axial MR scan through suprasellar cistern (600/15). Contrast-enhanced study. Section 16 in Fig. 2-12.

2/Brain, Axial MRI

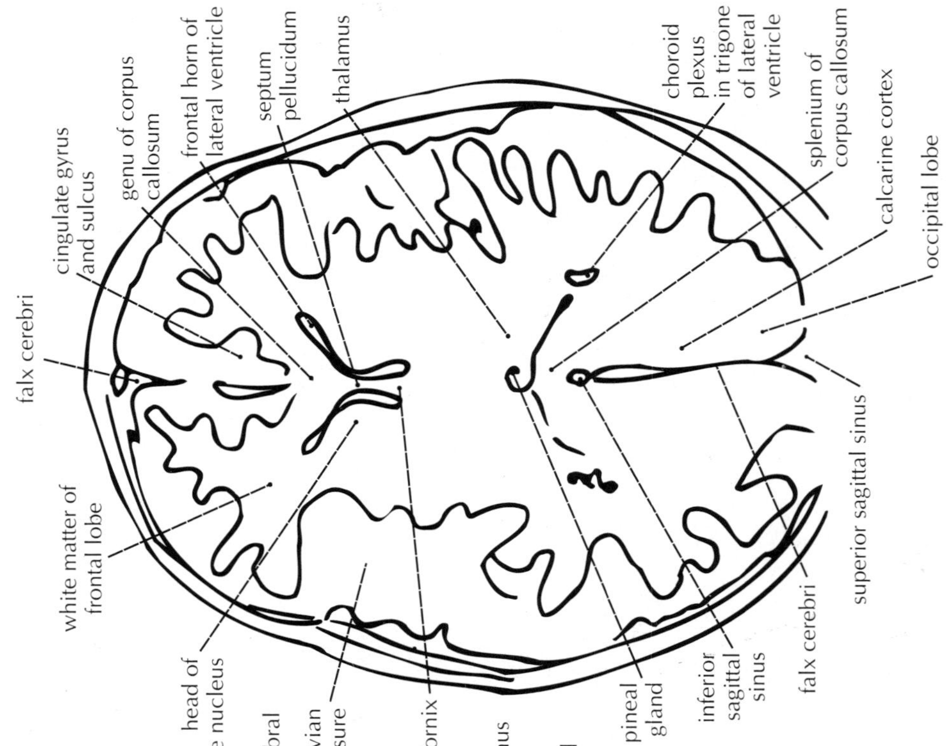

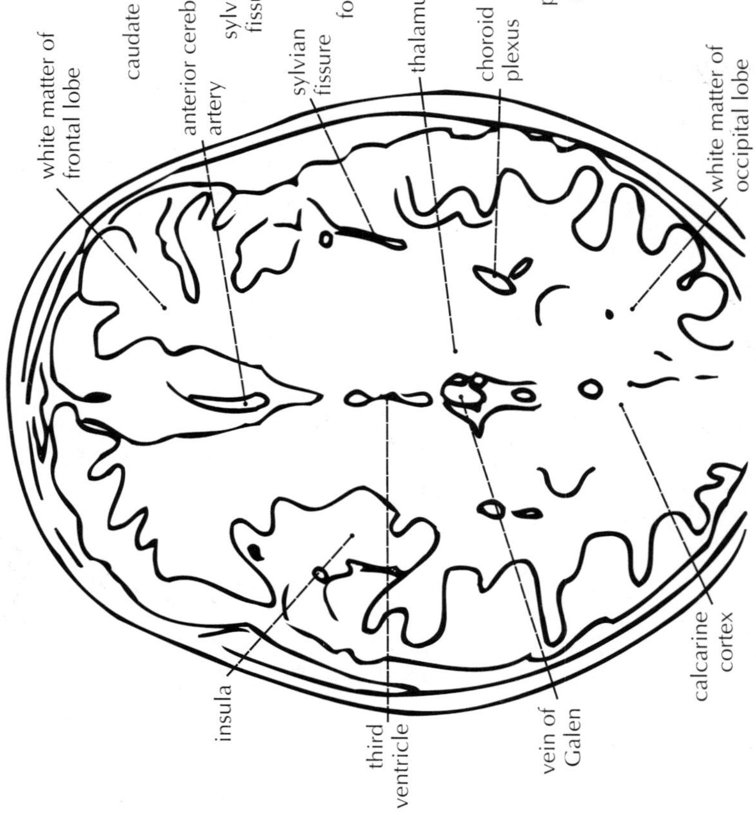

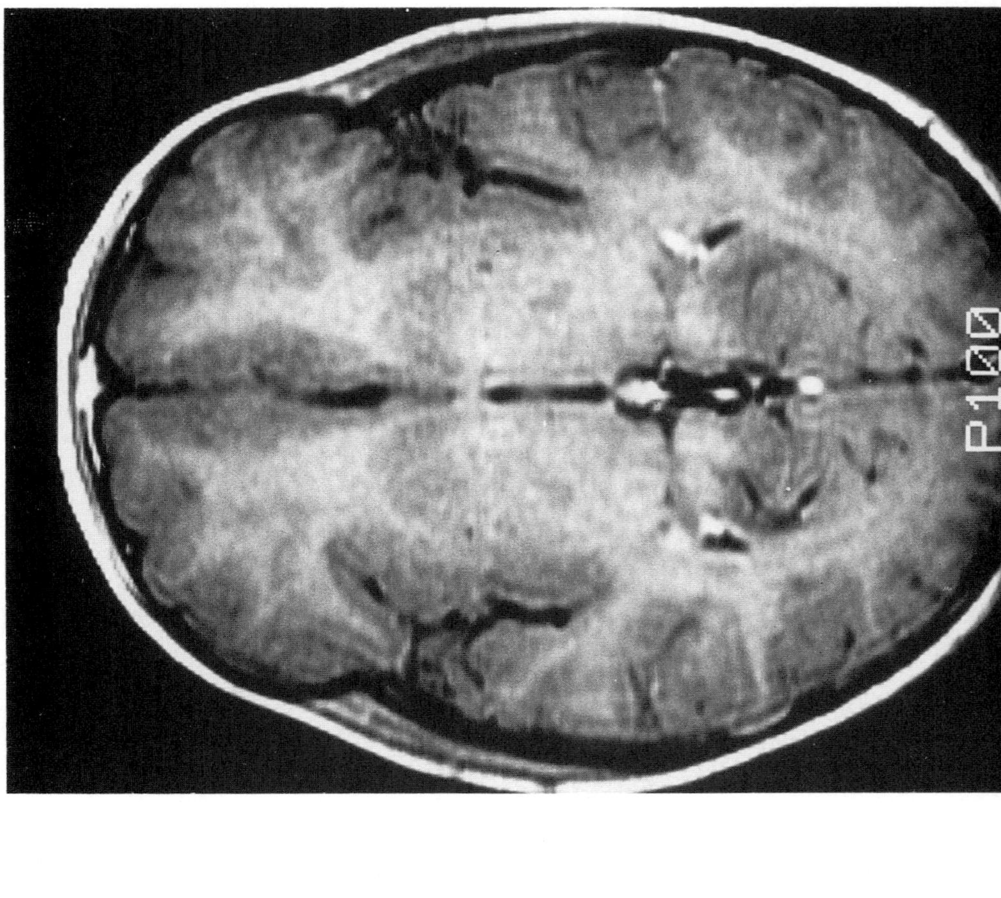

2-19 Axial MR scan through third ventricle (600/15). Contrast-enhanced study. Section 20 in Fig. 2-12.

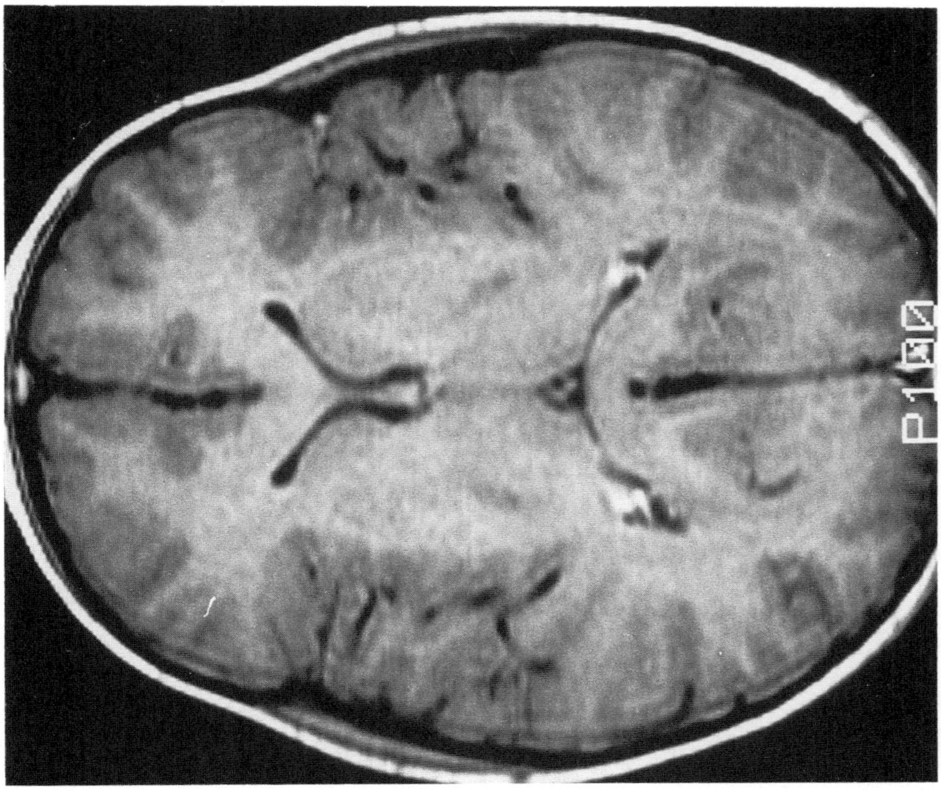

2-20 Axial MR scan through lateral ventricles (600/15). Contrast-enhanced study. Section 22 in Fig. 2-12.

2/Brain, Axial MRI

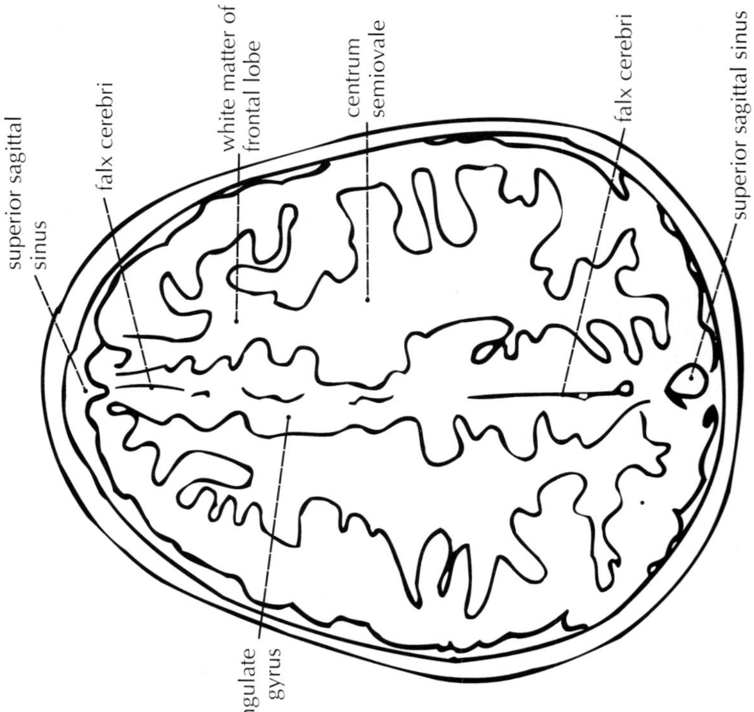

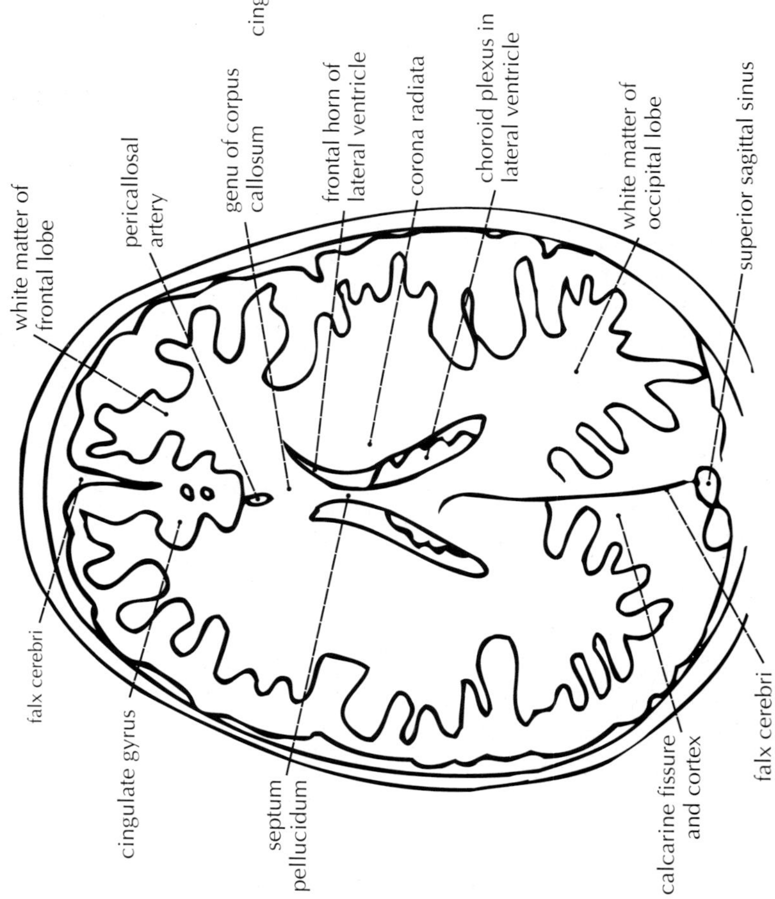

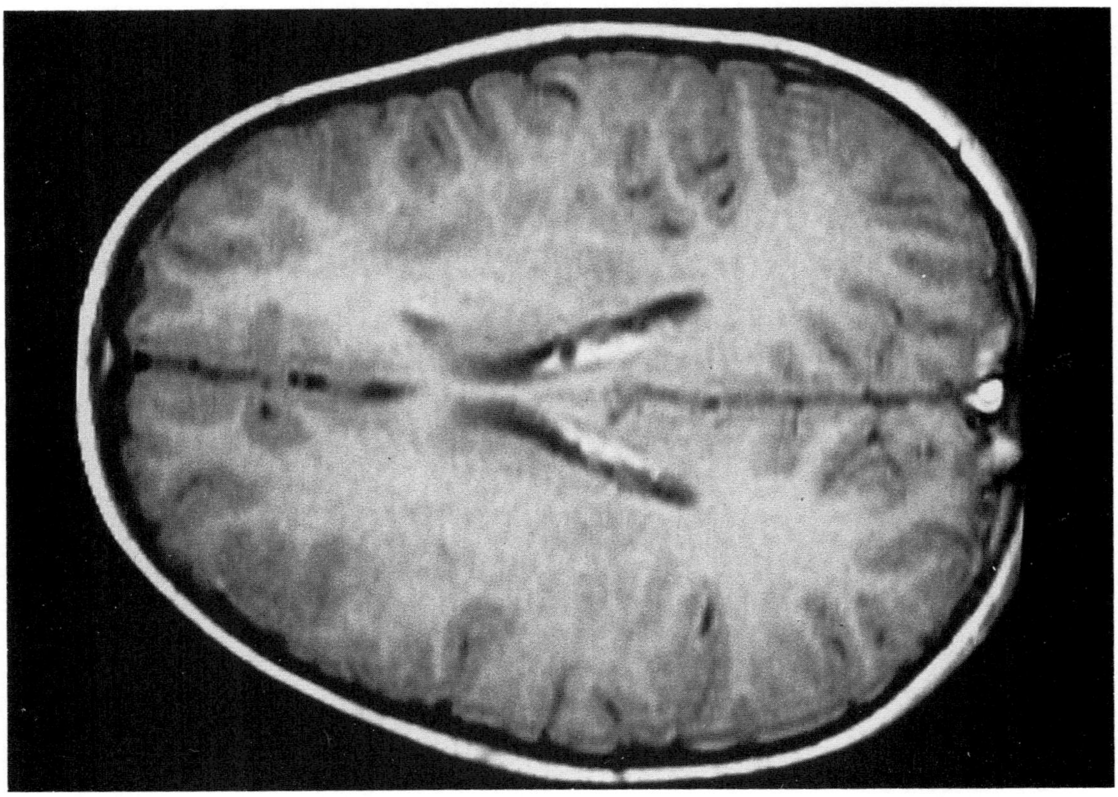

2-21 Axial MR scan through lateral ventricles (600/15). Contrast-enhanced study. Section 24 in Fig. 2-12.

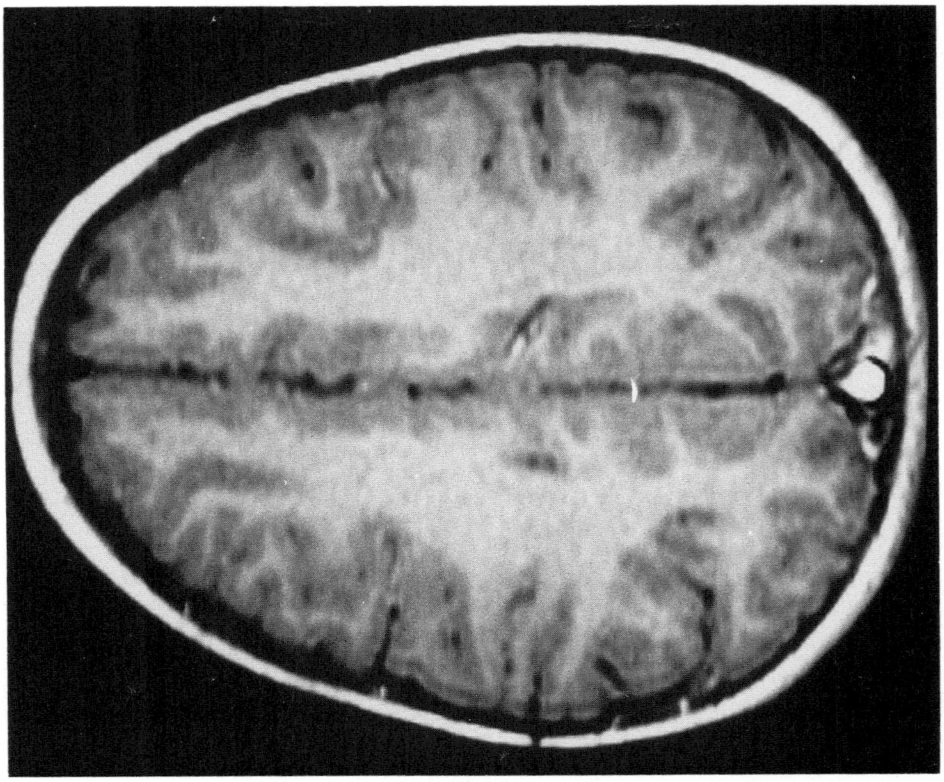

2-22 Axial MR scan through centrum semiovale (600/15). Contrast-enhanced study. Section 26 in Fig. 2-12.

2/Brain, Axial MRI

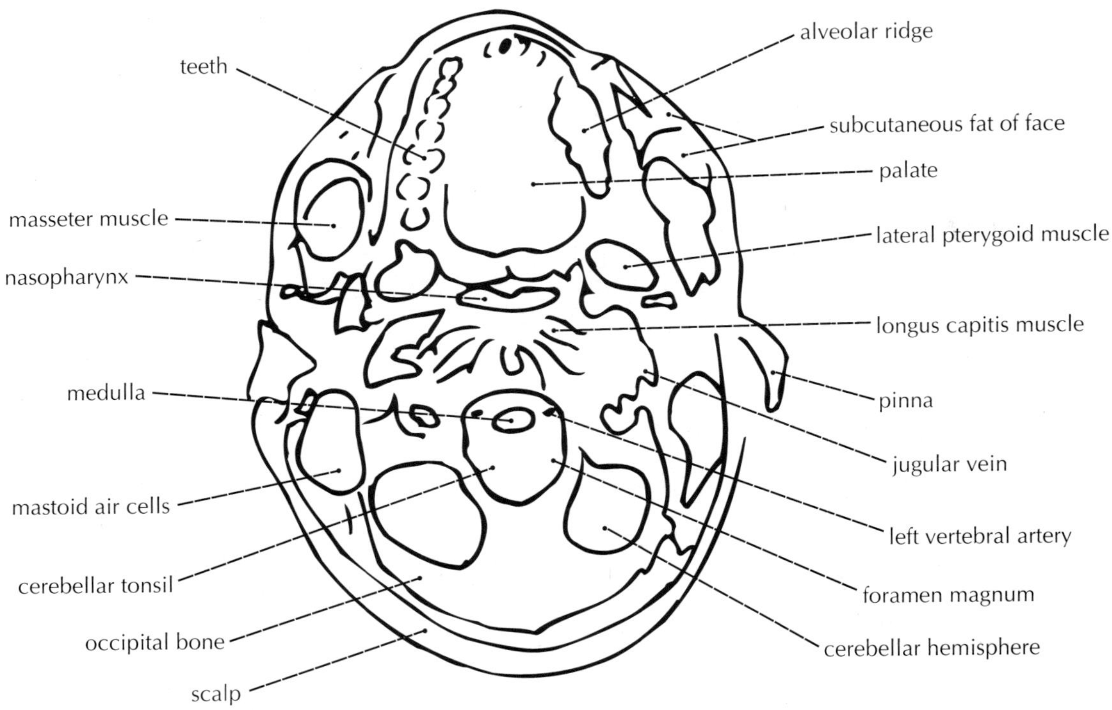

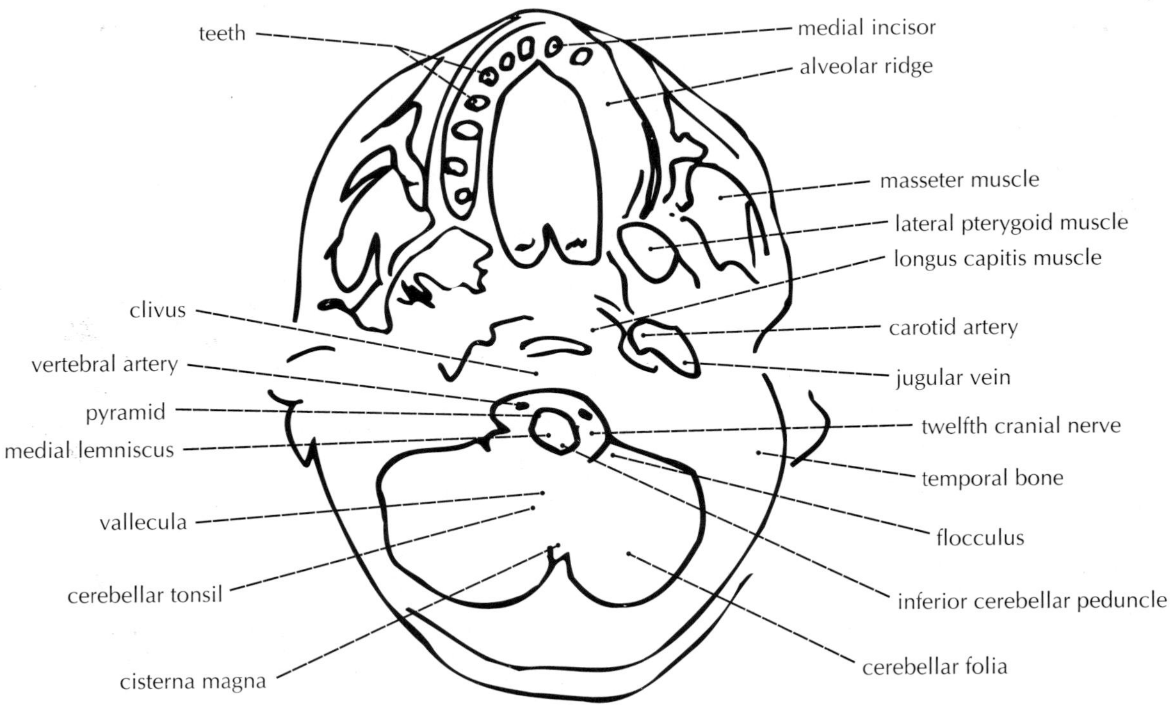

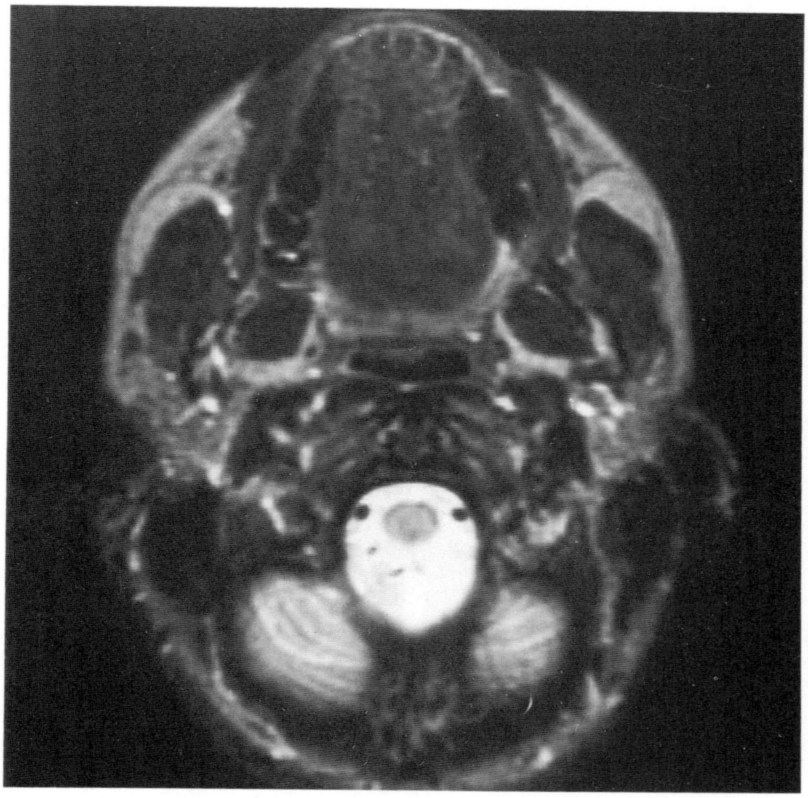

2-23 Axial MR scan through foramen magnum and lower posterior fossa (2000/90). Section 4 in Fig. 2-12.

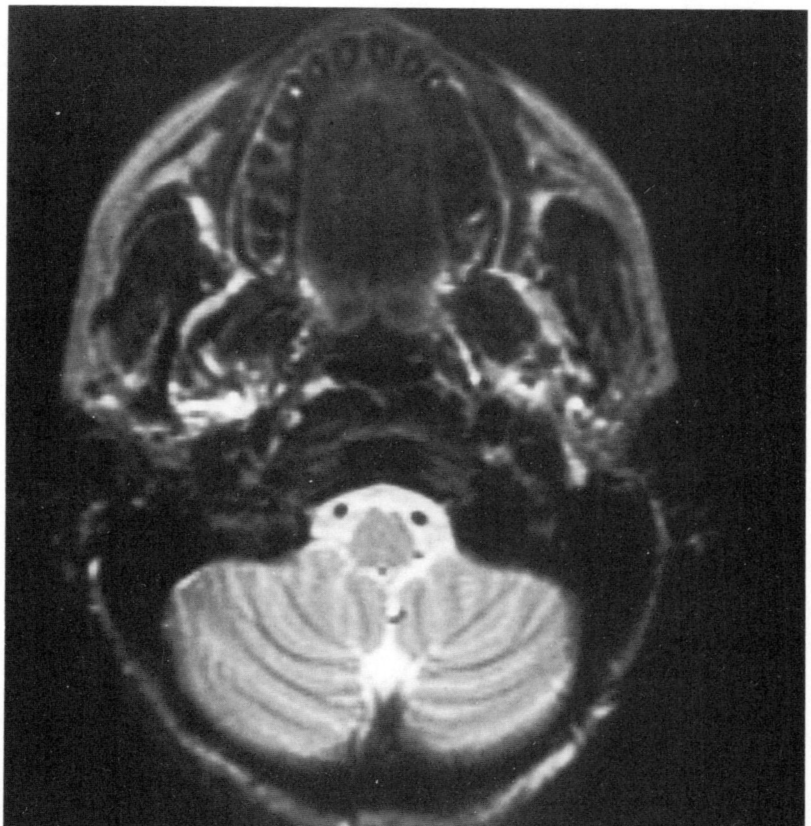

2-24 Axial MR scan through posterior fossa (2000/90). Section 6 in Fig. 2-12.

2/Brain, Axial MR

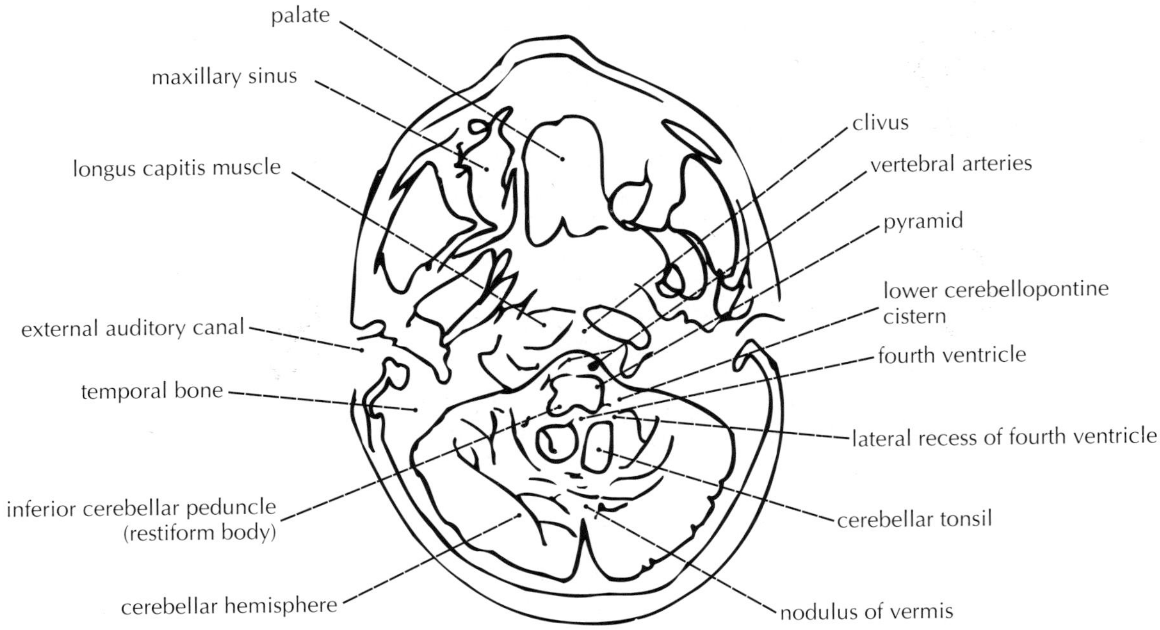

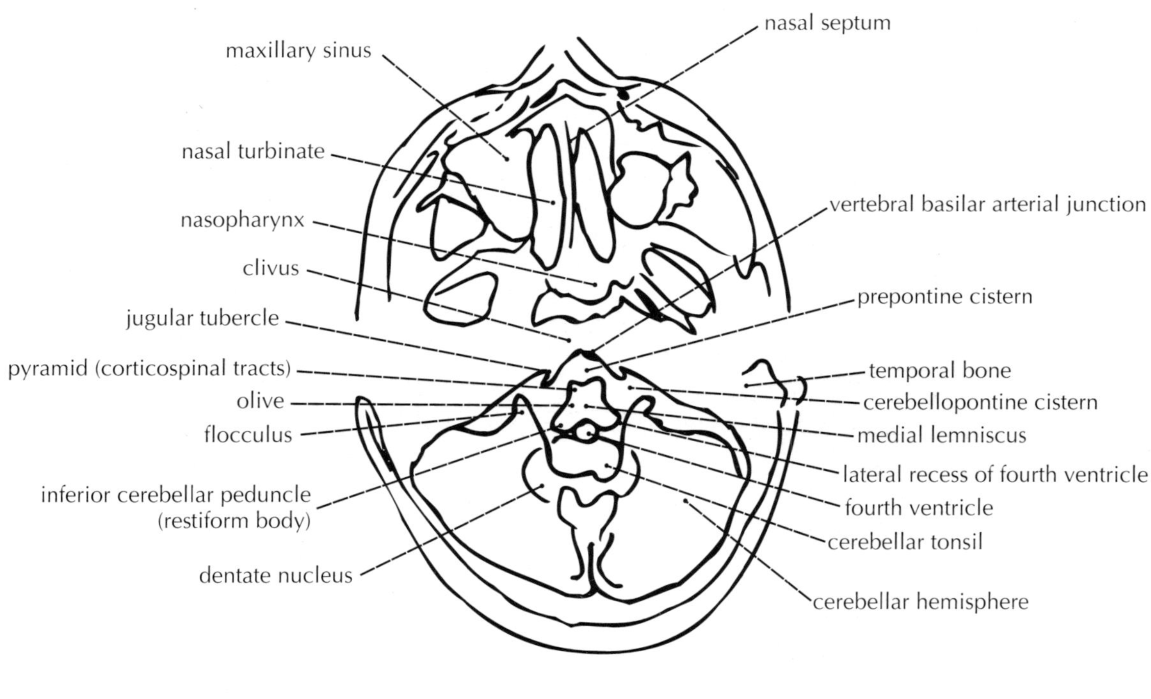

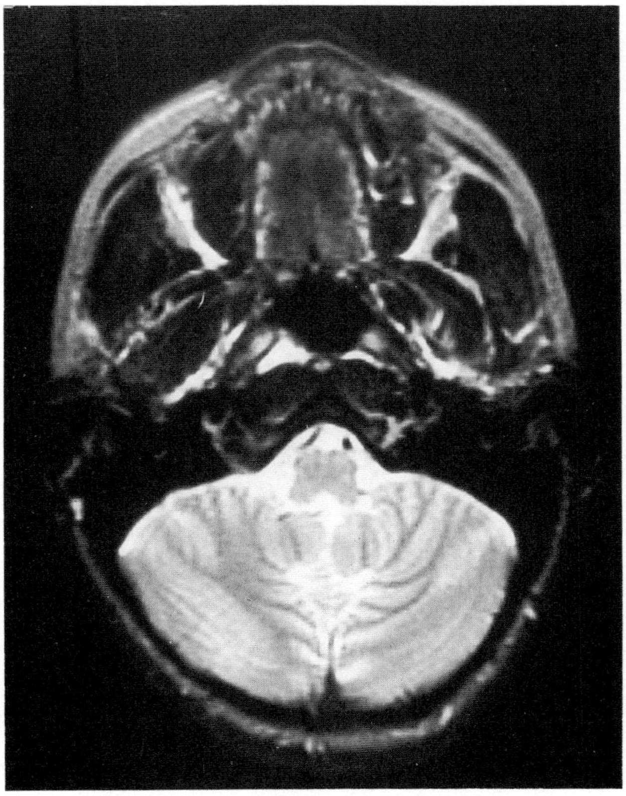

2-25 Axial MR scan through lower fourth ventricle and medulla (2000/90). Section 8 in Fig. 2-12.

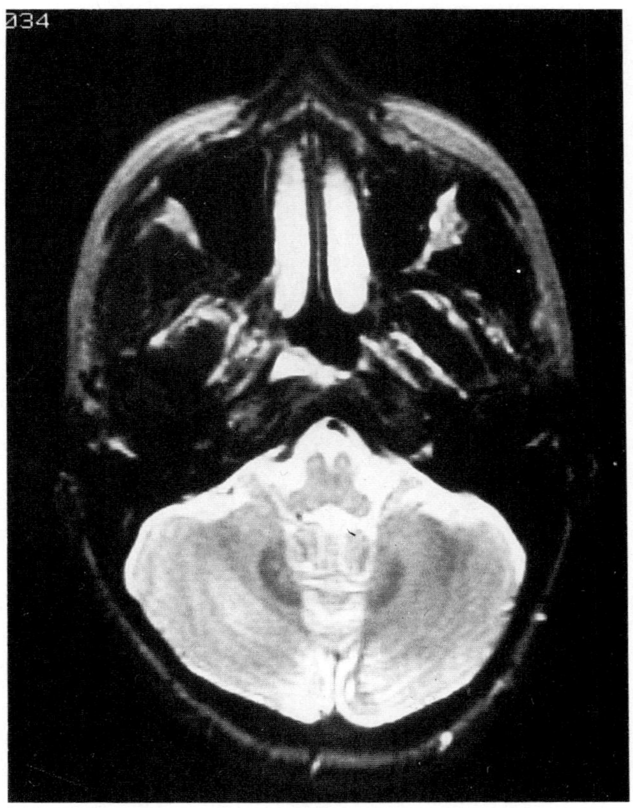

2-26 Axial MR scan through lower fourth ventricle and medulla (2000/90). Section 10 in Fig. 2-12.

2/Brain, Axial MRI

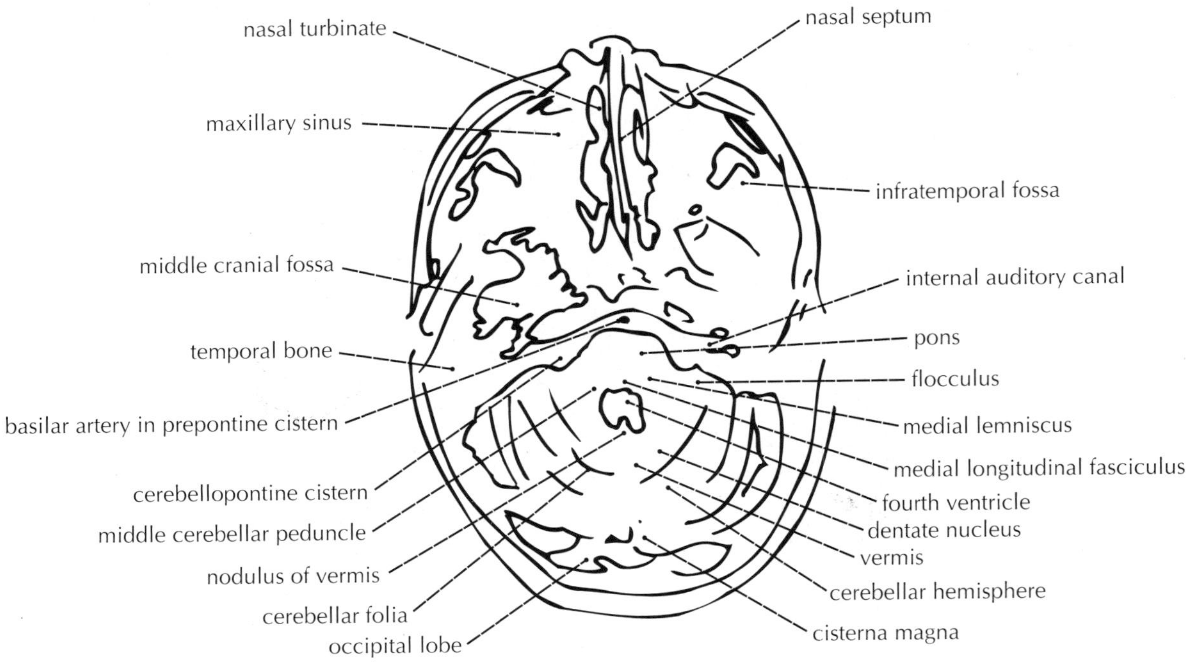

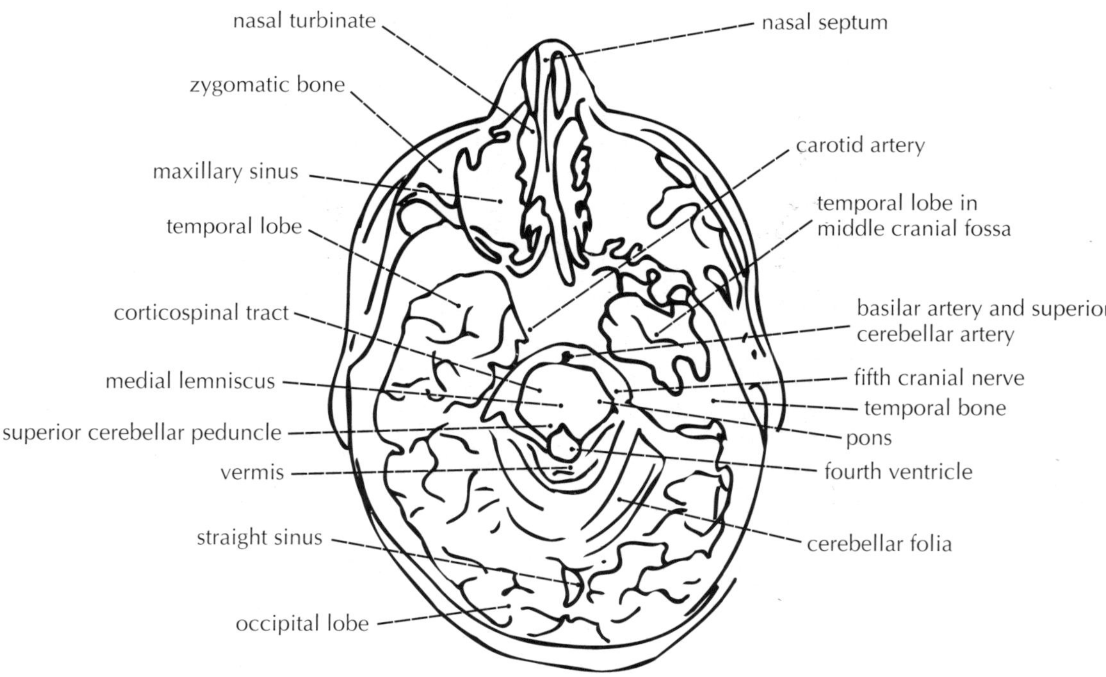

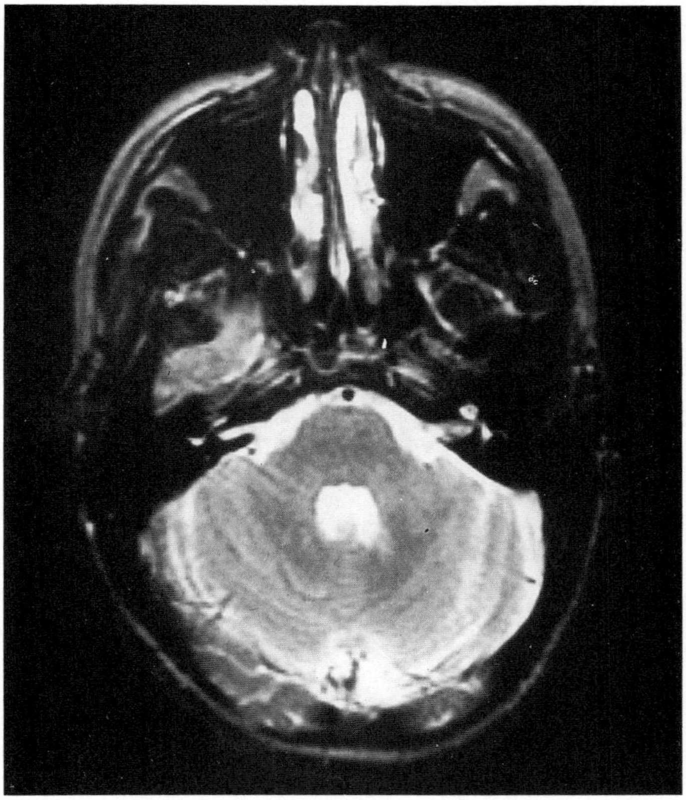

2-27 Axial MR scan through fourth ventricle (2000/90). Section 12 in Fig. 2-12.

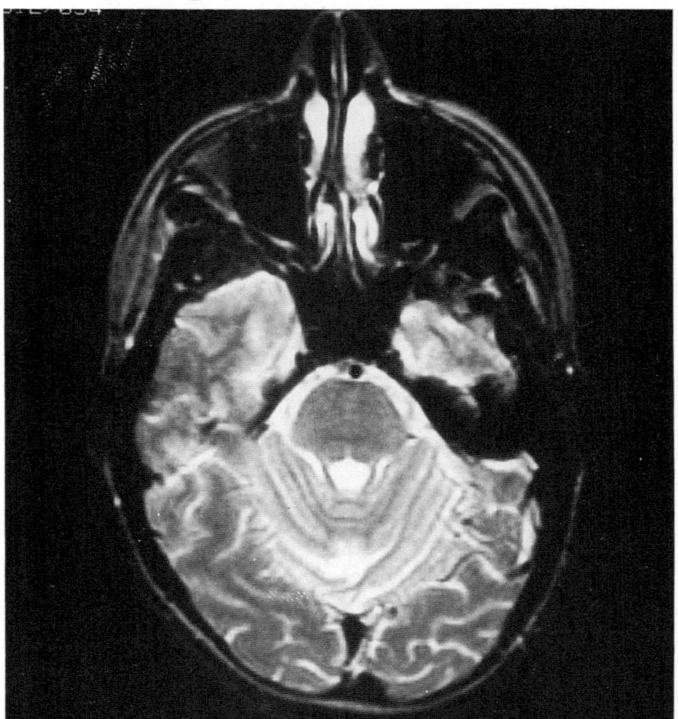

2-28 Axial MR scan through fourth ventricle (2000/90). Section 14 in Fig. 2-12.

2/Brain, Axial MRI

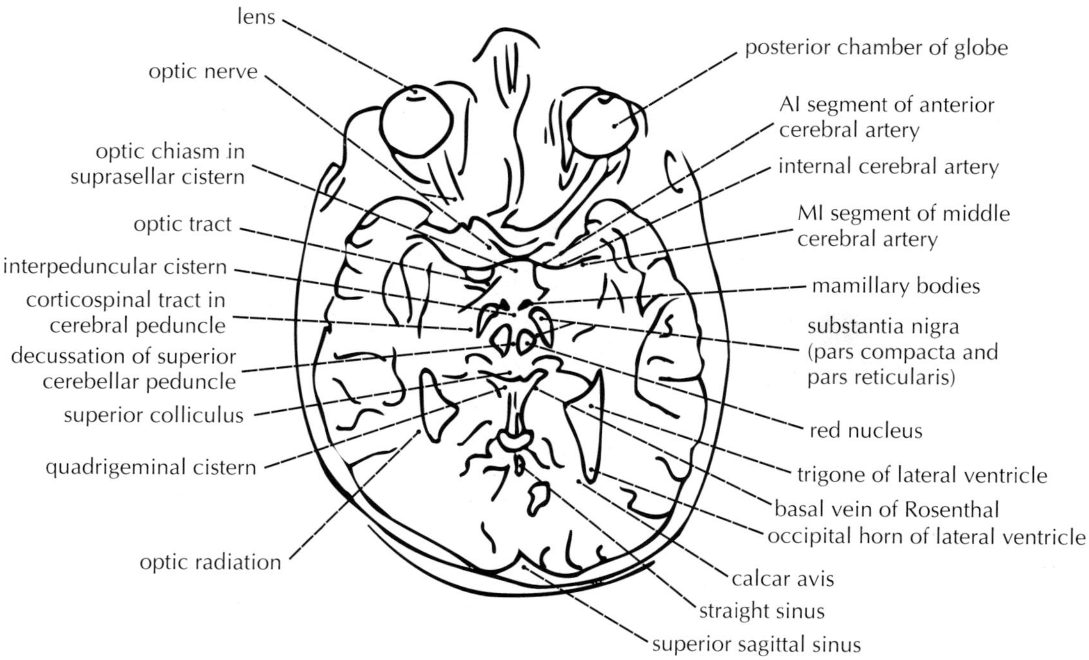

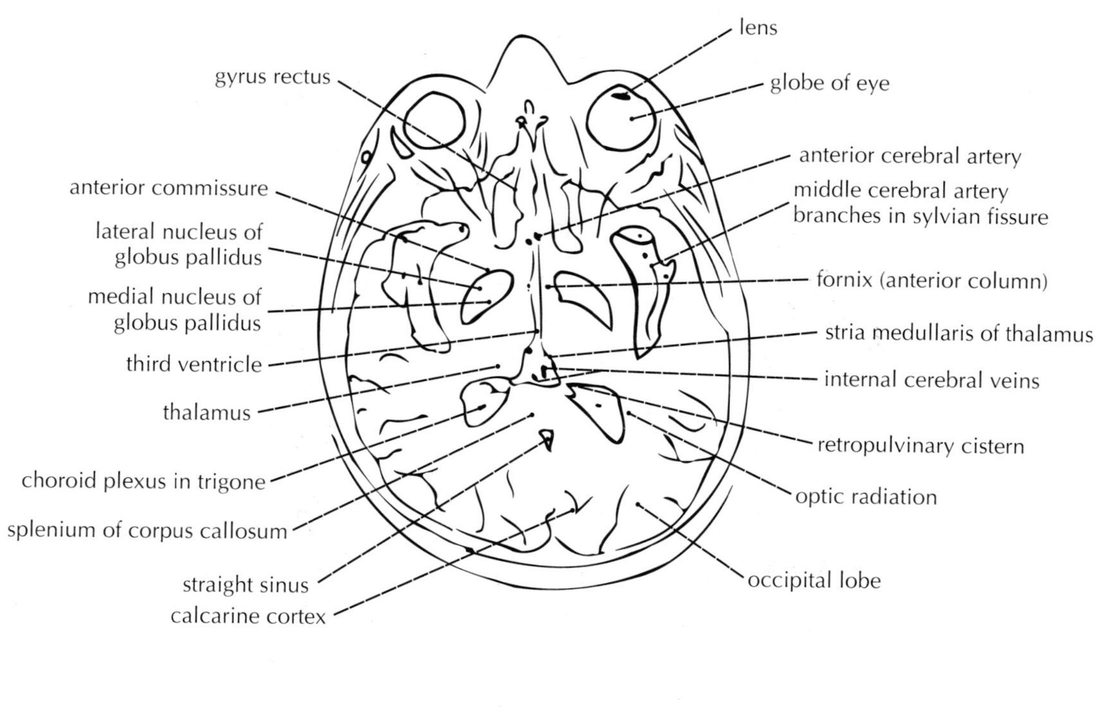

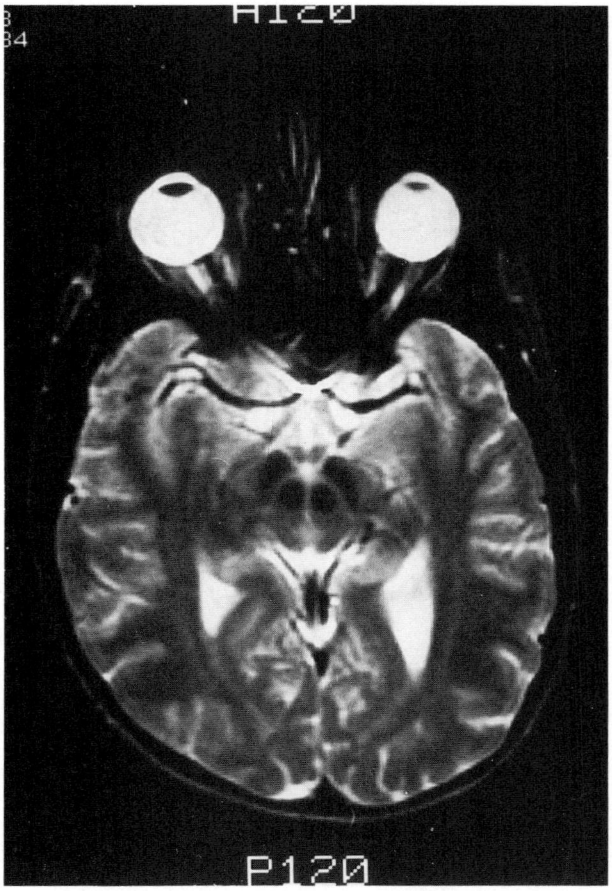

2-29 Axial MR scan through midbrain (2000/90). Section 16 in Fig. 2-12.

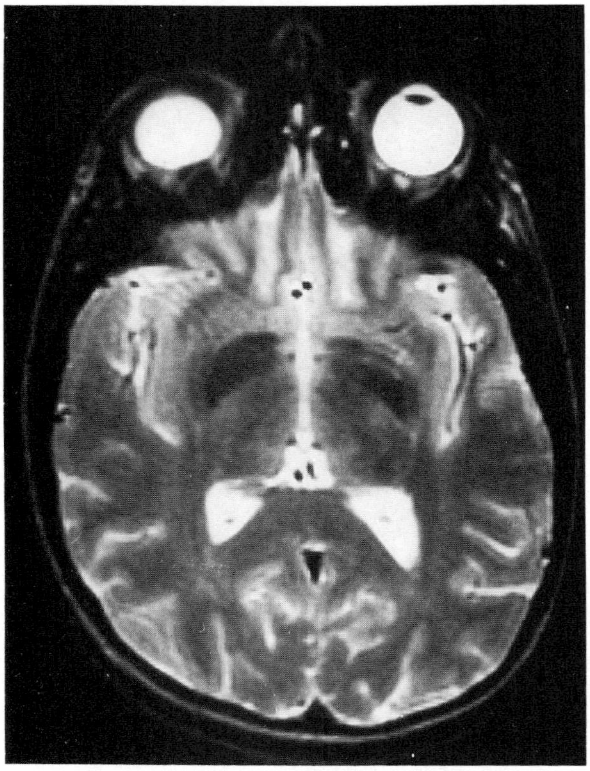

2-30 Axial MR scan through third ventricle (2000/90). Section 20 in Fig. 2-12.

2/Brain, Axial MRI

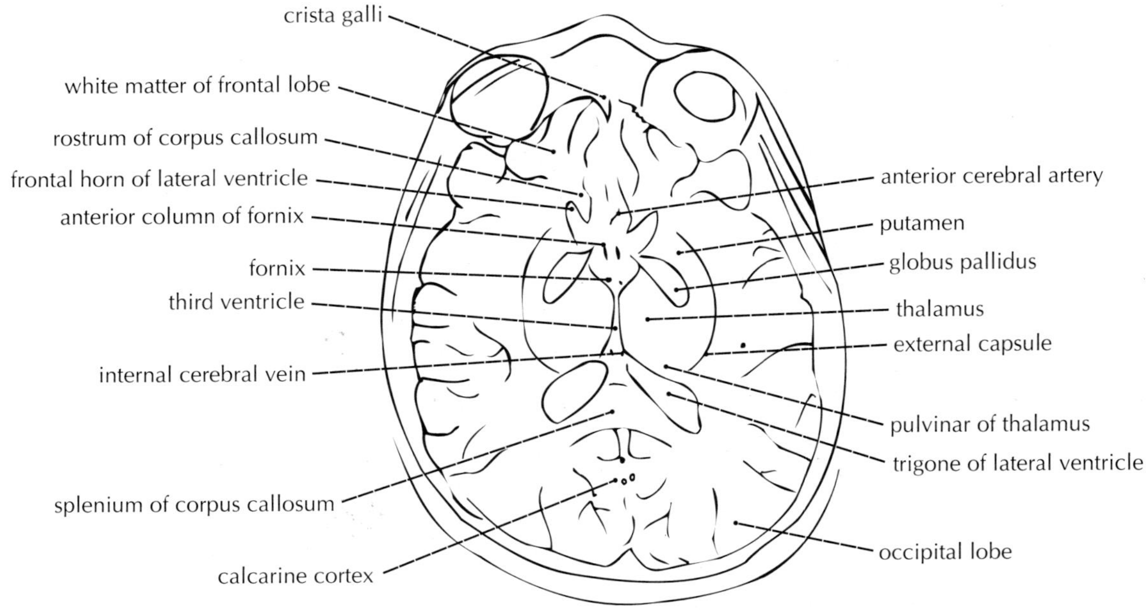

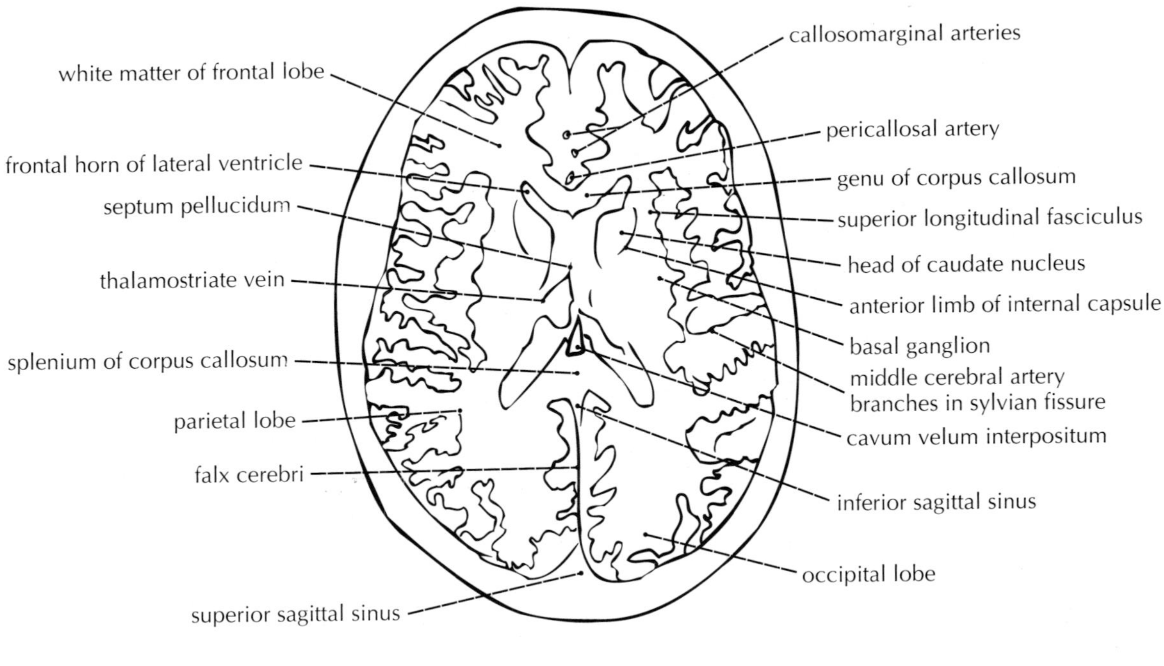

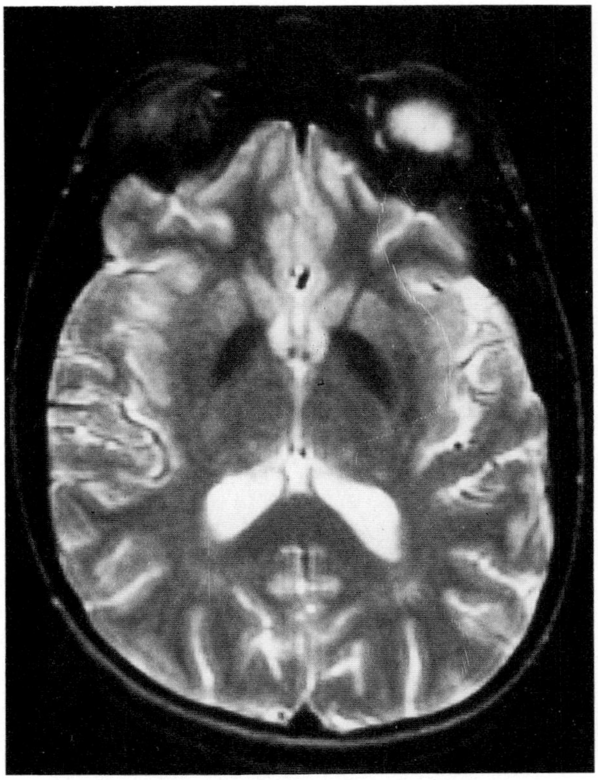

2-31 Axial MR scan through third ventricle (2000/90). Section 22 in Fig. 2-12.

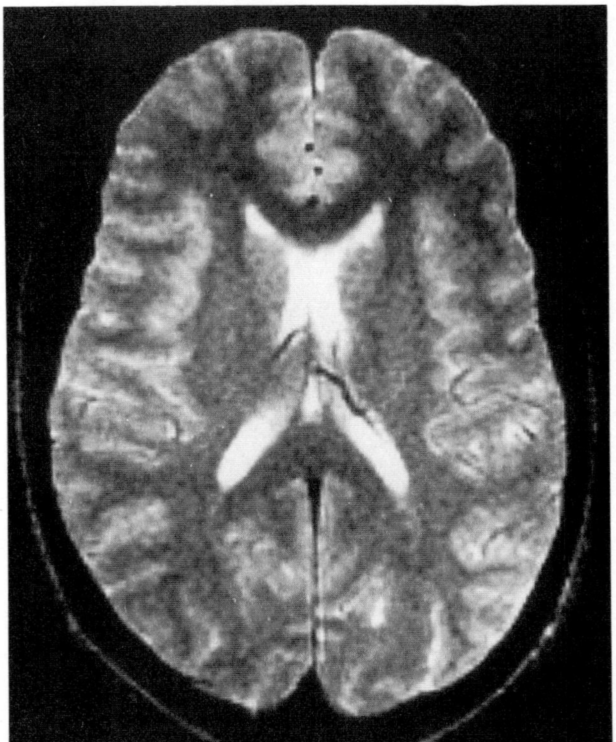

2-32 Axial MR scan through lateral ventricles (2000/90). Section 24 in Fig. 2-12.

2/Brain, Axial MRI

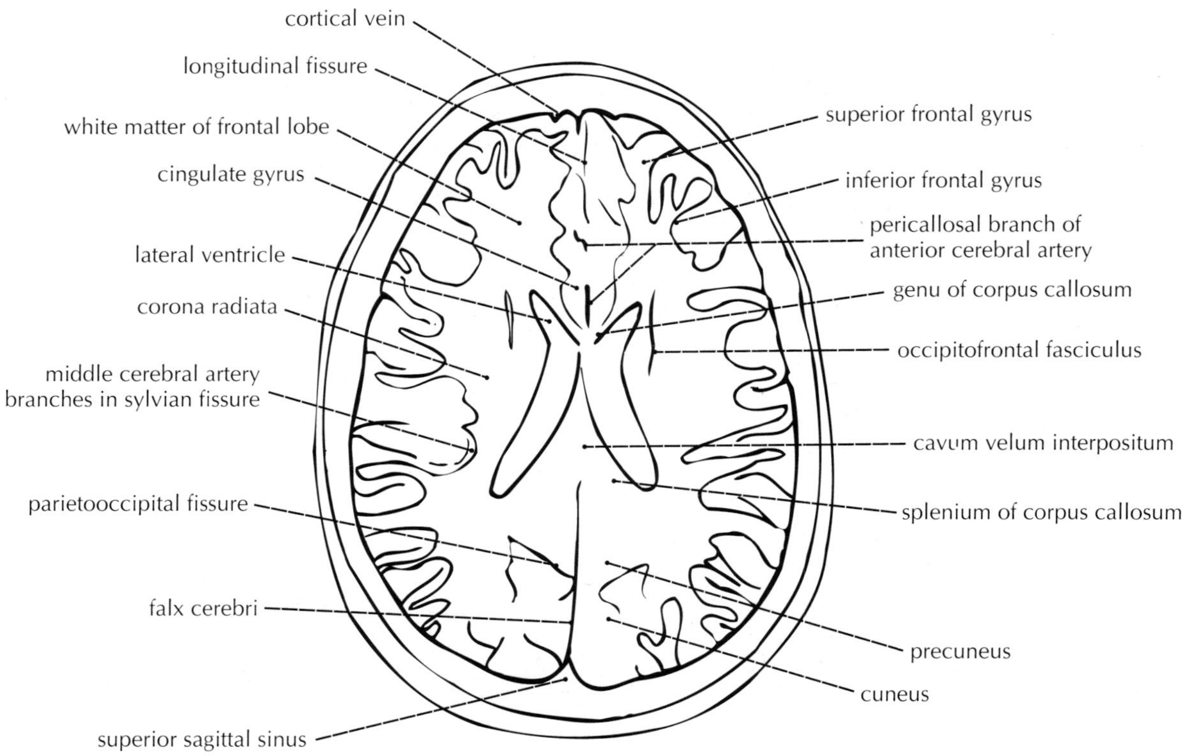

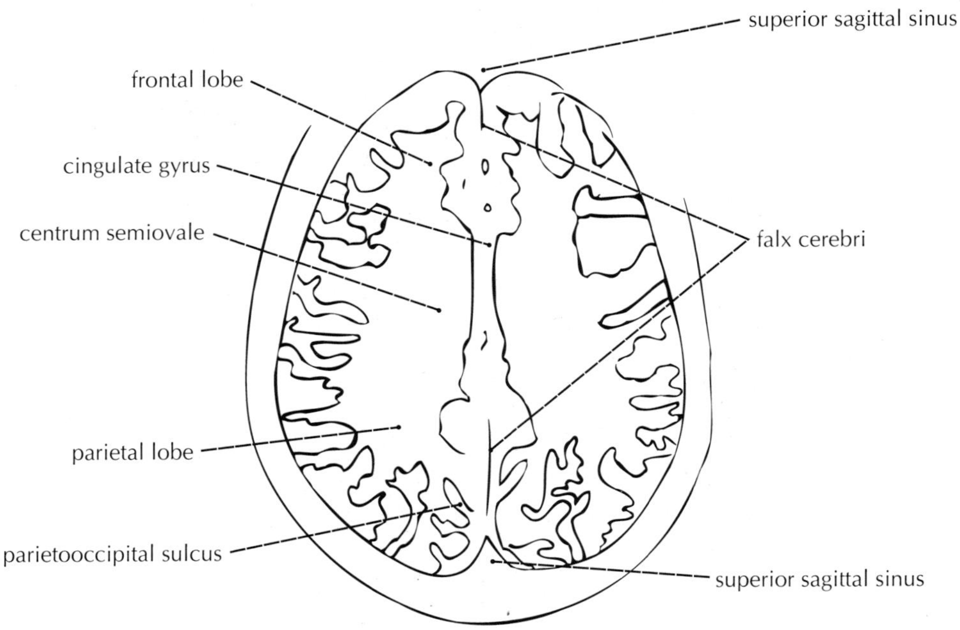

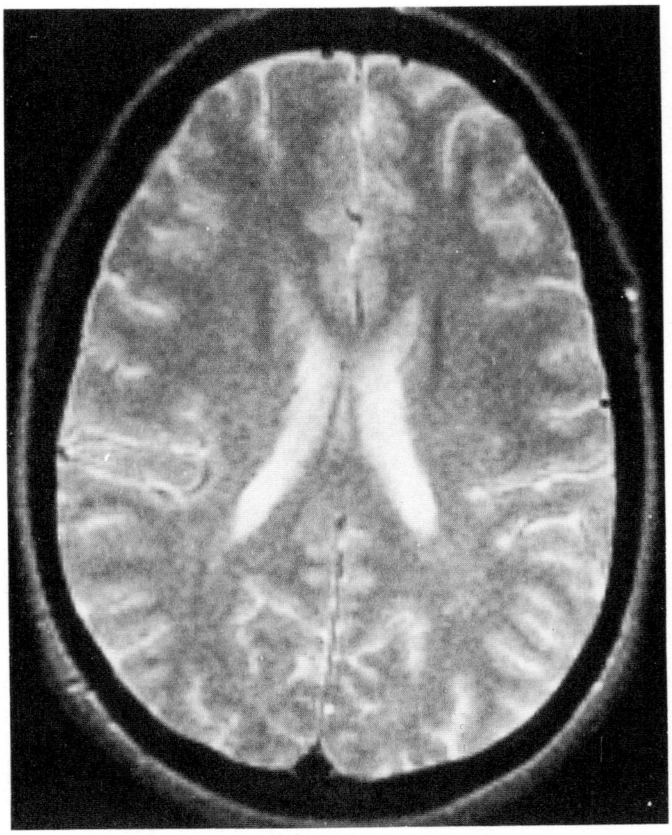

2-33 Axial MR scan through lateral ventricles (2000/90). Section 26 in Fig. 2-12.

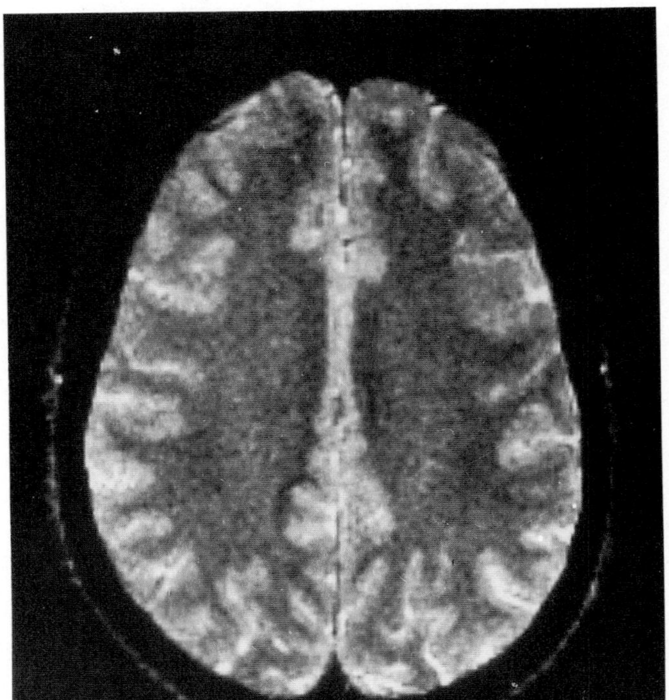

2-34 Axial MR scan through parietal lobe above the ventricles (2000/90). Section 28 in Fig. 2-12.

2/Brain, Axial MRI

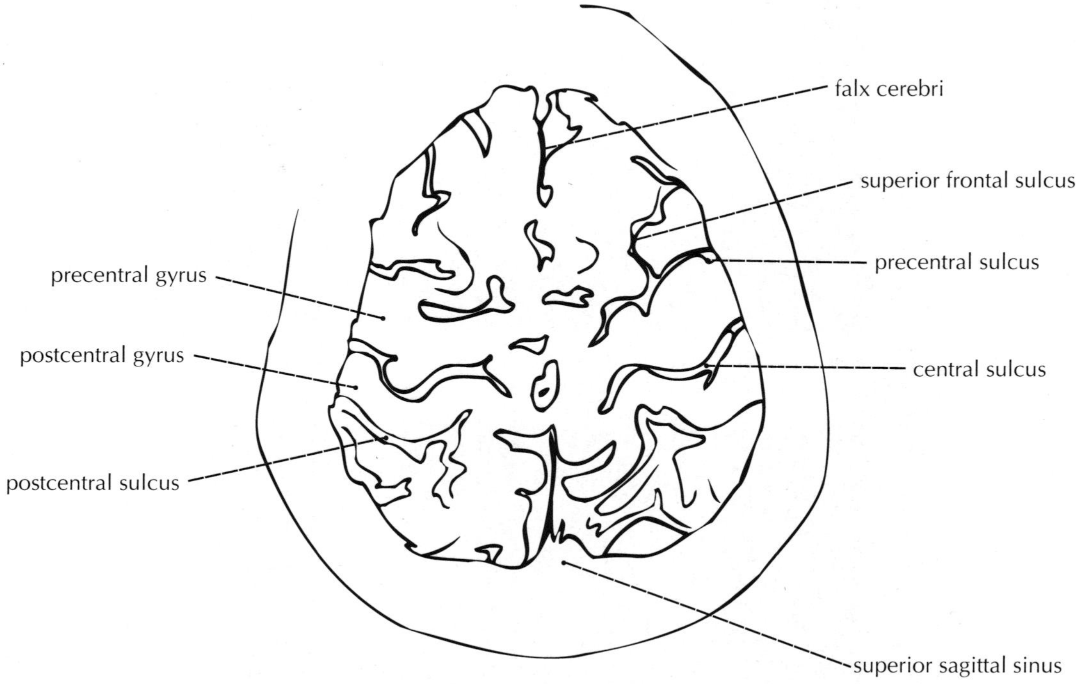

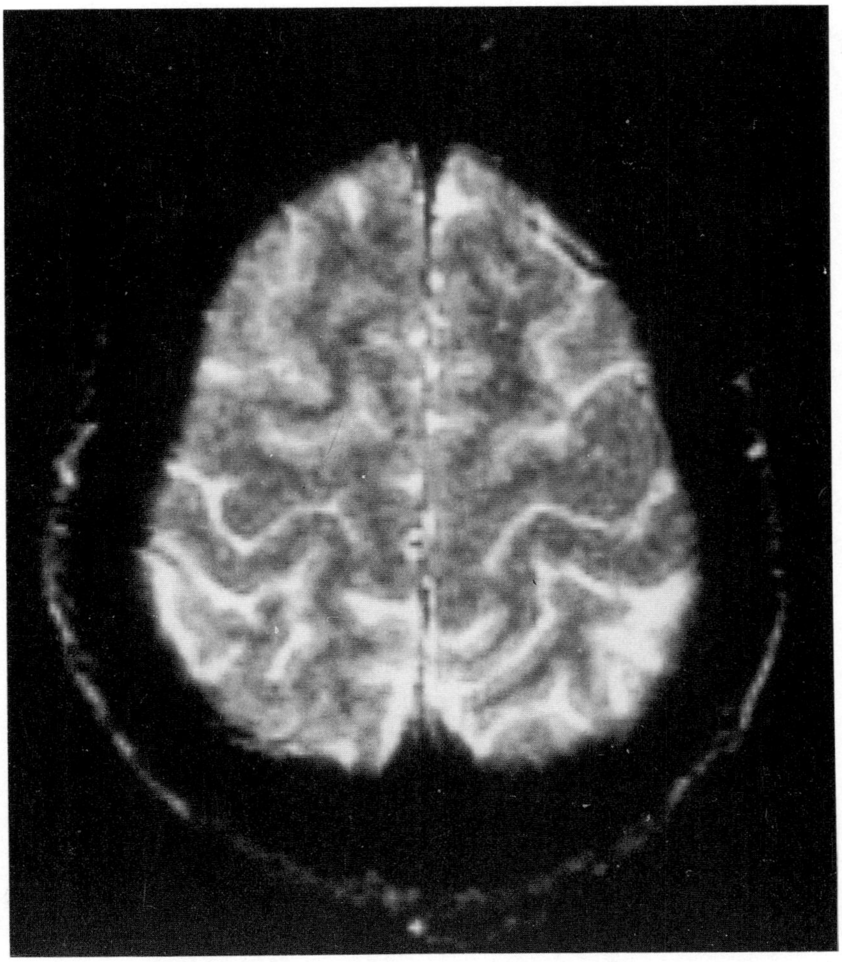

2-35 Axial MR scan through vertex (2000/90). Section 34 in Fig. 2-12.

2/Brain, Sagittal Scout MRI and Coronal MRI

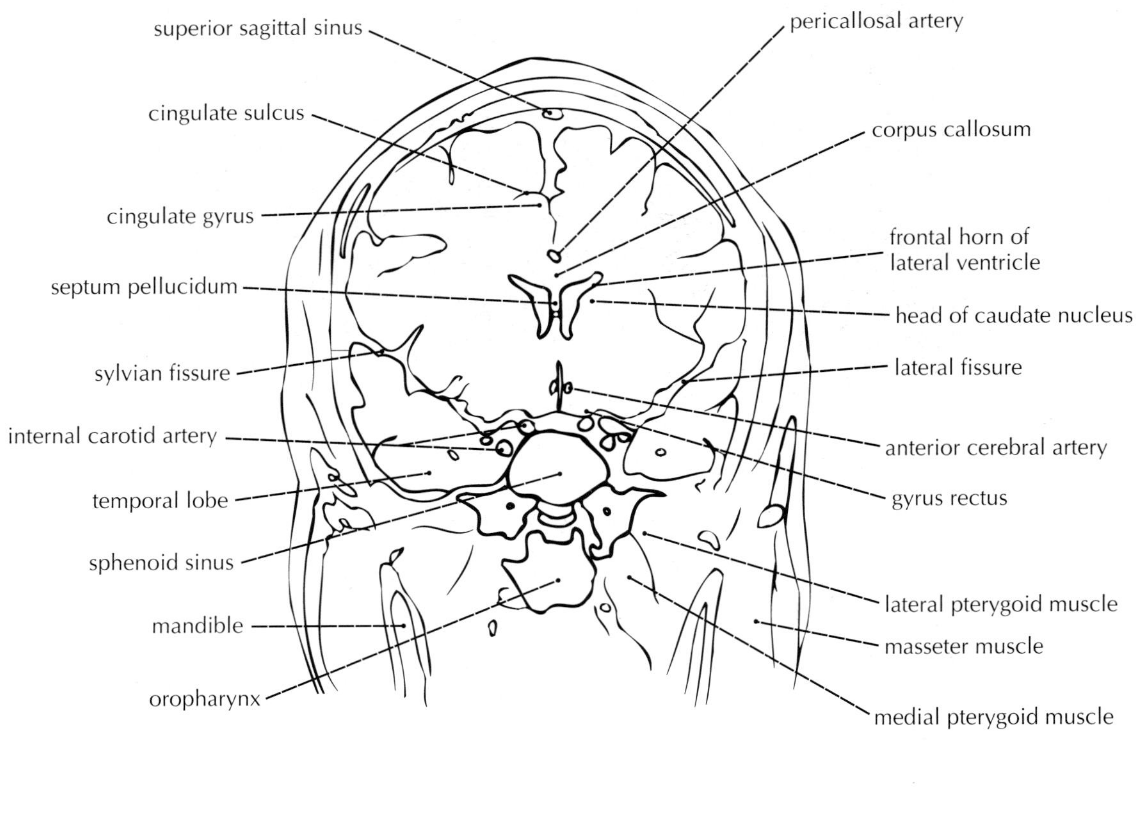

2/Brain, Sagittal Scout MRI and Coronal MRI

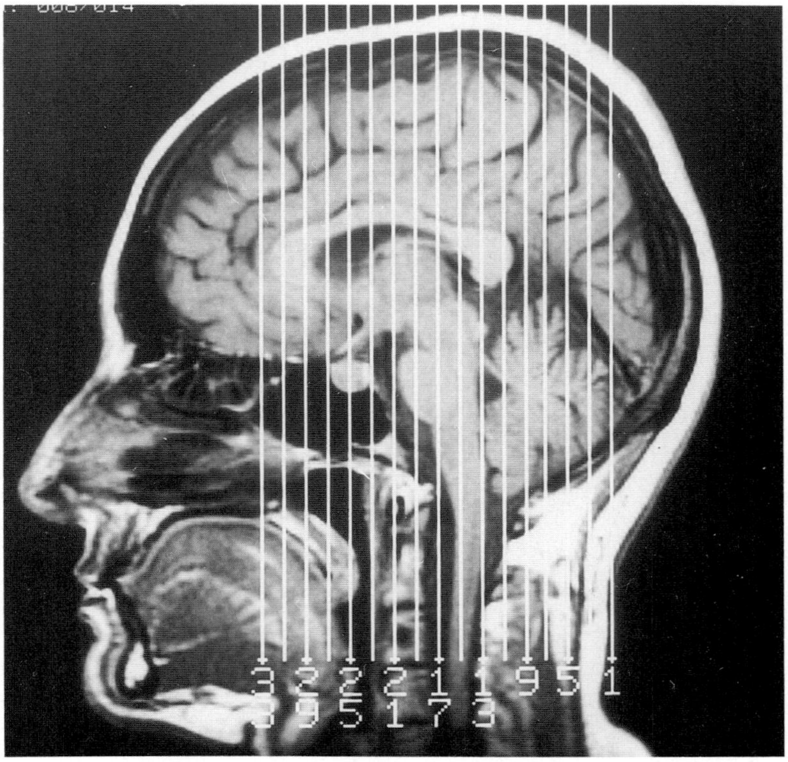

2-36 Sagittal MR scout scan demonstrating coronal MR sections obtained with various techniques (Fig. 2-37 through 2-49).

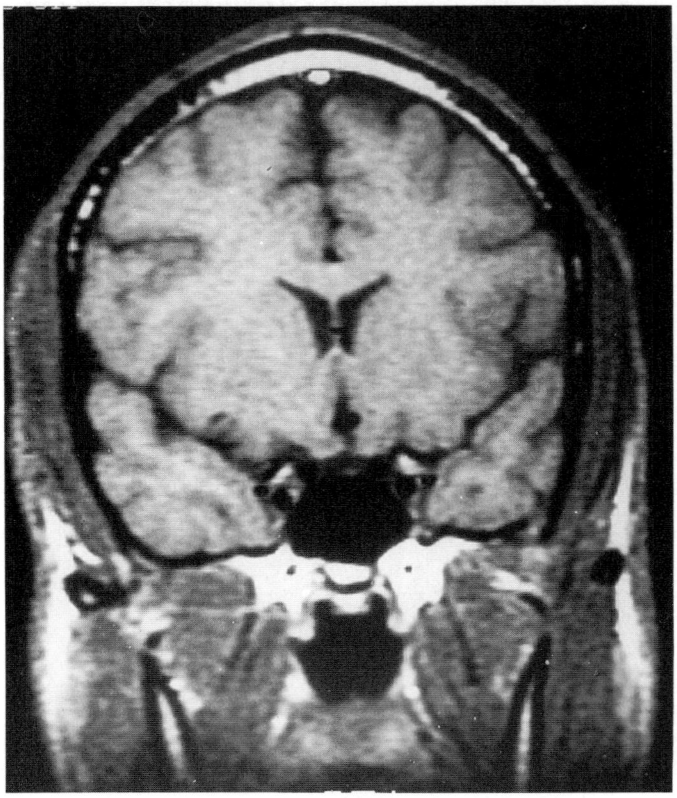

2-37 Coronal MR scan through frontal lobes (800/20). Section 29 in Fig. 2-36.

2/Brain, Coronal MRI

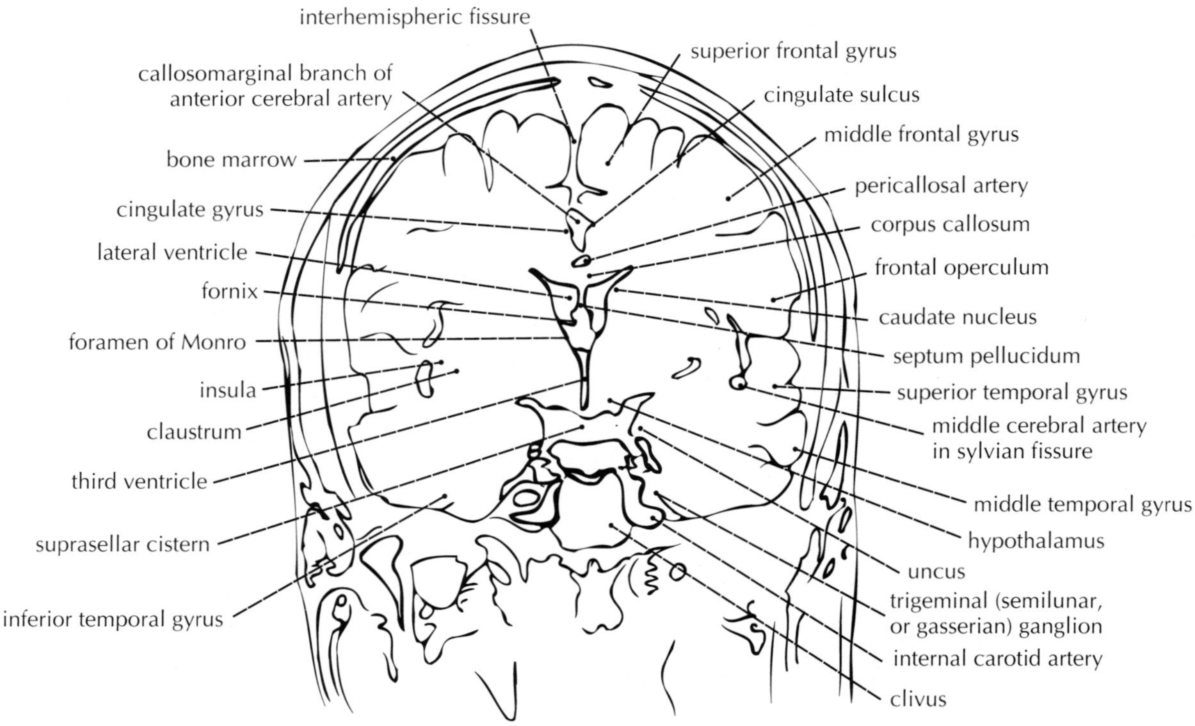

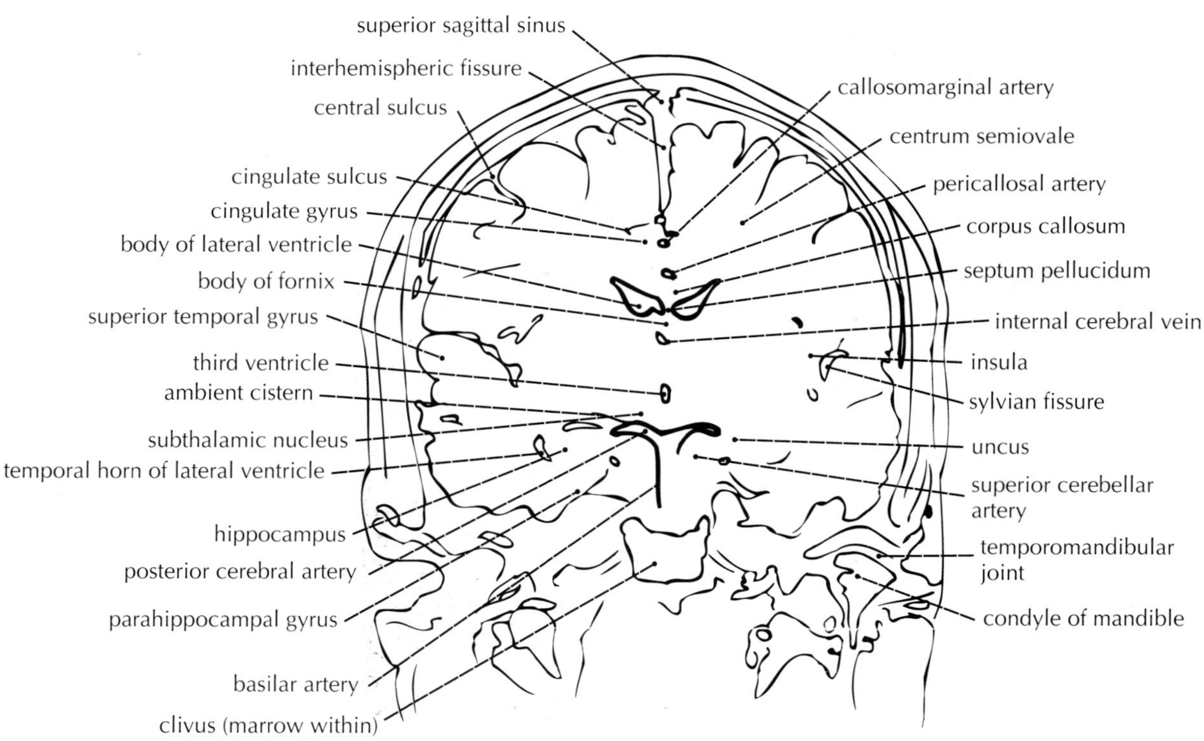

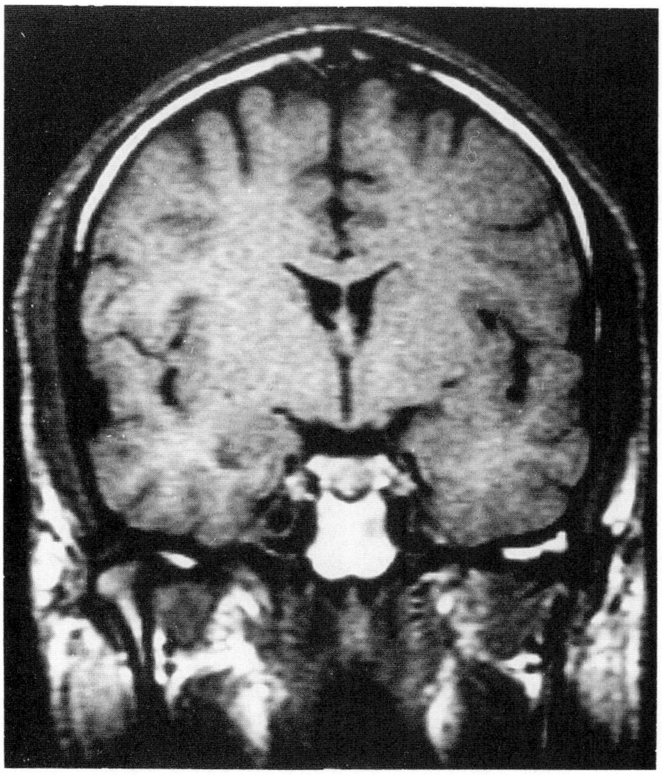

2-38 Coronal MR scan through third ventricle (600/20). Section 23 in Fig. 2-36.

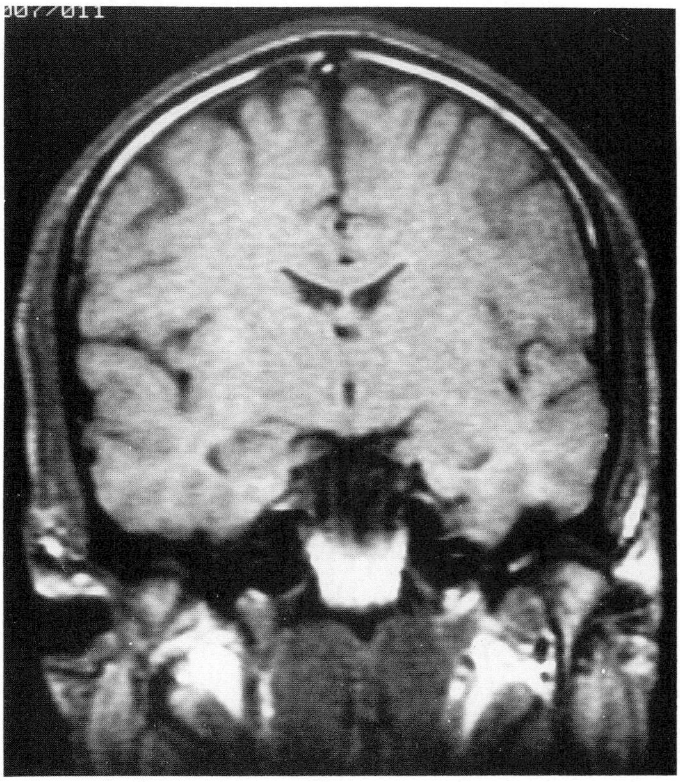

2-39 Coronal MR scan through third ventricle and clivus (600/20). Section 21 in Fig. 2-36.

2/Brain, Coronal MRI

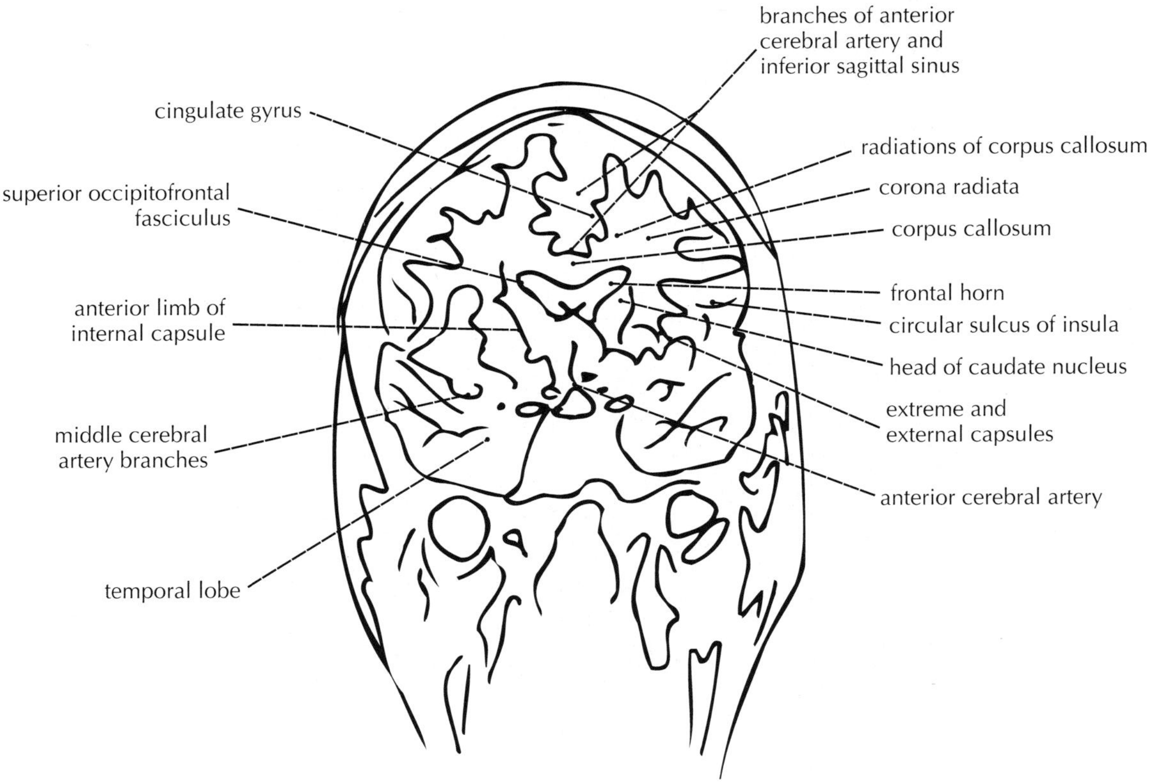

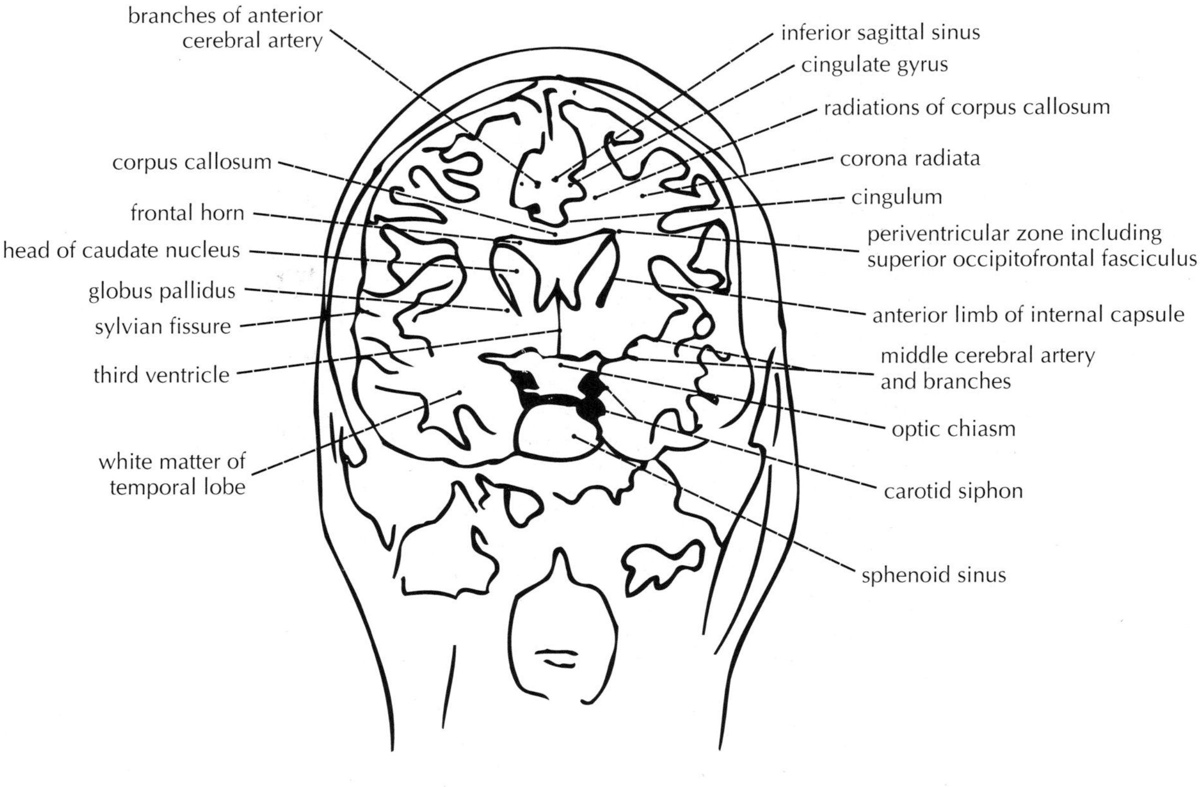

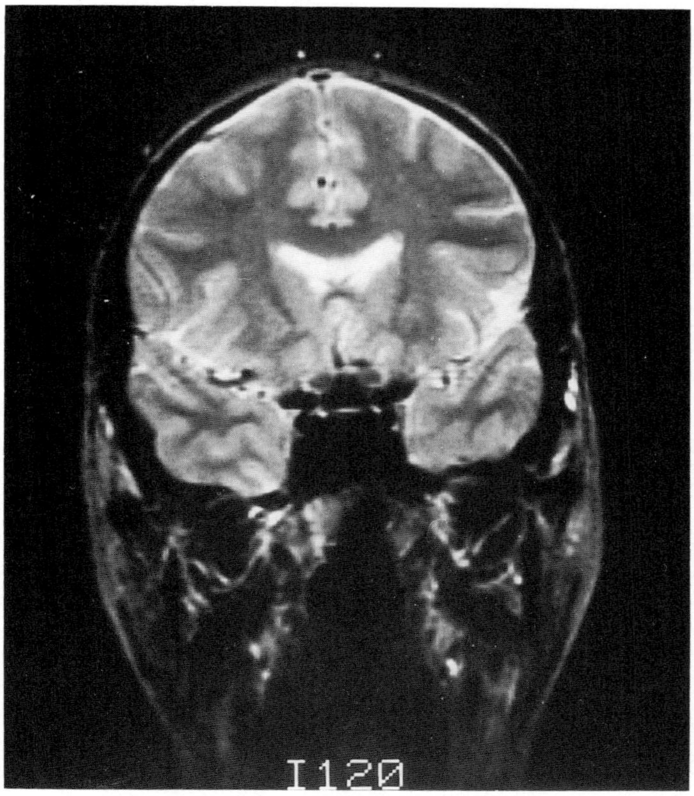

2-40 Coronal MR scan through frontal horns (2000/90). Section 29 in Fig. 2-36.

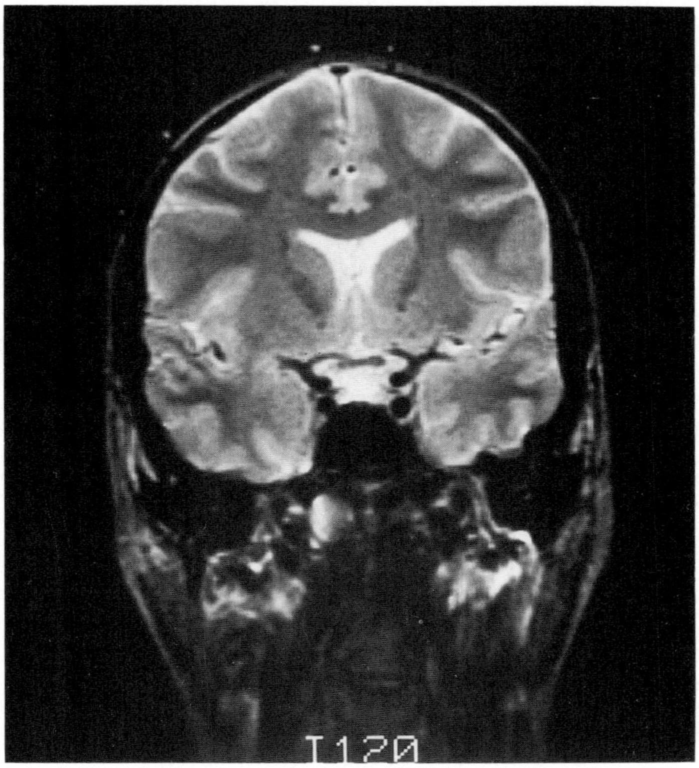

2-41 Coronal MR scan through frontal horns (2000/90). Section 25 in Fig. 2-36.

2/Brain, Coronal MRI

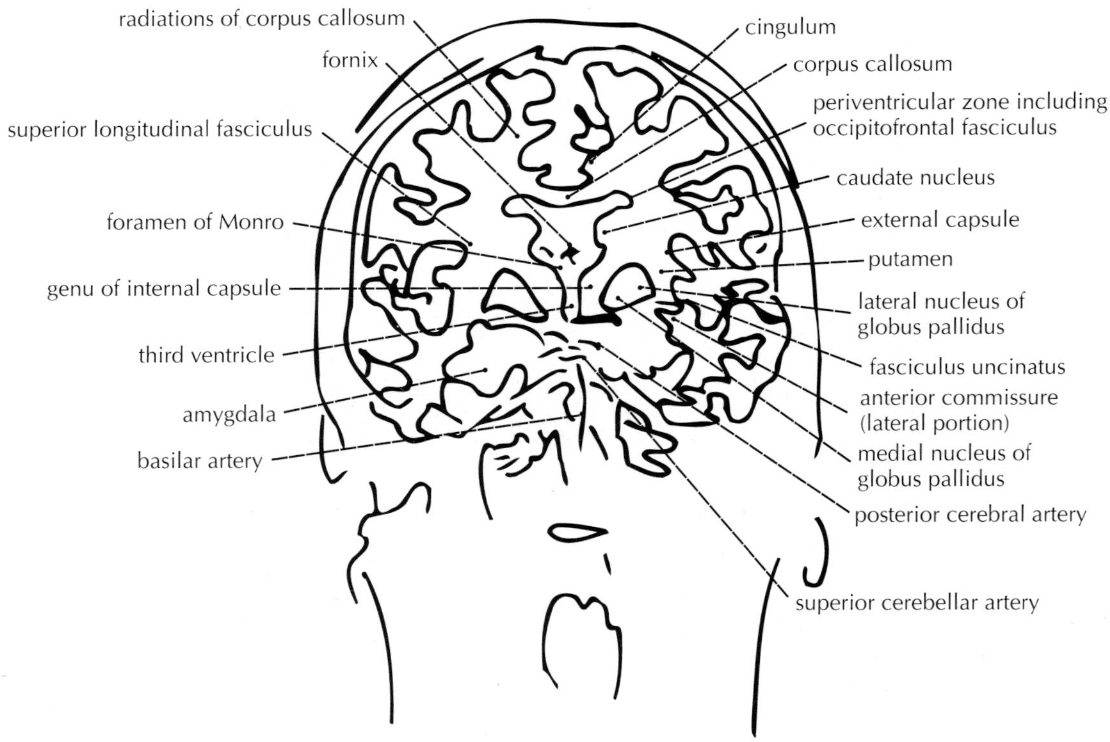

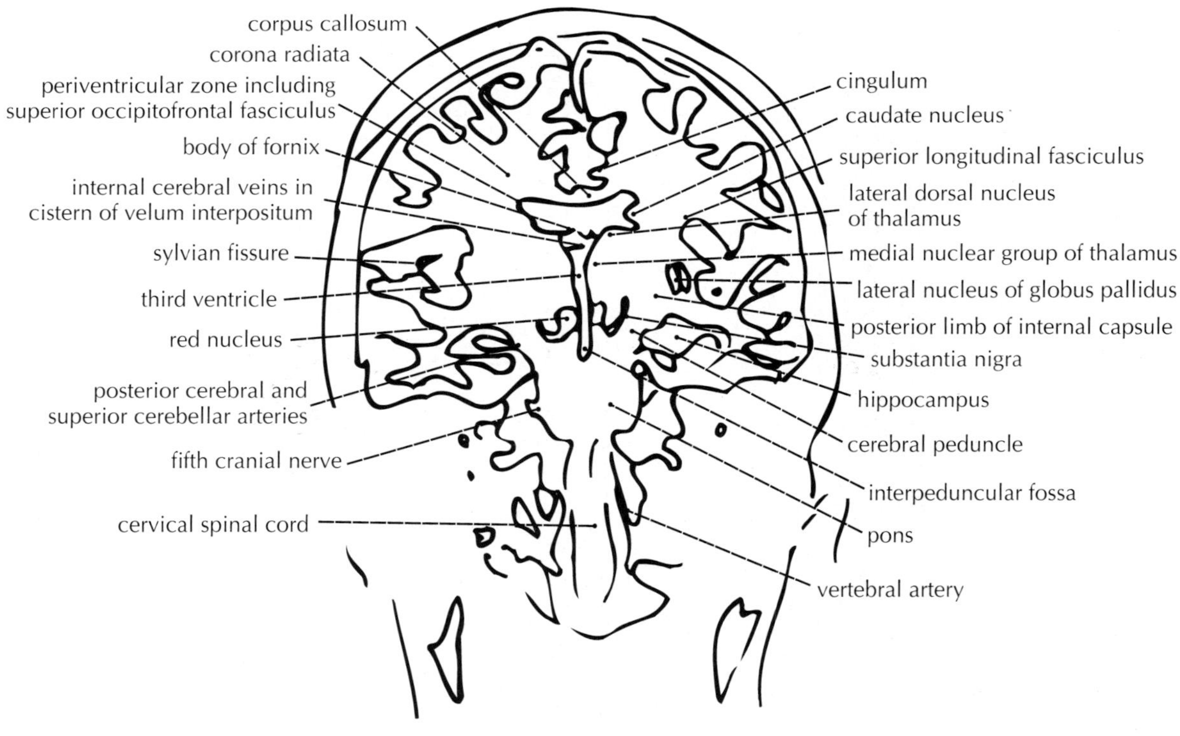

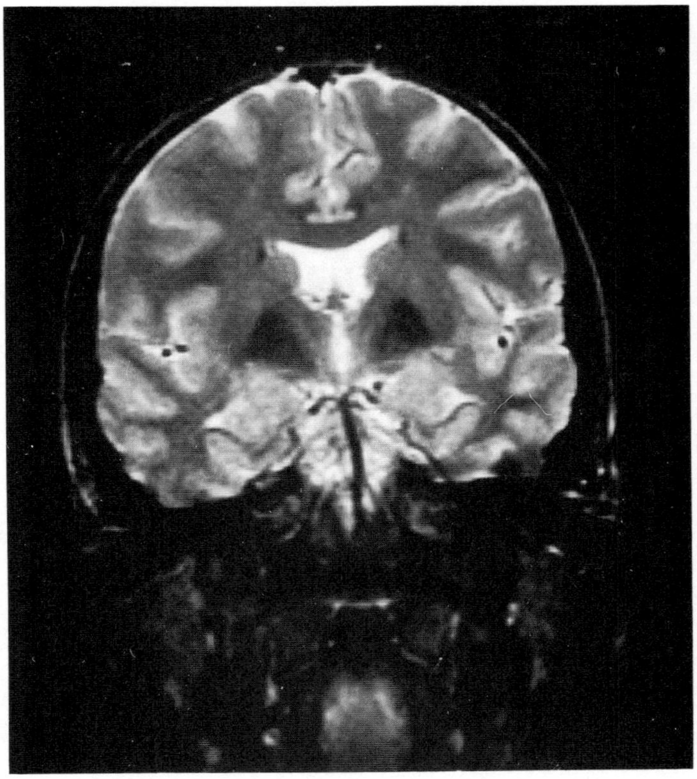

2-42 Coronal MR scan through third ventricle and basal ganglia (2000/90). Section 21 in Fig. 2-36.

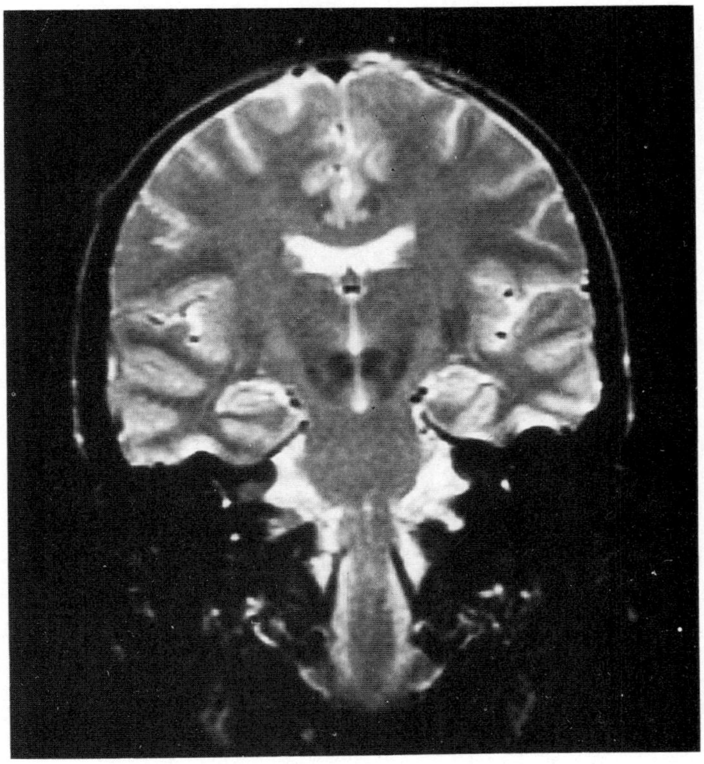

2-43 Coronal MR scan through red nucleus (2000/90). Section 17 in Fig. 2-36.

2/Brain, Coronal MRI

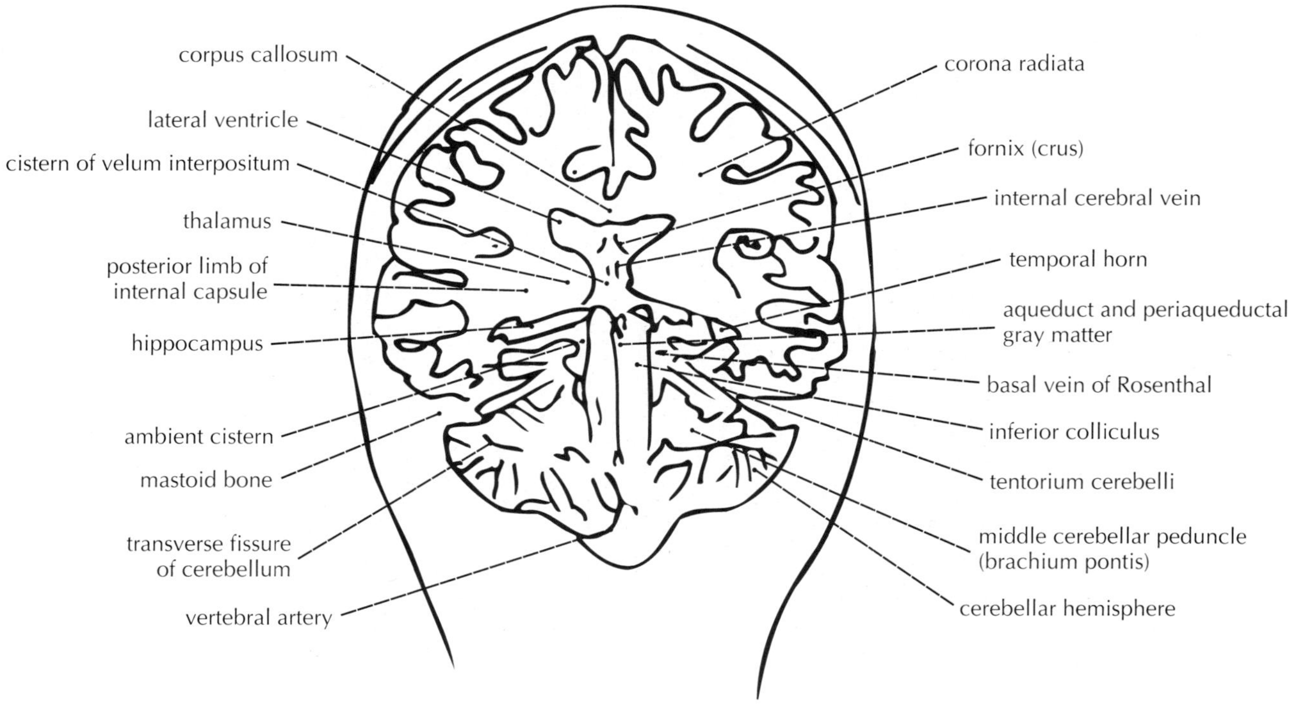

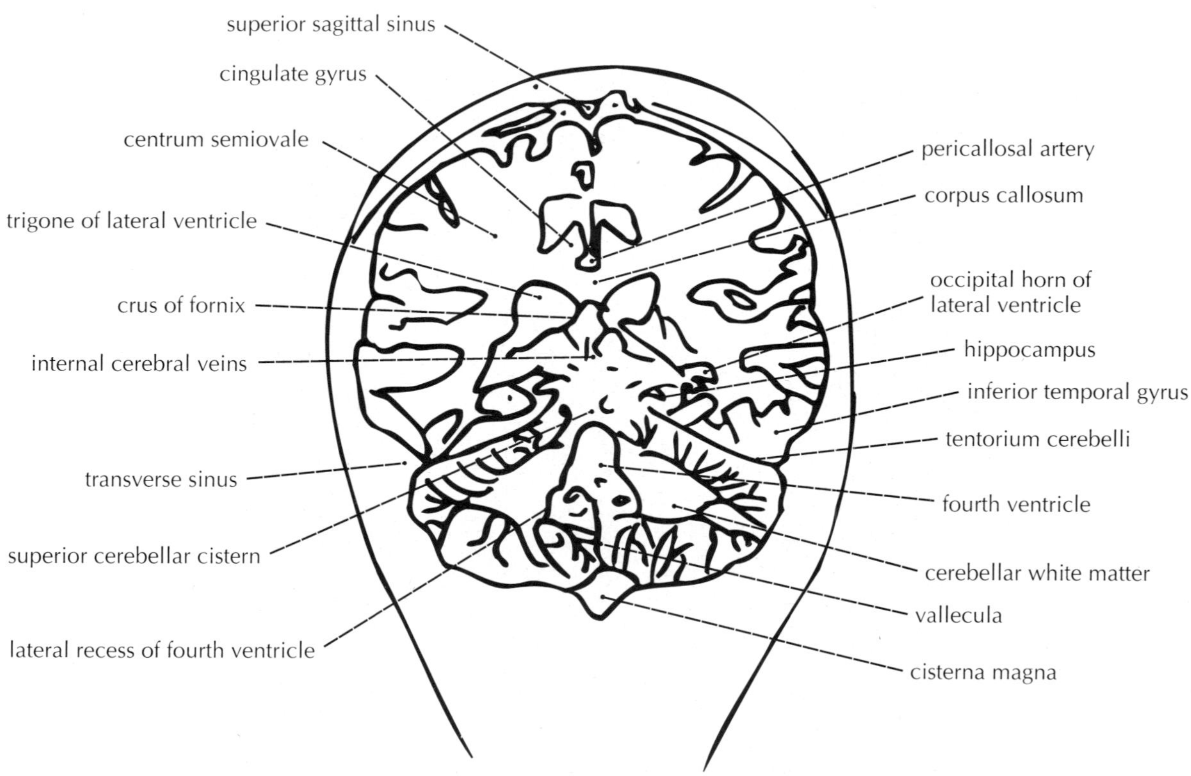

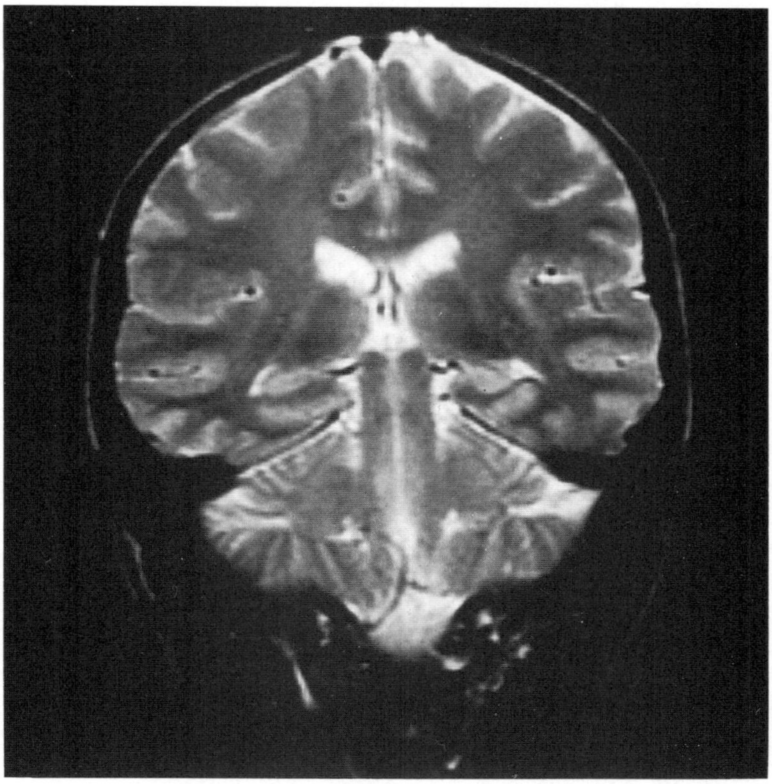

2-44 Coronal MR scan through posterior body of corpus callosum (2000/90). Section 15 in Fig. 2-36.

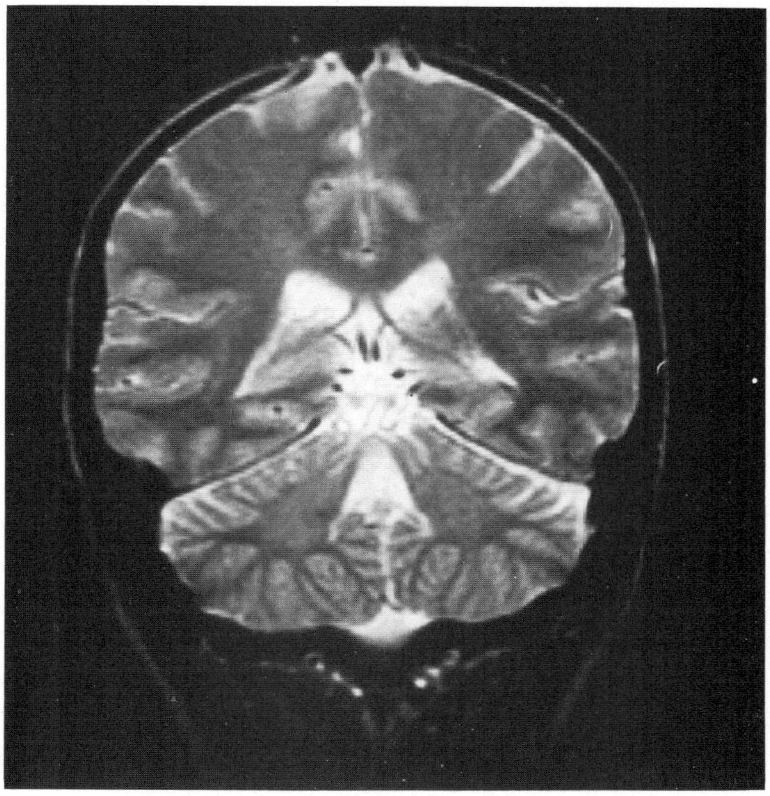

2-45 Coronal MR scan through fourth ventricle (2000/90). Section 13 in Fig. 2-36.

2/Brain, Coronal MRI

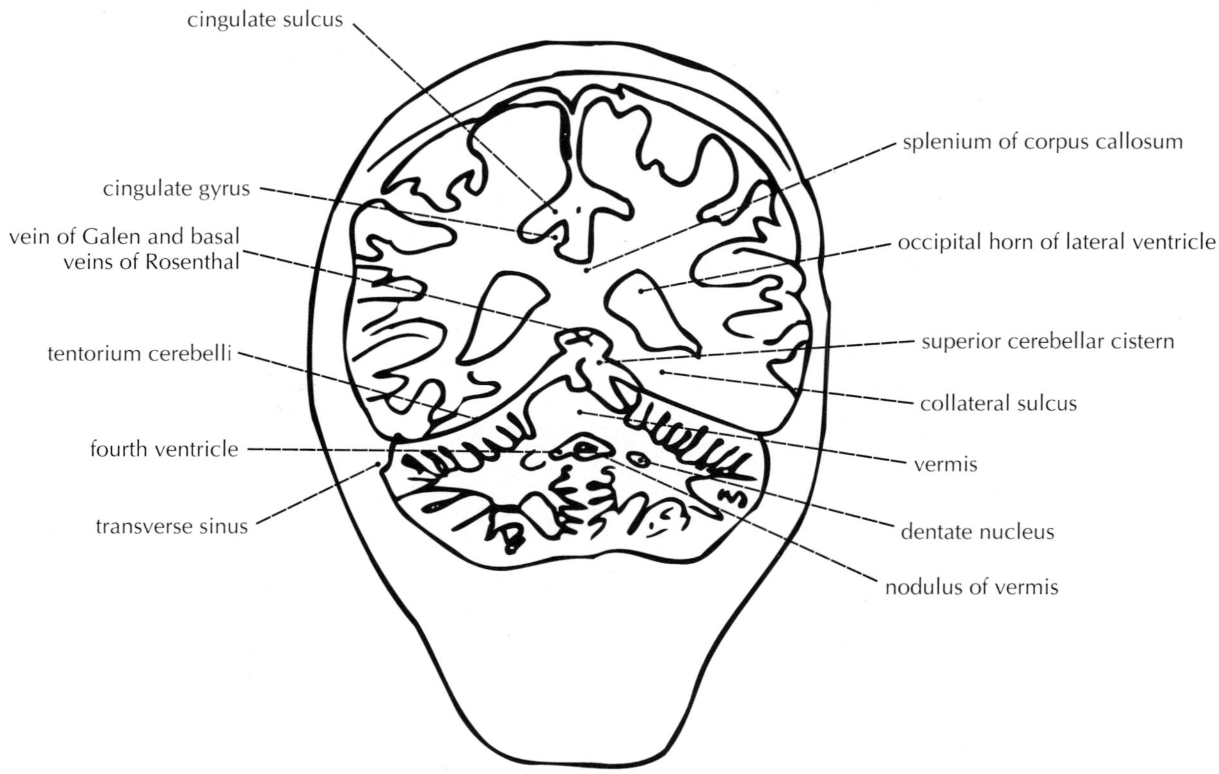

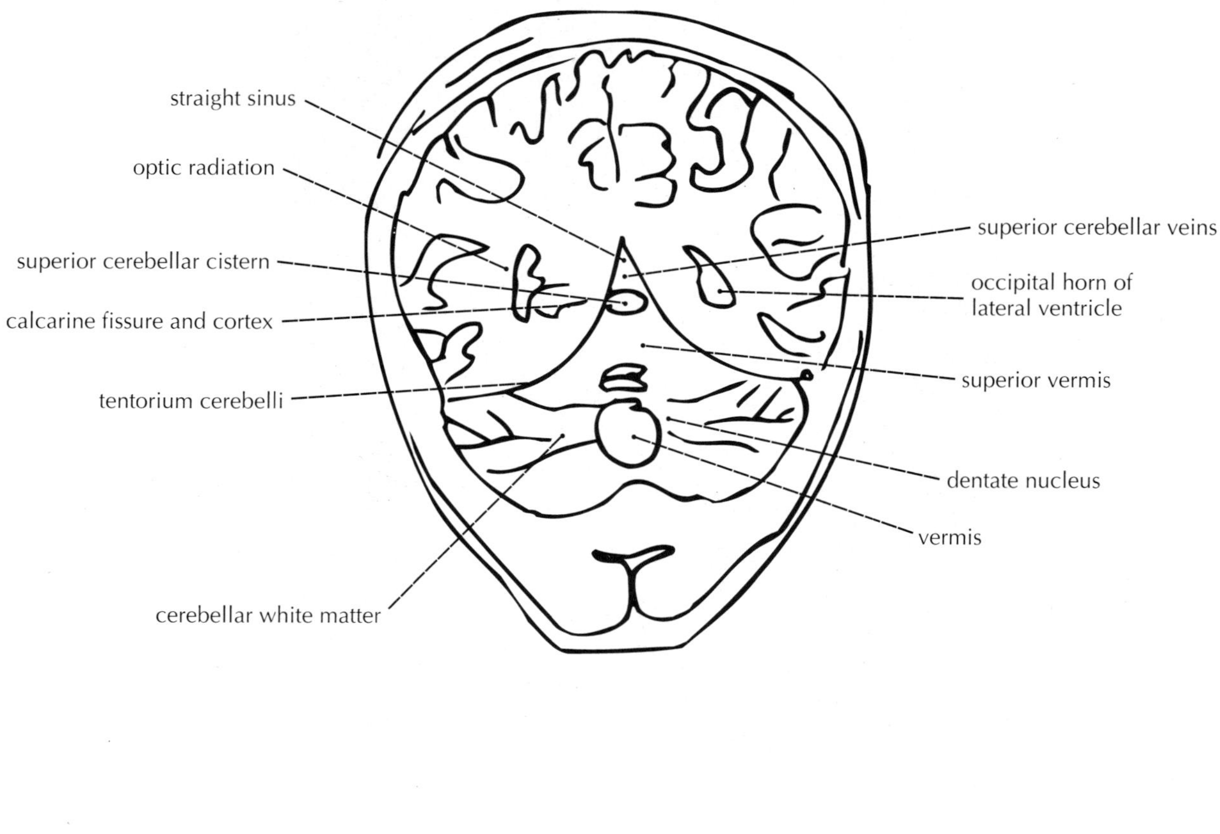

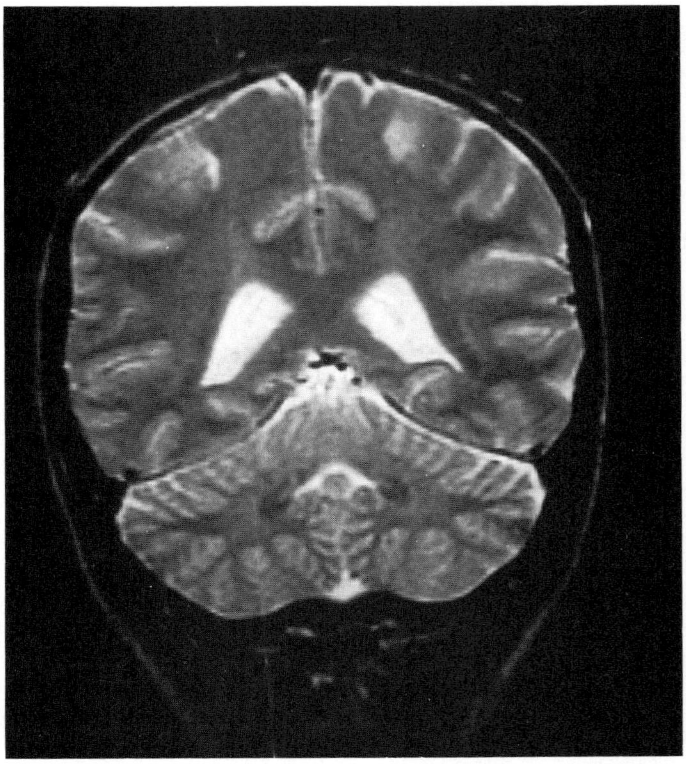

2-46 Coronal MR scan through fourth ventricle (2000/90). Section 11 in Fig. 2-36.

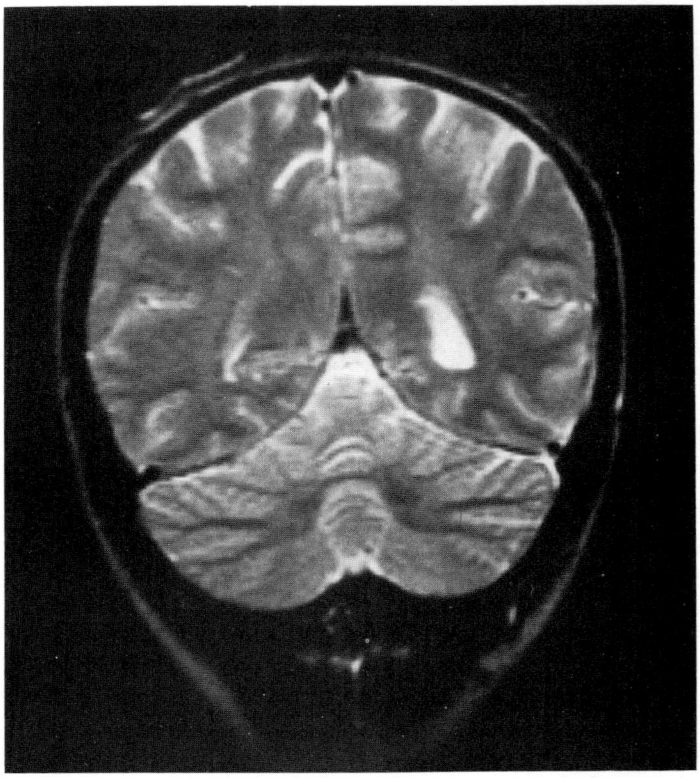

2-47 Coronal MR scan through posterior fossa (2000/90). Section 5 in Fig. 2-36.

2/Brain, Coronal MRI

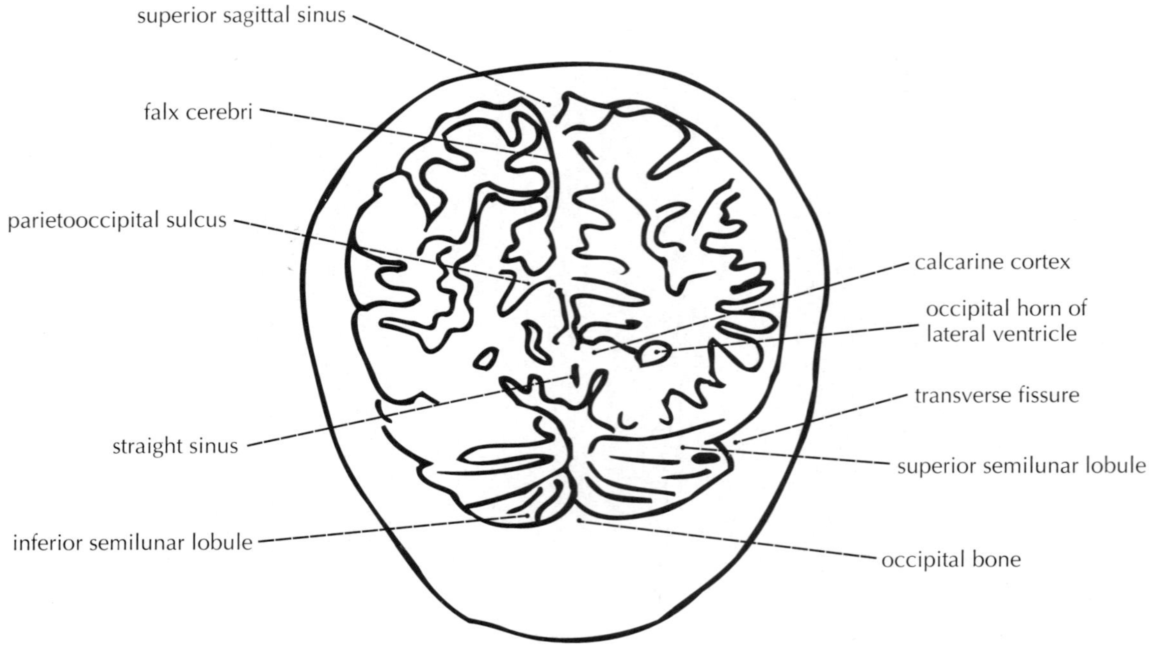

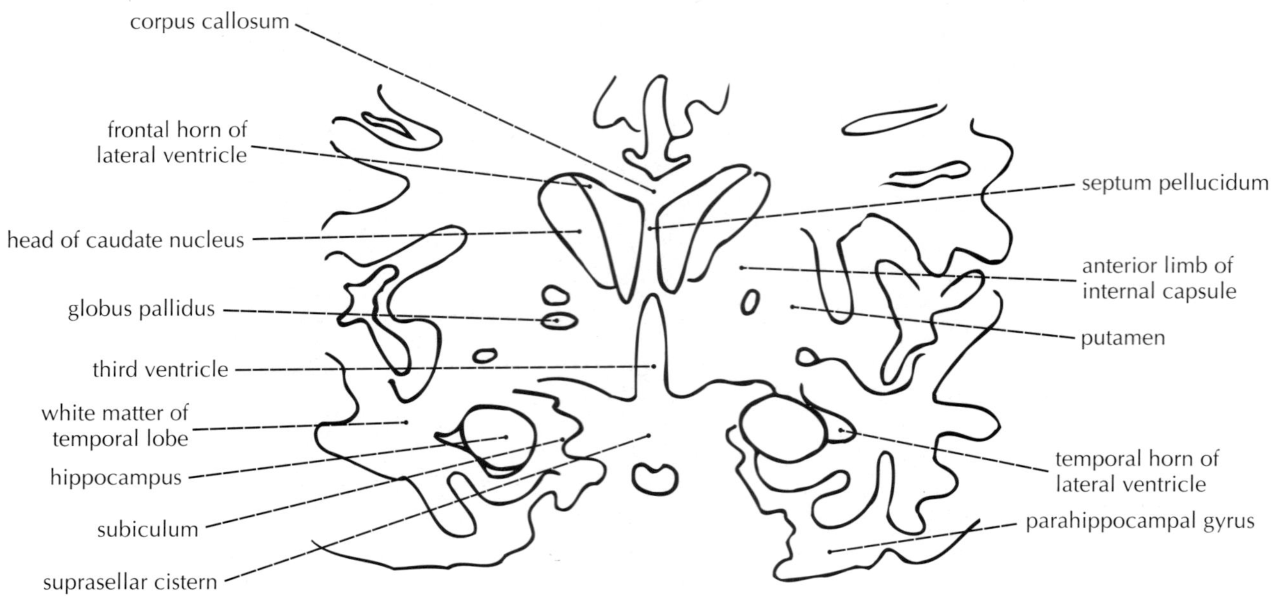

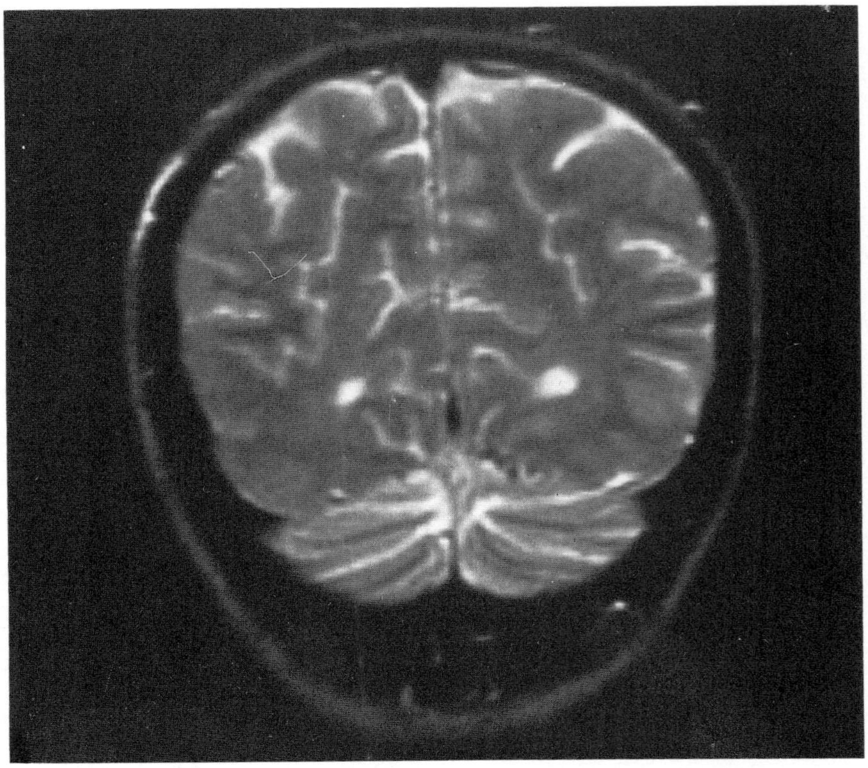

2-48 Coronal MR scan through posterior fossa (2000/90). Section 3 in Fig. 2-36.

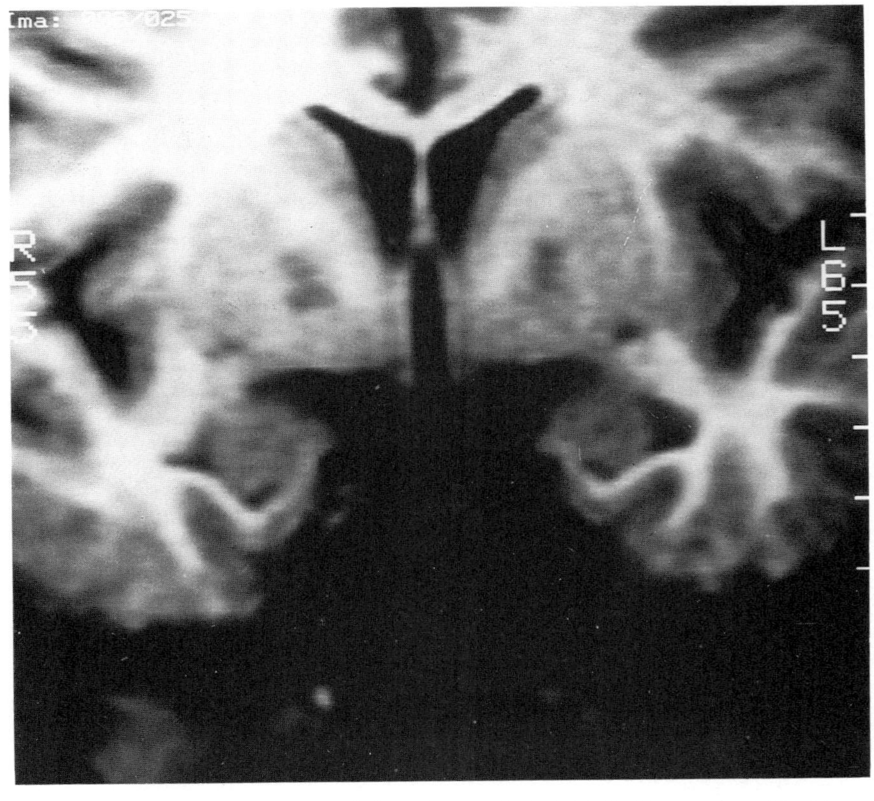

2-49 Coronal MR scan through basal ganglia (150/10, flip angle 60°). Magnified section through level 27 in Fig. 2-36.

2/Brain, Axial Scout and Sagittal MRI

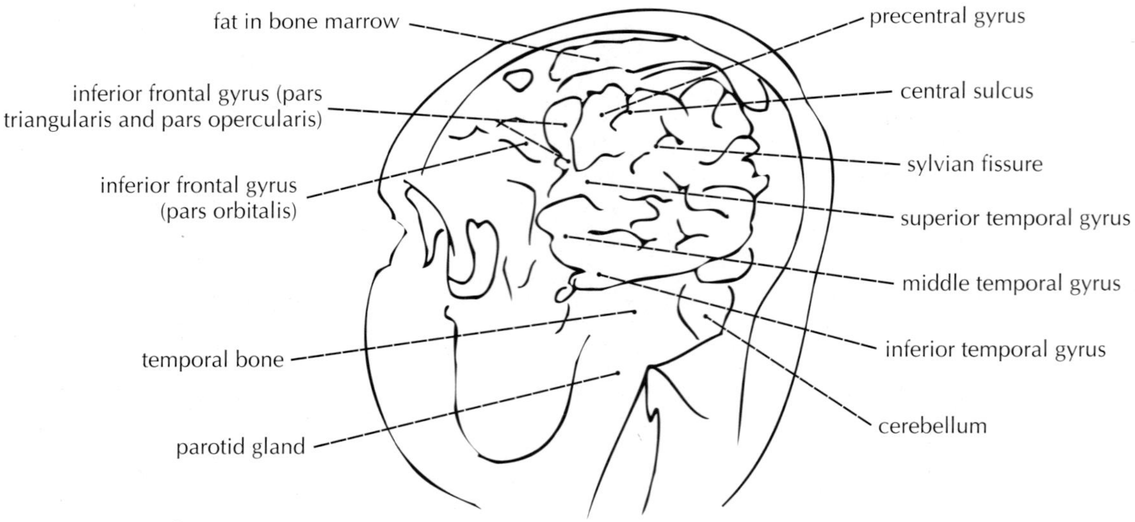

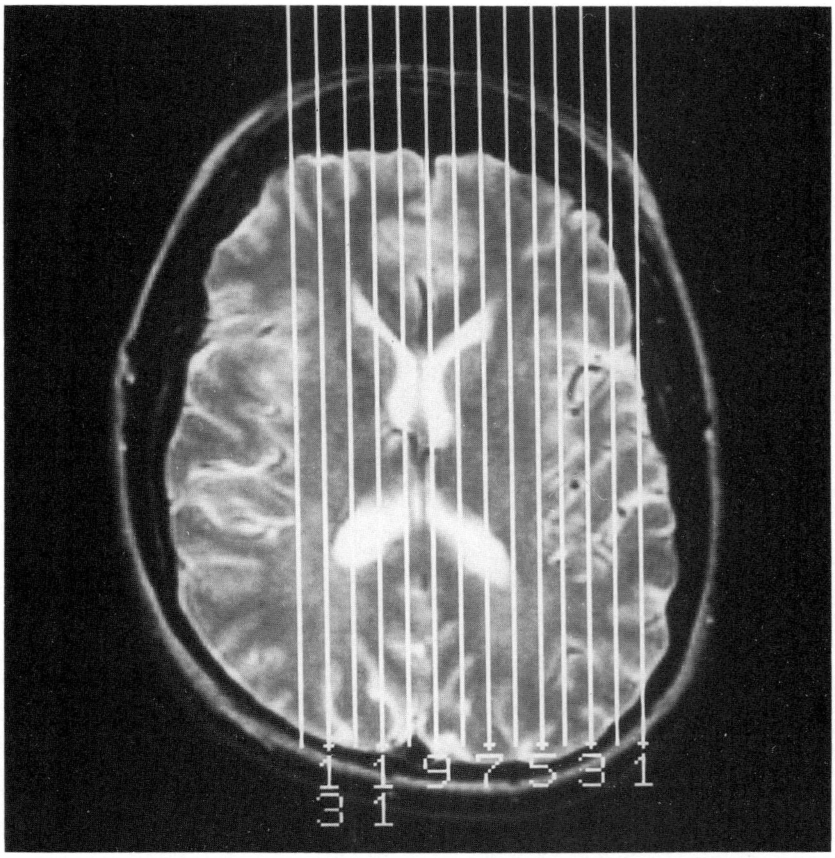

2-50 This axial scout MR scan is used to illustrate the locations of sagittal MR sections. Sections 1, 2, 3, 5, 6, 7, 8, and 9 will be shown.

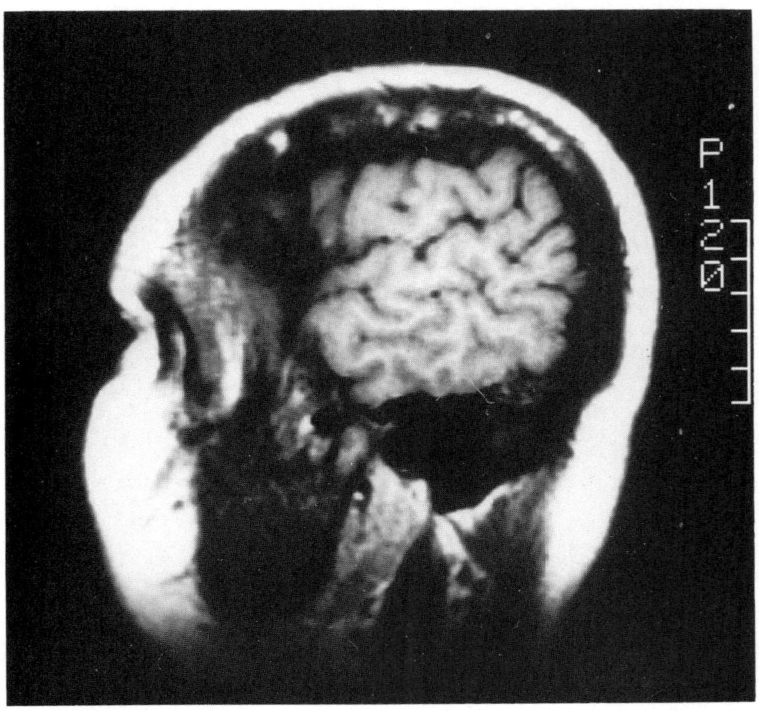

2-51 Sagittal MR scan through temporal lobe (600/15). Section 1 in Fig. 2-50.

2/Brain, Sagittal MRI

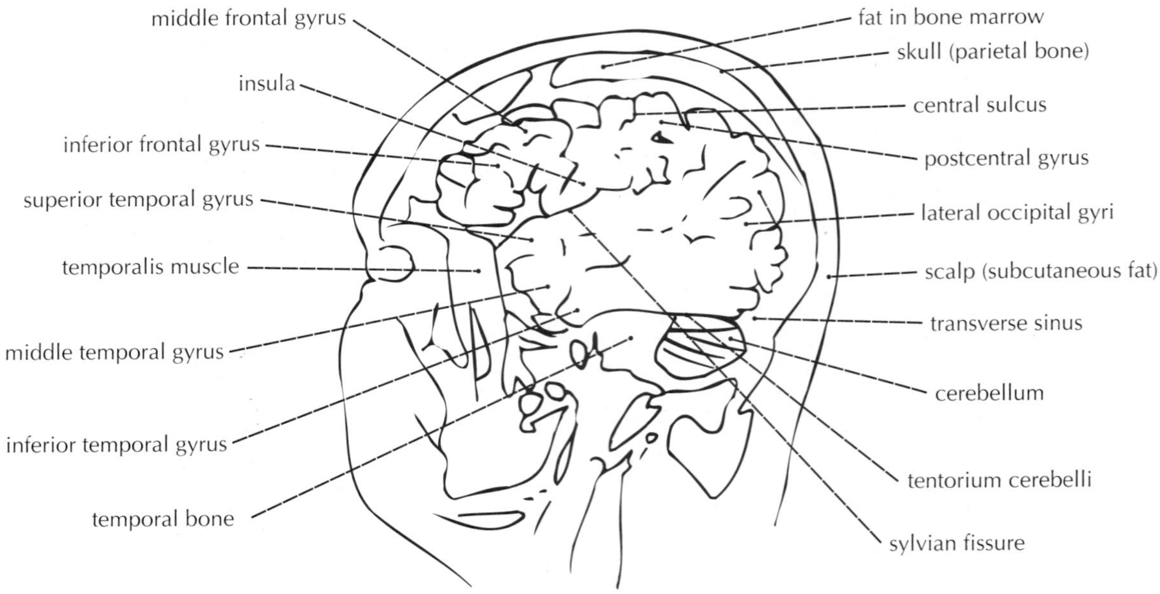

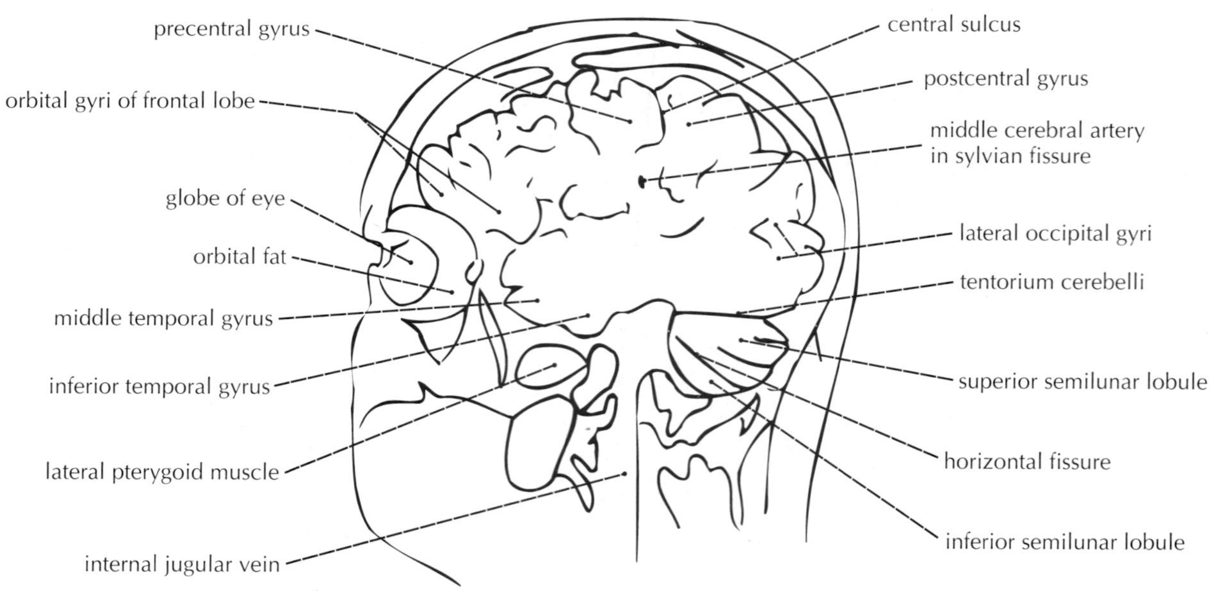

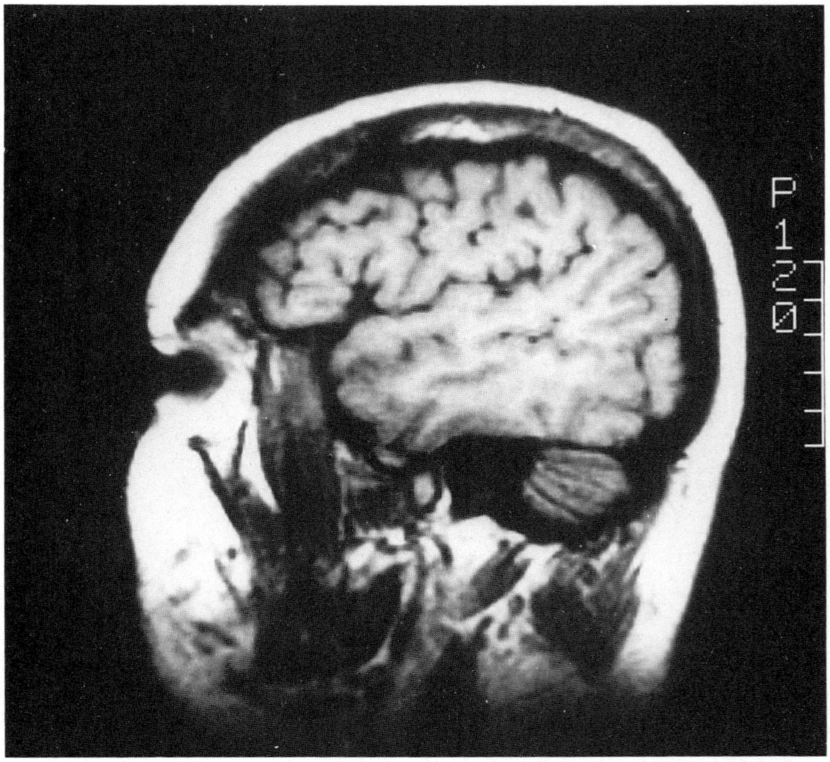

2-52 Sagittal MR scan through temporal lobe (600/15). Section 2 in Fig. 2-50.

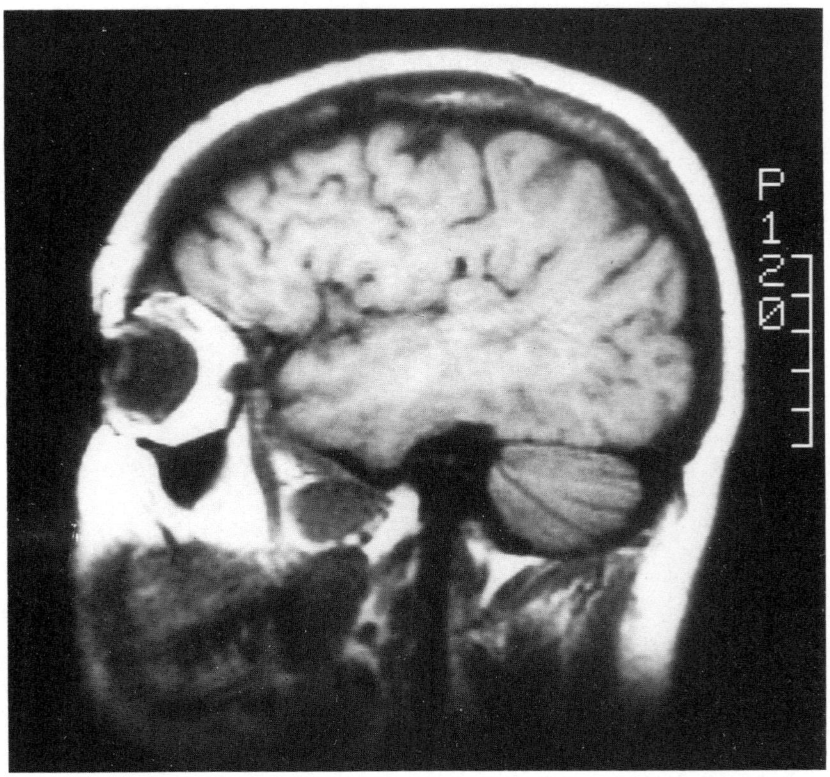

2-53 Sagittal MR scan through temporal lobe (600/15). Section 3 in Fig. 2-50.

2/Brain, Sagittal MRI

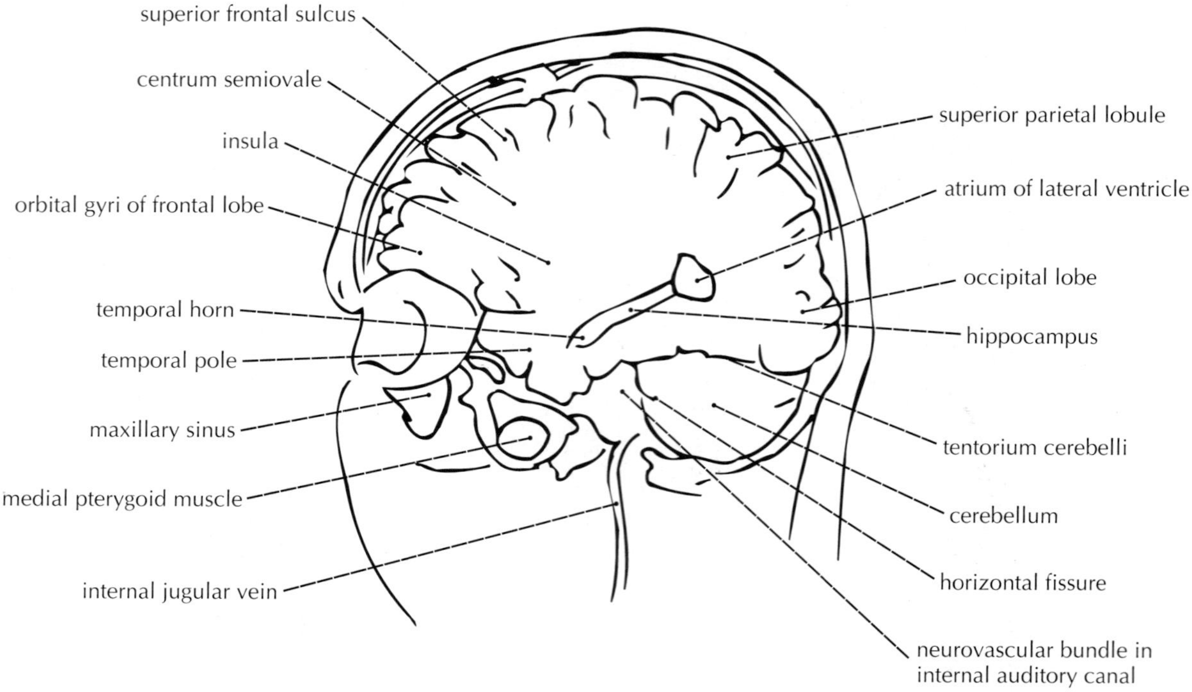

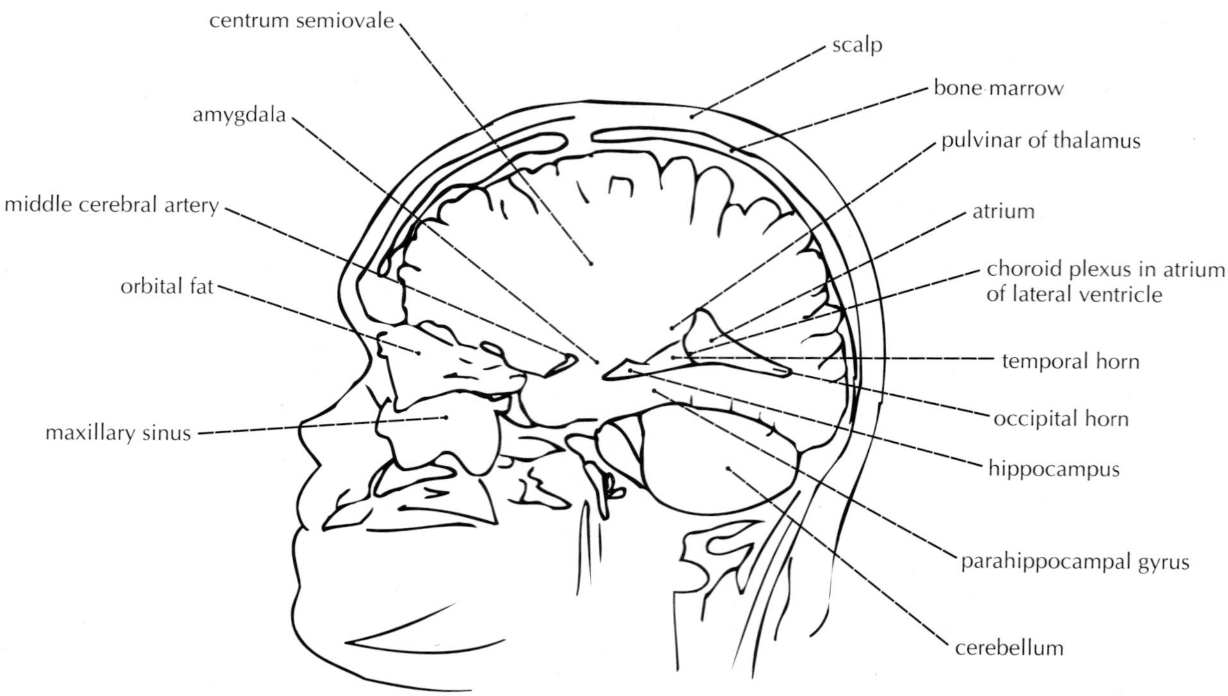

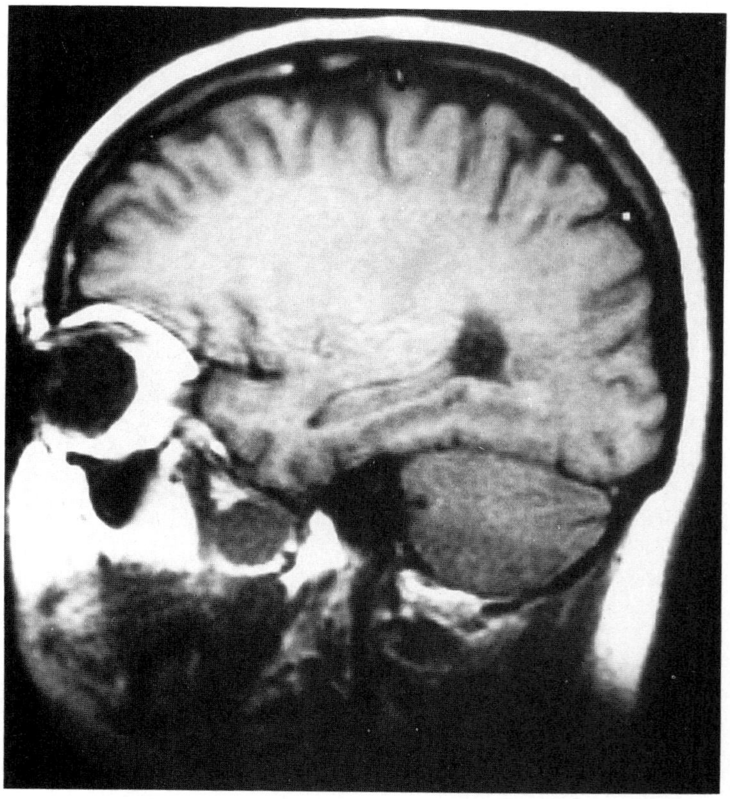

2-54 Sagittal MR scan through atrium and temporal horn (600/15). Section 5 in Fig. 2-50.

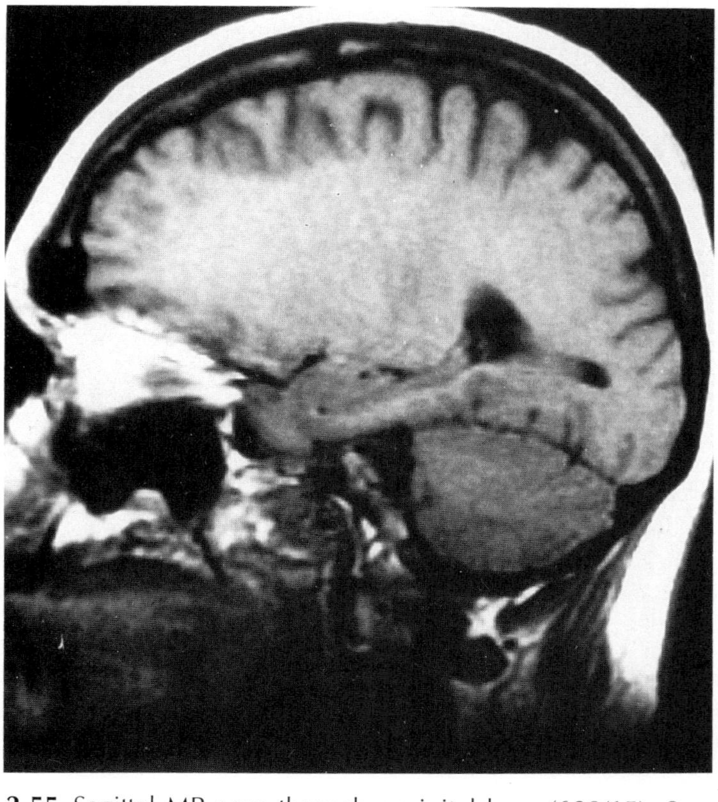

2-55 Sagittal MR scan through occipital horn (600/15). Section 6 in Fig. 2-50.

2/Brain, Sagittal MRI

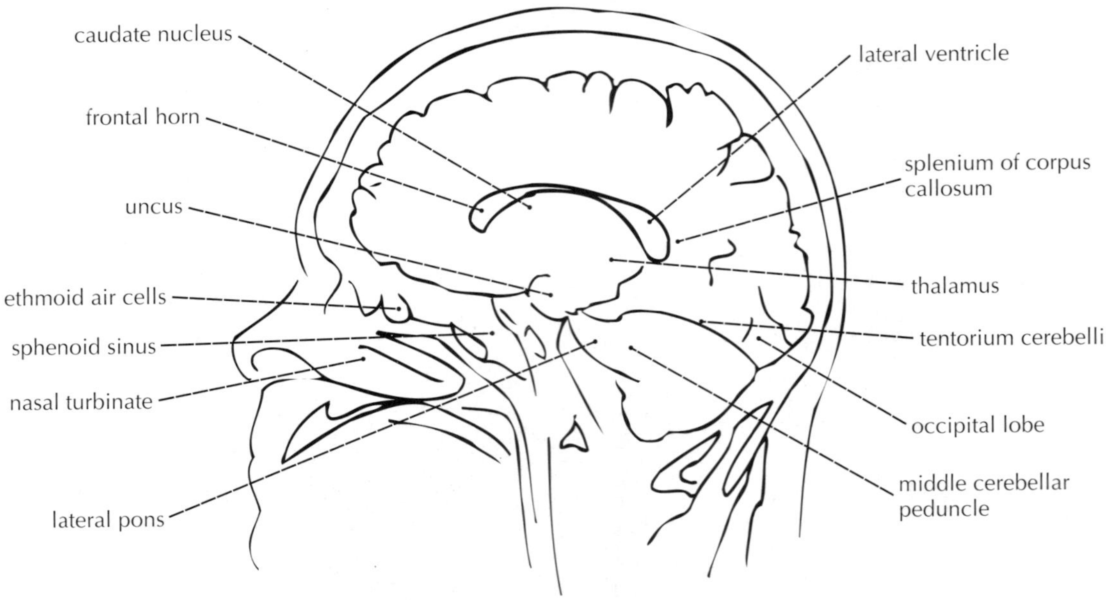

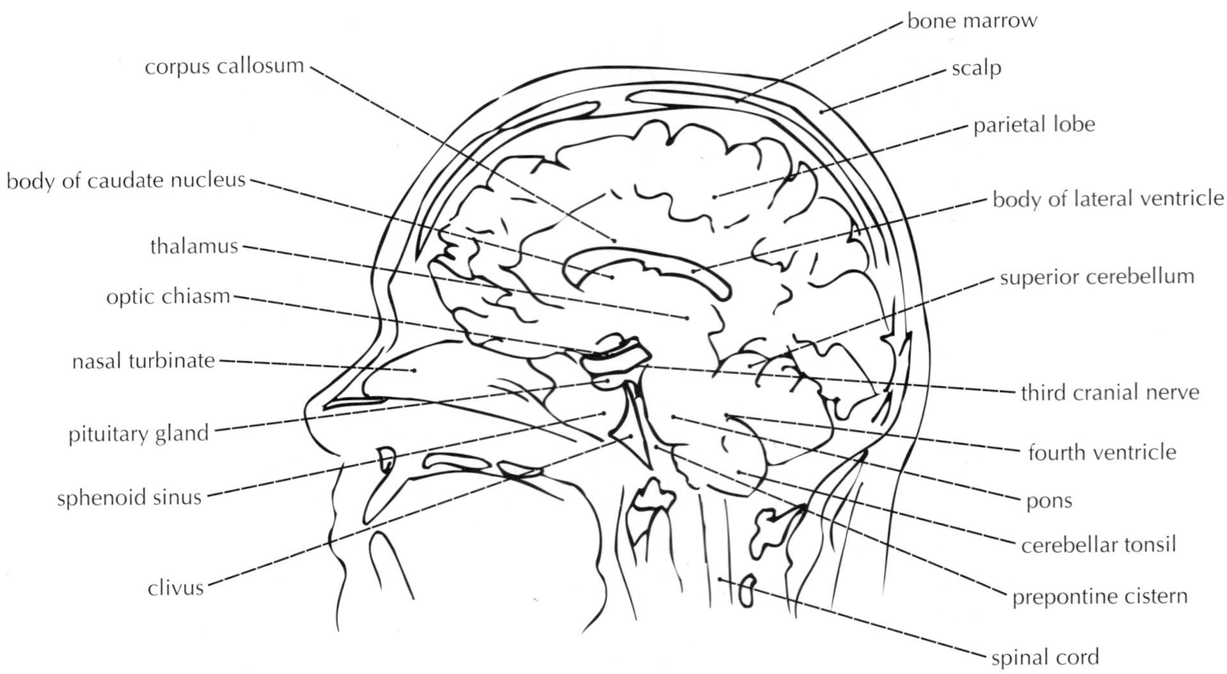

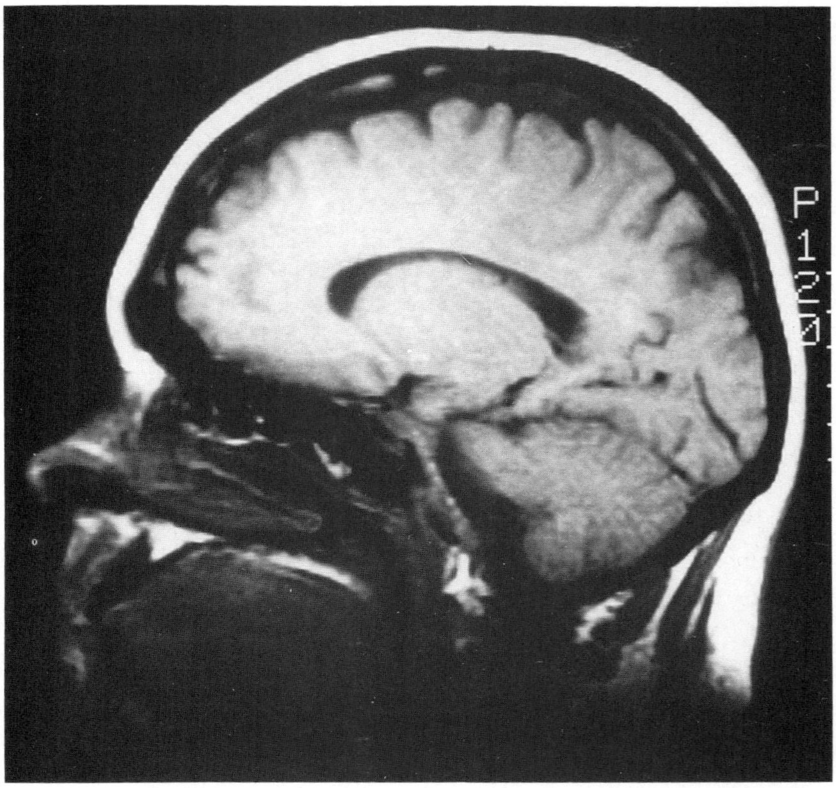

2-56 Sagittal MR scan through lateral ventricle and thalamus (600/15). Section 7 in Fig. 2-50.

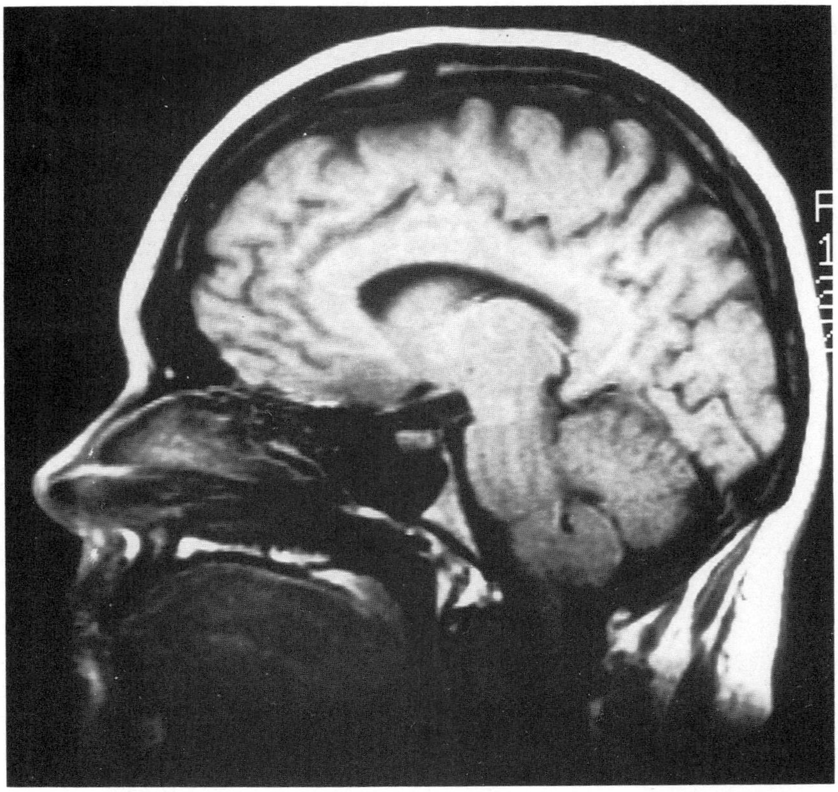

2-57 Sagittal MR scan through lateral ventricle and thalamus (600/15). Section 8 in Fig. 2-50.

2/Brain, Sagittal MRI

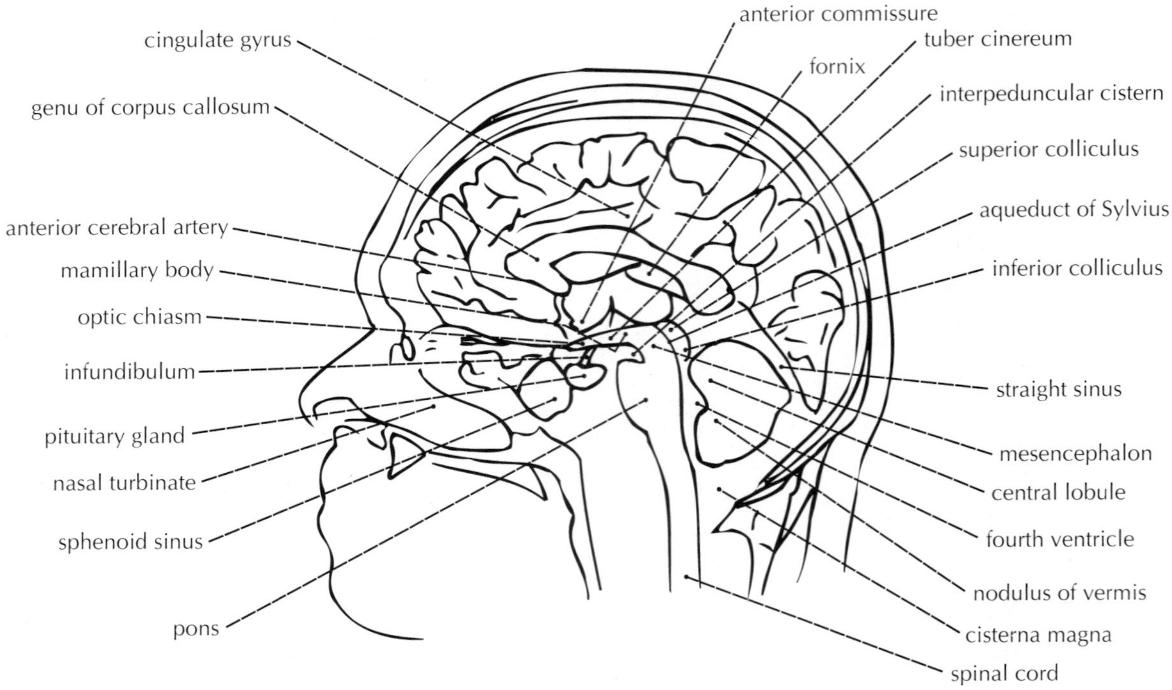

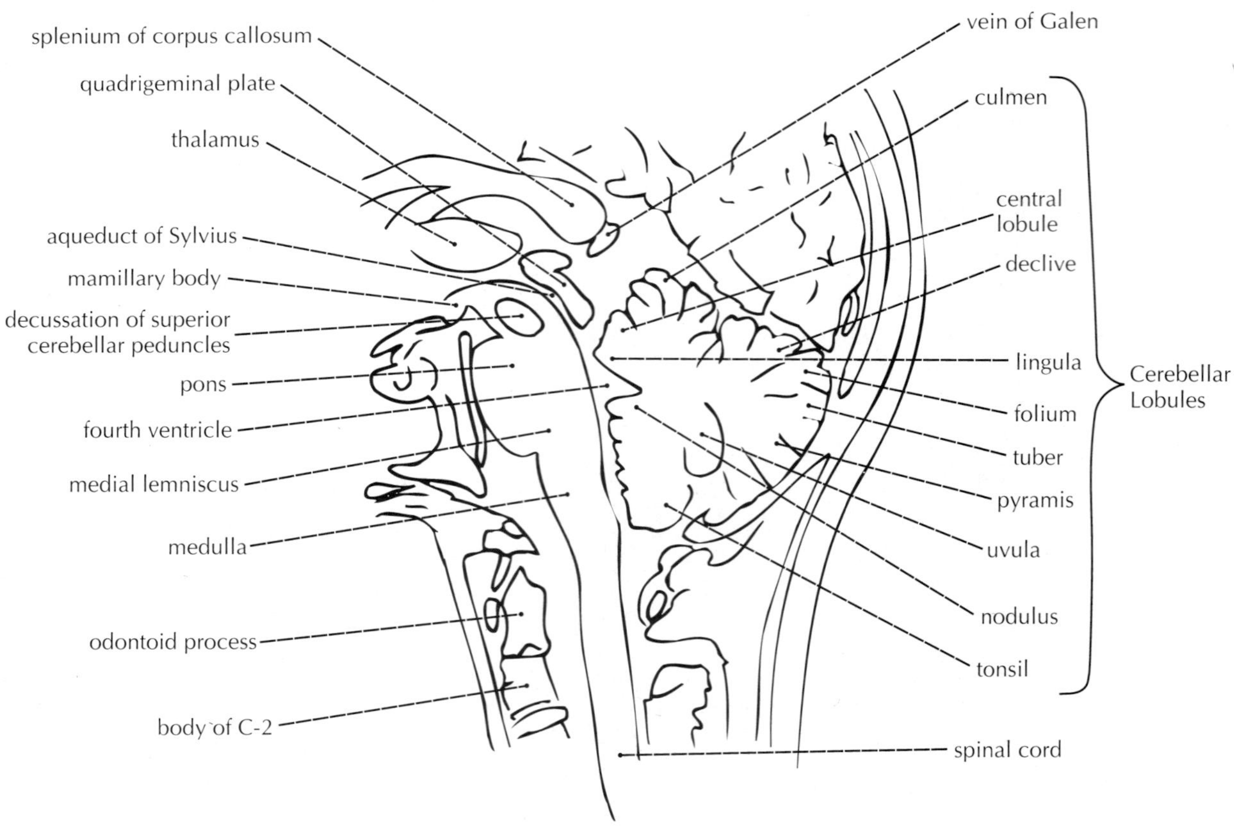

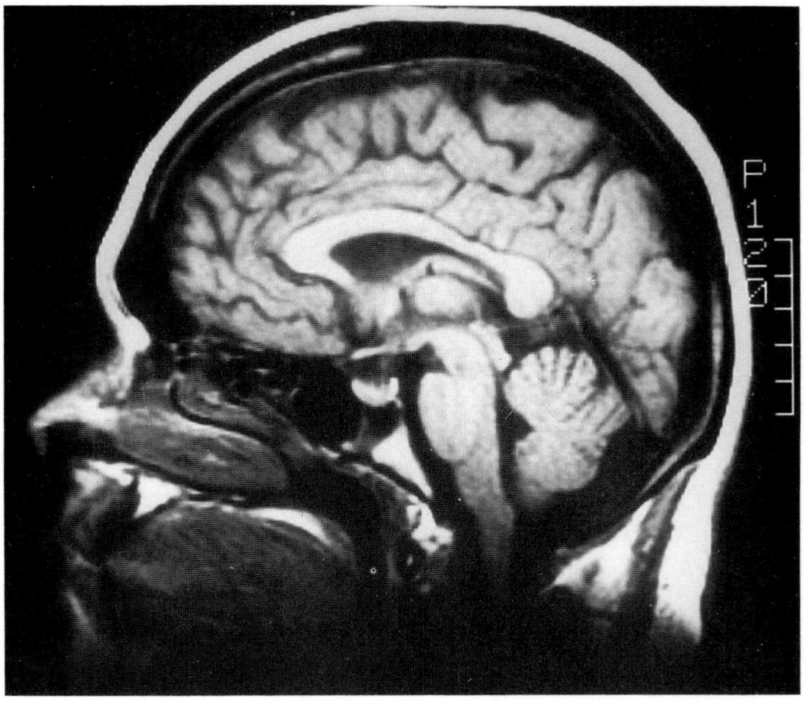

2-58 Sagittal MR scan of the midline (600/15). Section 9 in Fig. 2-50.

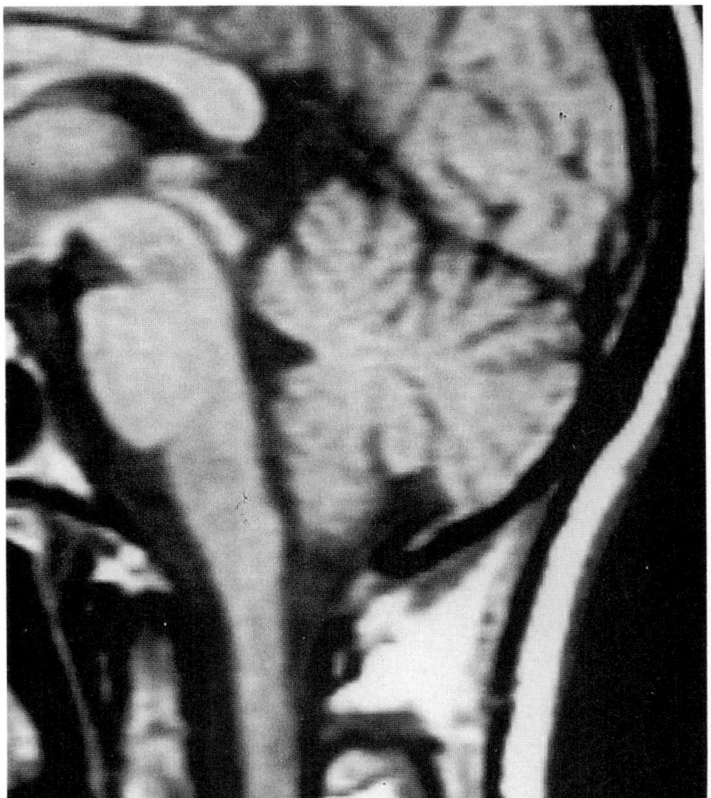

2-59 Sagittal MR scan through cerebellum, midline section (600/15).

2/Brain, Sagittal Scout MRI and Axial MRI (Infant)

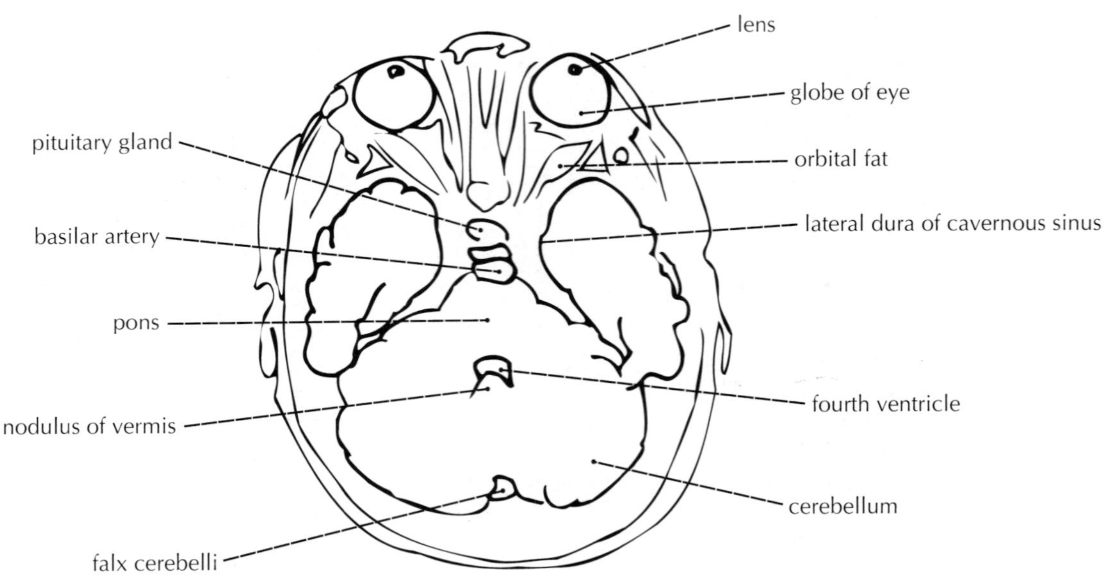

2/Brain, Sagittal Scout MRI and Axial MRI (Infant)

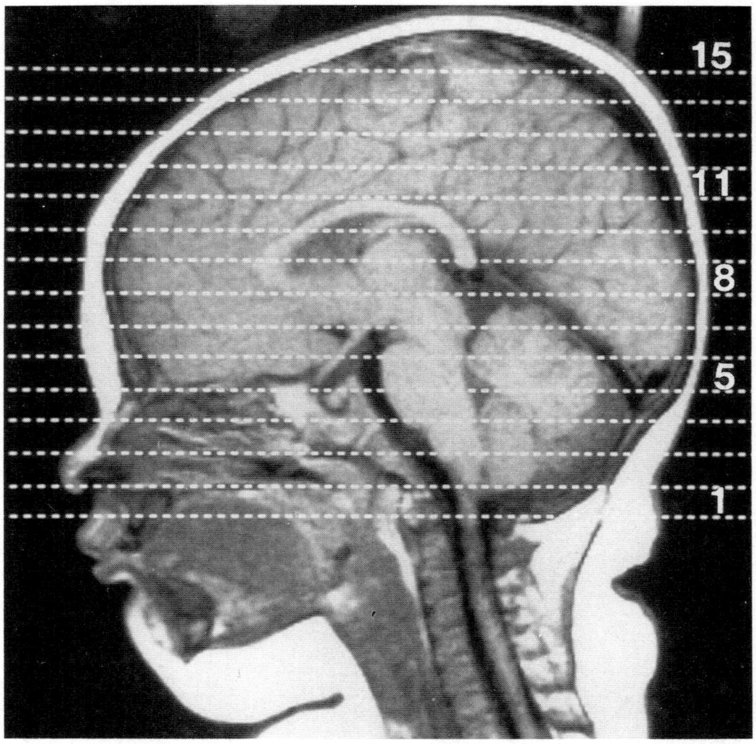

2-60 Sagittal scout MR scan for demonstration of the axial MR sections. Sections 5, 8, and 11 will be shown.

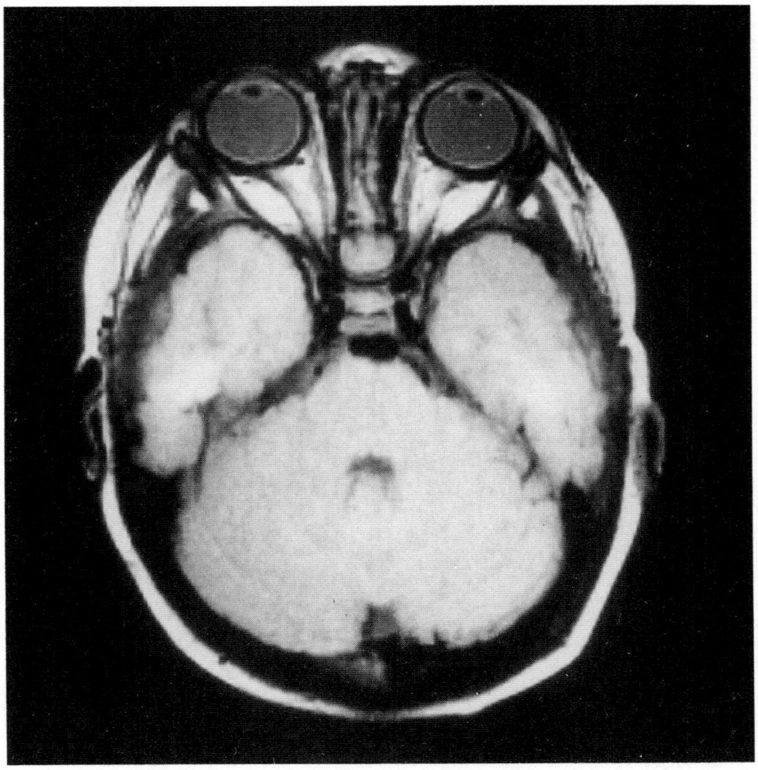

2-61 Axial MR scan of a 5-month-old infant (2000/30). Section 5 in Fig. 2-60.

2/Brain, Axial MRI (Infant)

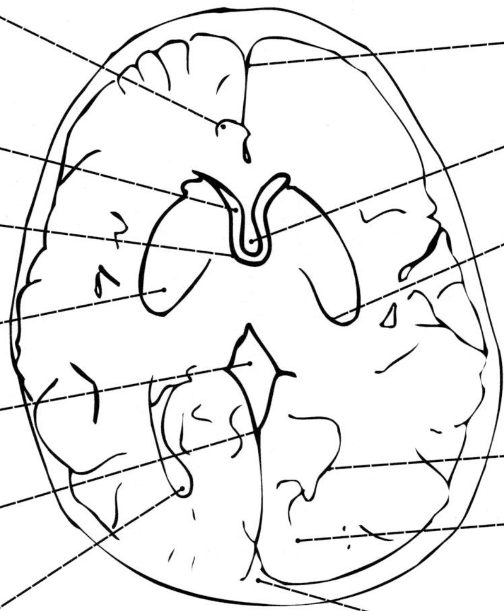

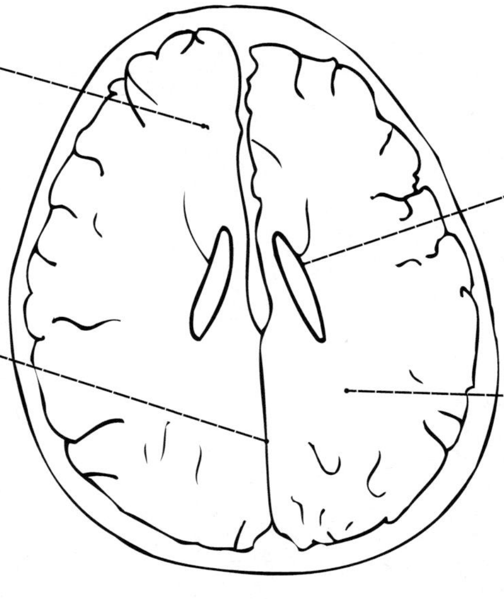

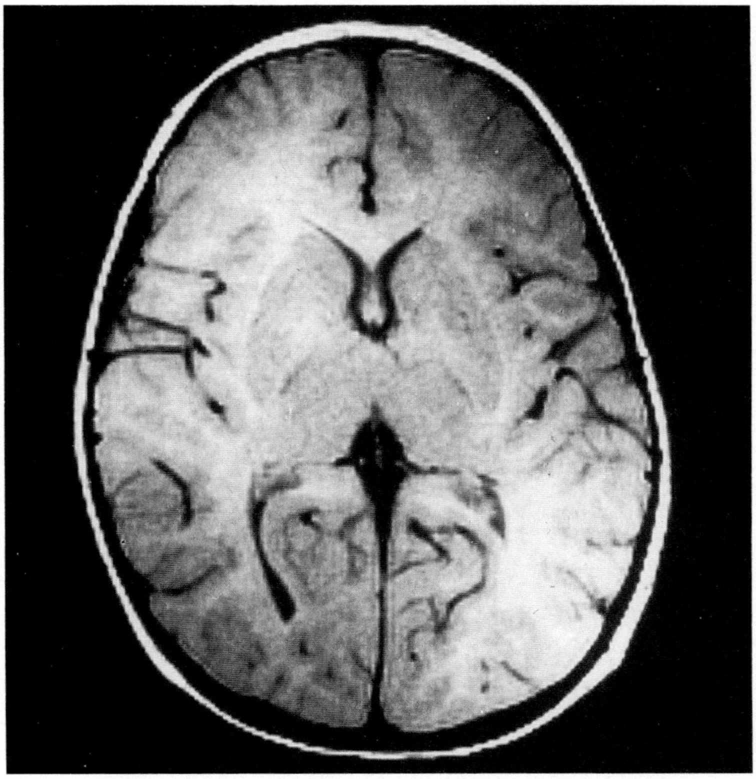

2-62 Axial MR scan of a 5-month-old infant (2000/30). Section 8 in Fig. 2-60.

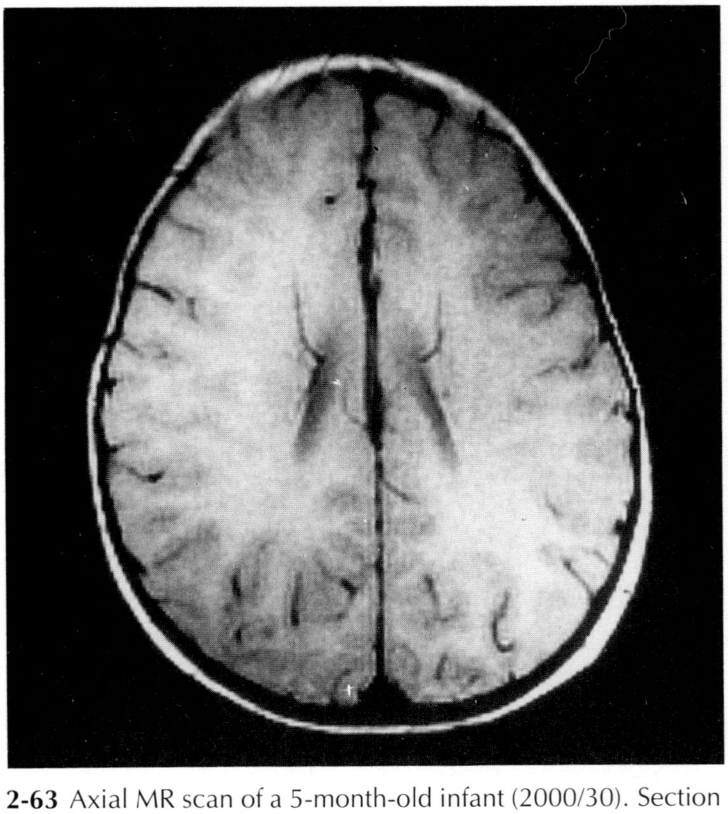

2-63 Axial MR scan of a 5-month-old infant (2000/30). Section 11 in Fig. 2-60.

2/Brain, Axial MRI (Infant)

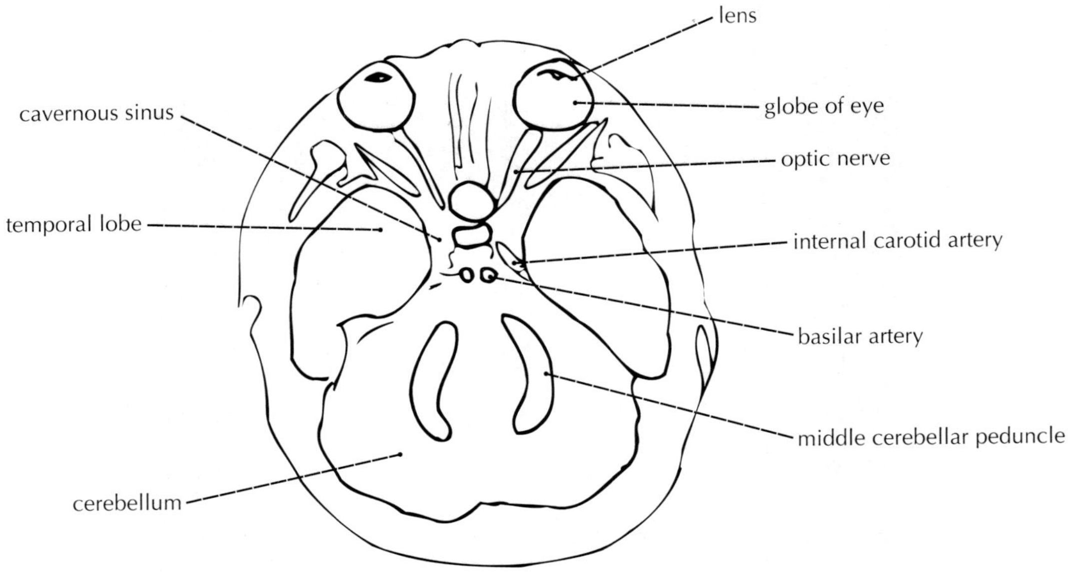

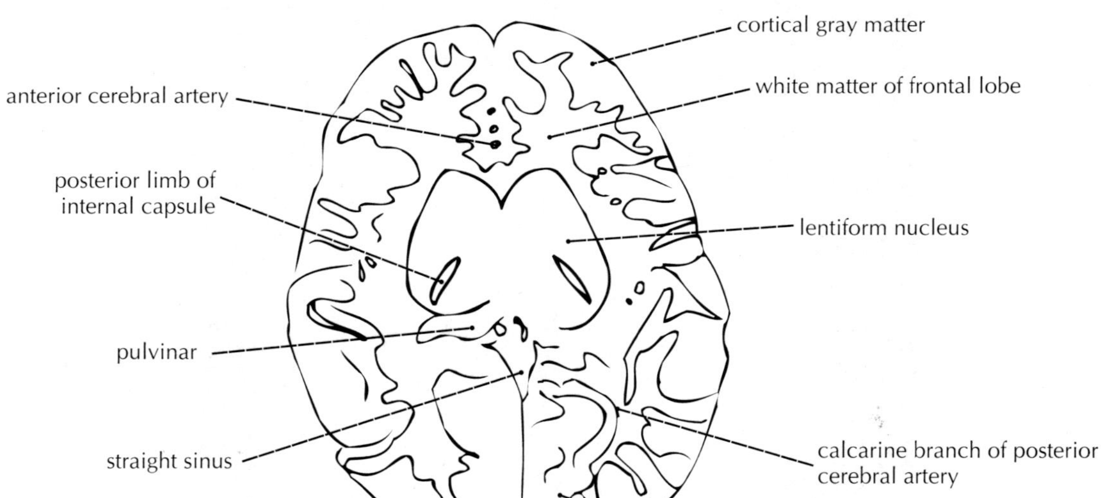

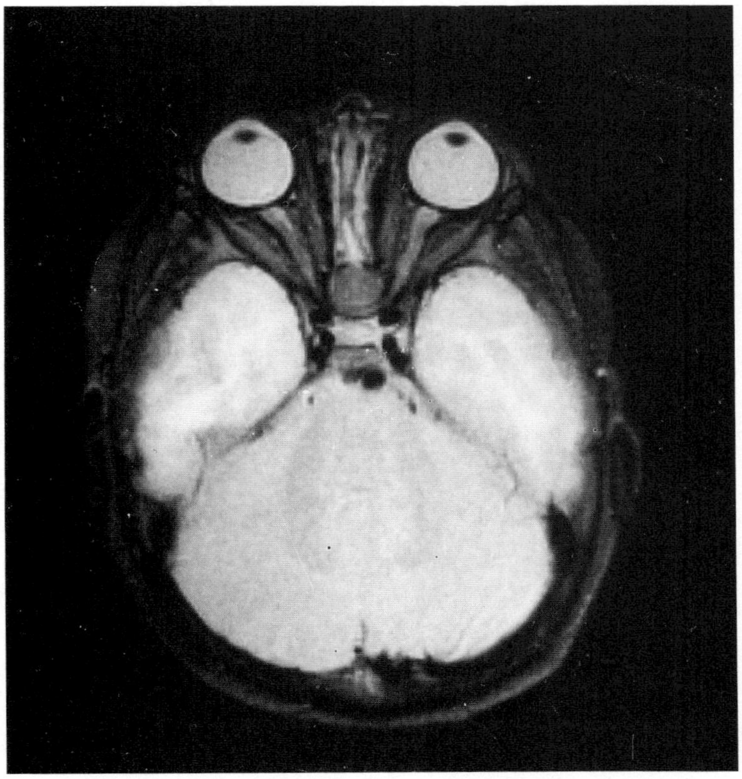

2-64 Axial MR scan of a 5-month-old infant (2000/60). Section 5 in Fig. 2-60.

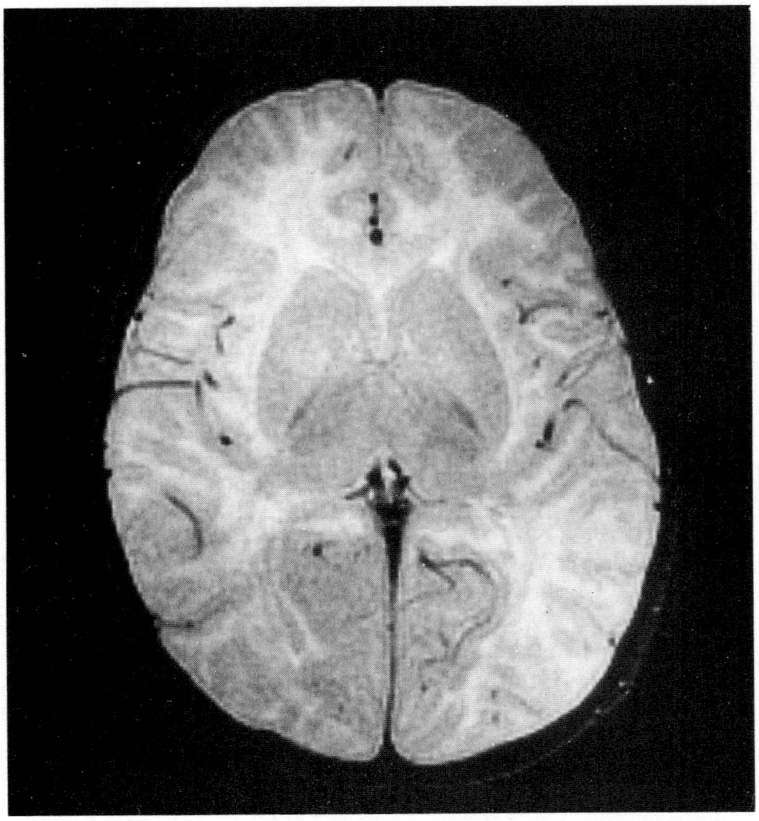

2-65 Axial MR scan of a 5-month-old infant (2000/60). Section 8 in Fig. 2-60.

2/Brain, Axial MRI (Infant)

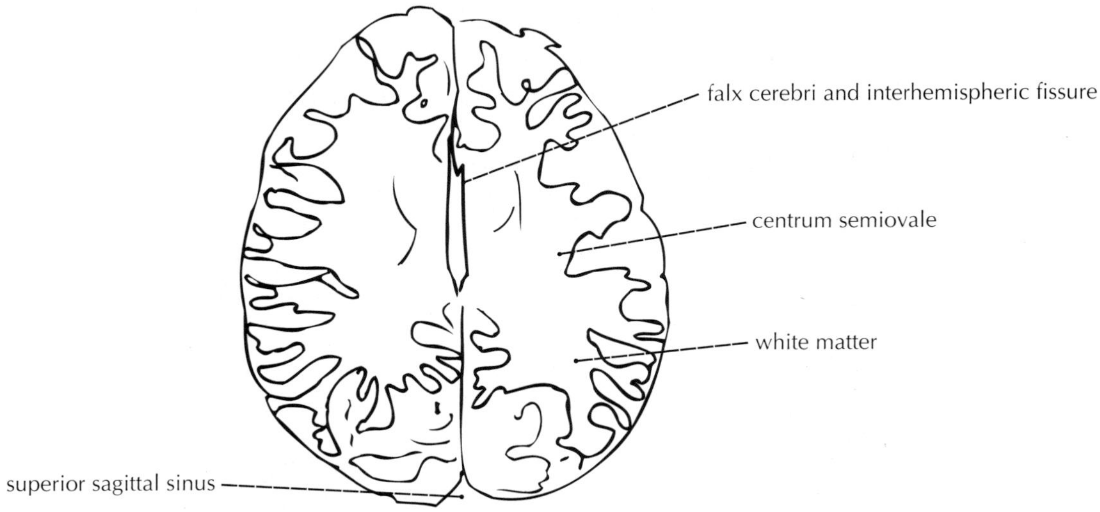

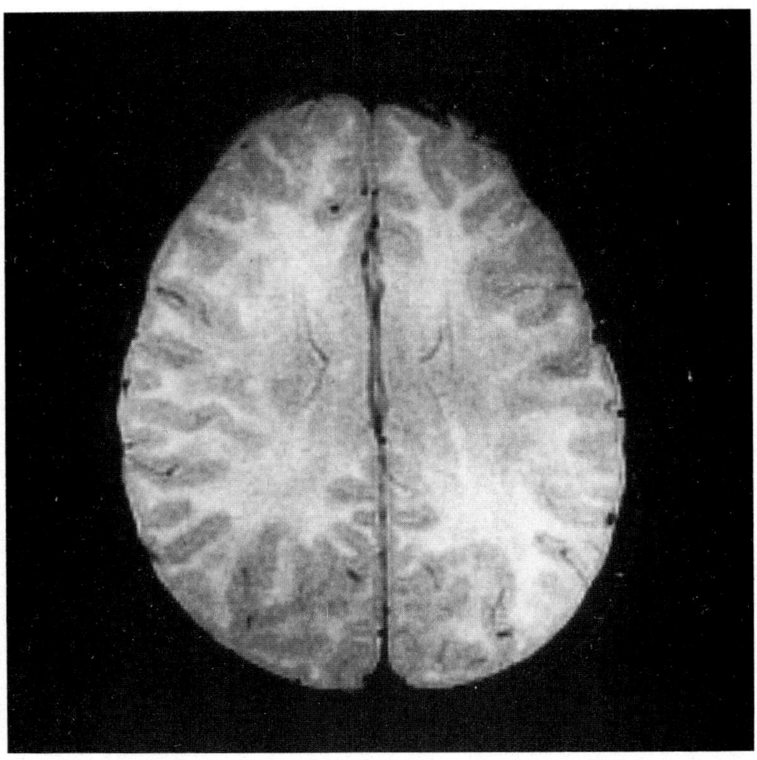

2-66 Axial MR scan of a 5-month-old infant (2000/60). Section 11 in Fig. 2-60.

2/Brain, Axial Scout MRI

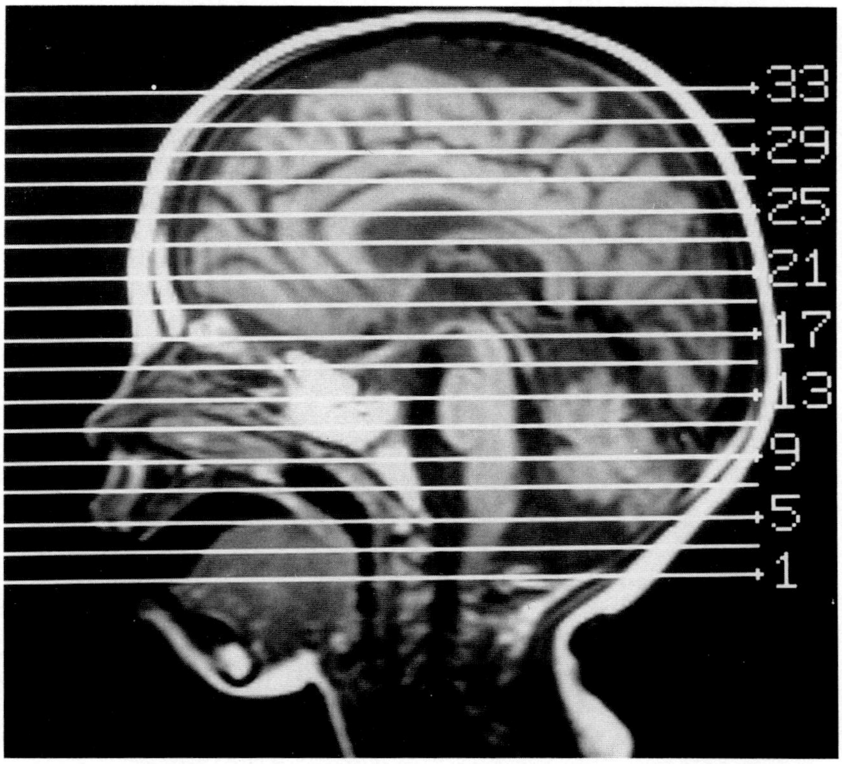

2-67 Sagittal scout MR scan for demonstration of axial MR sections. Sections 9, 15, 19, 21, and 25 will be shown.

2/Brain, Axial MRI (Infant)

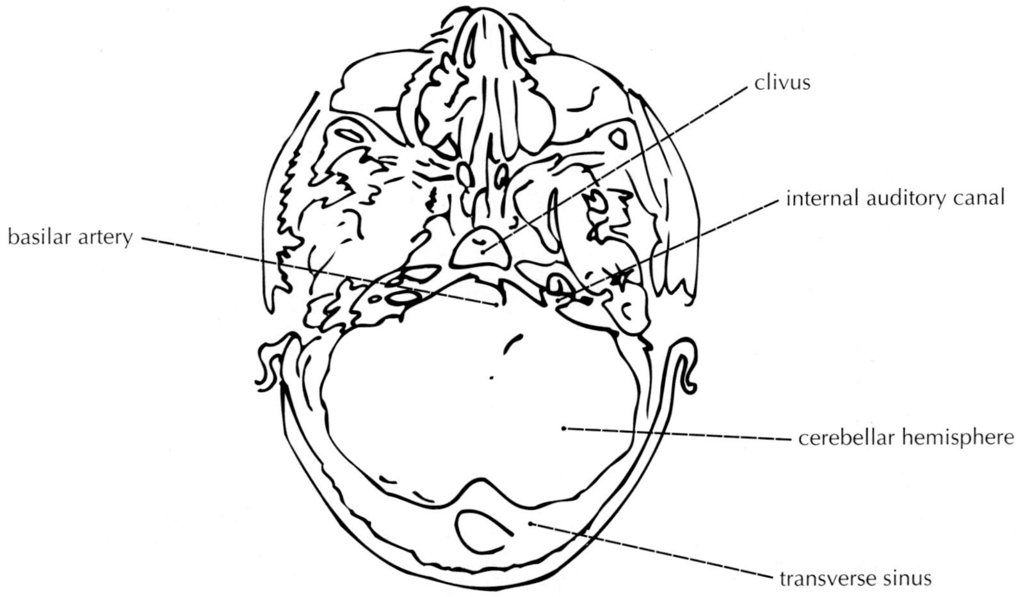

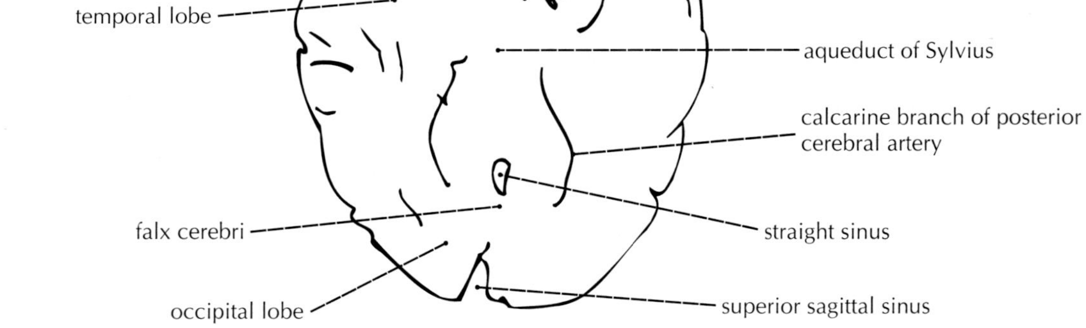

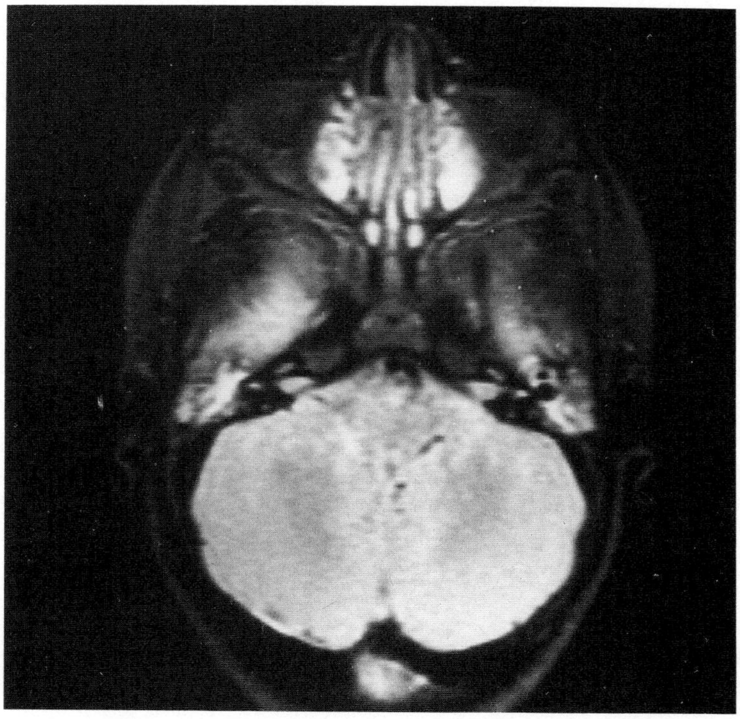

2-68 Axial MR scan of a 9-month-old infant (2000/80). Section 9 in Fig. 2-67.

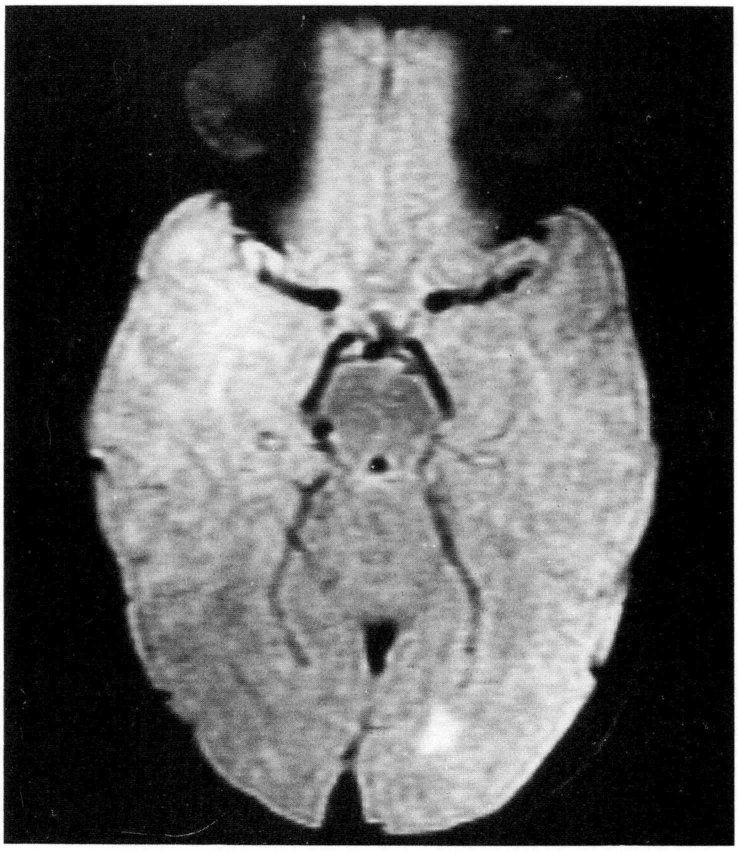

2-69 Axial MR scan of a 9-month-old infant (2000/80). Section 15 in Fig. 2-67.

2/Brain, Axial MRI (Infant)

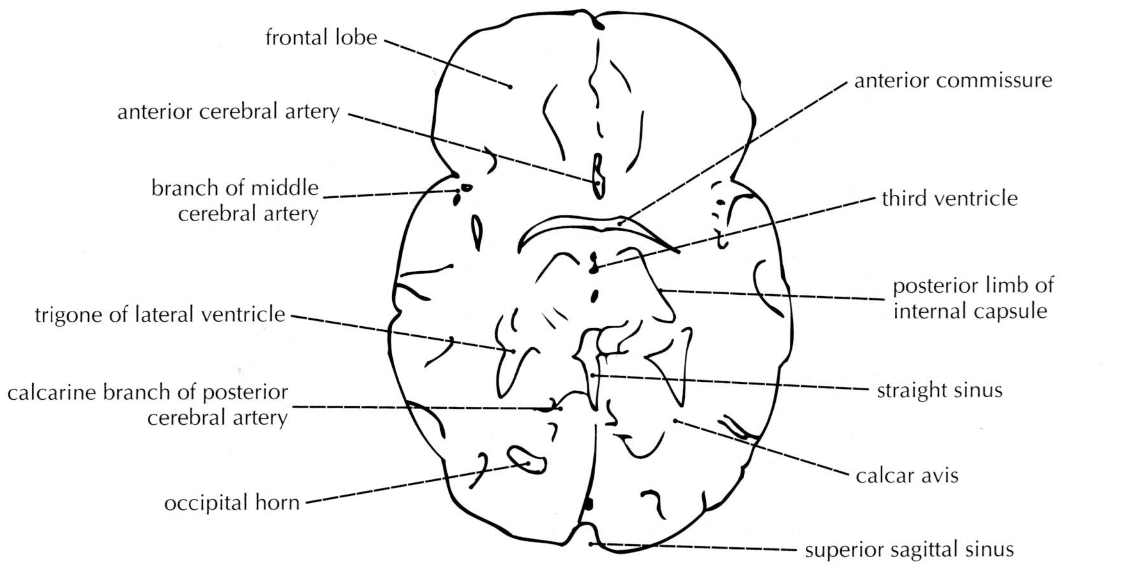

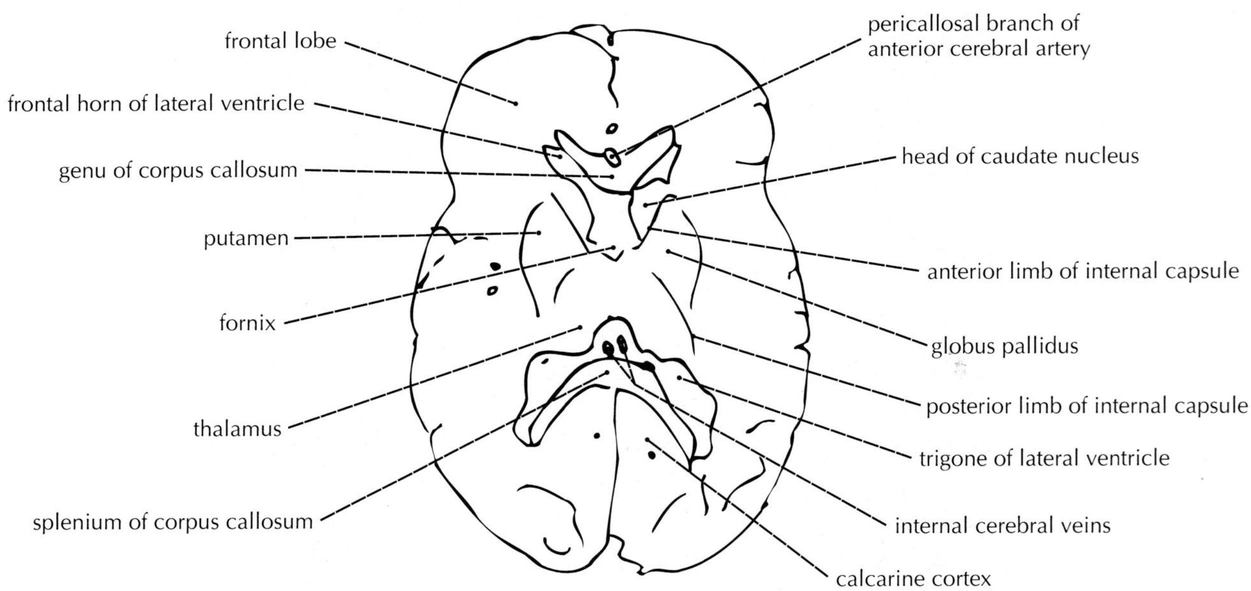

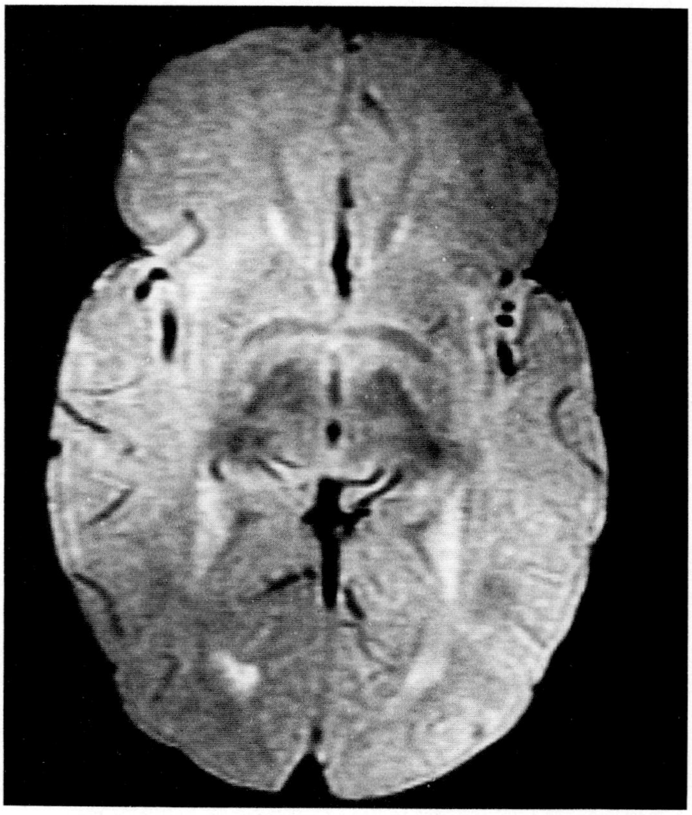

2-70 Axial MR scan of a 9-month-old infant (2000/80). Section 19 in Fig. 2-67.

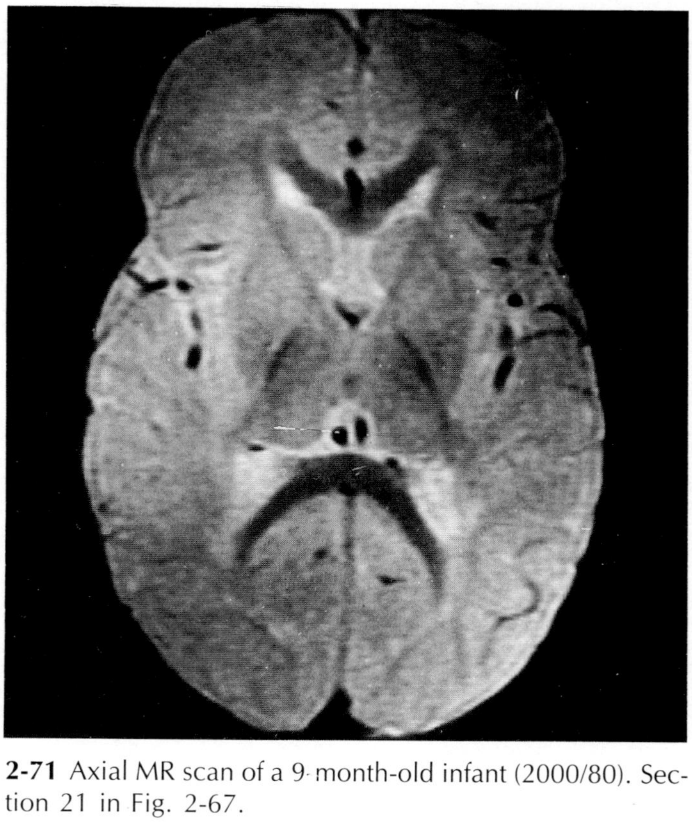

2-71 Axial MR scan of a 9-month-old infant (2000/80). Section 21 in Fig. 2-67.

2/Brain, Axial MRI (Infant)

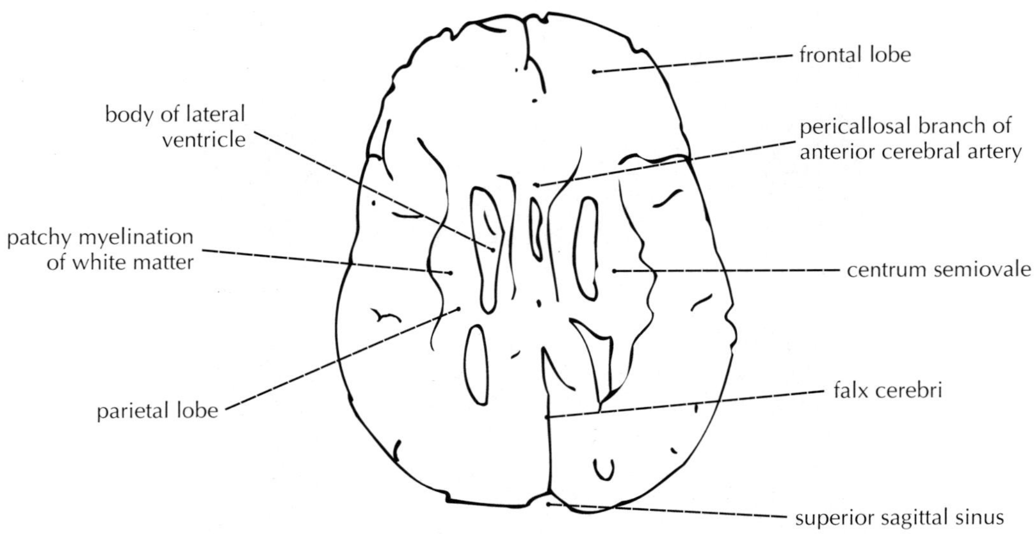

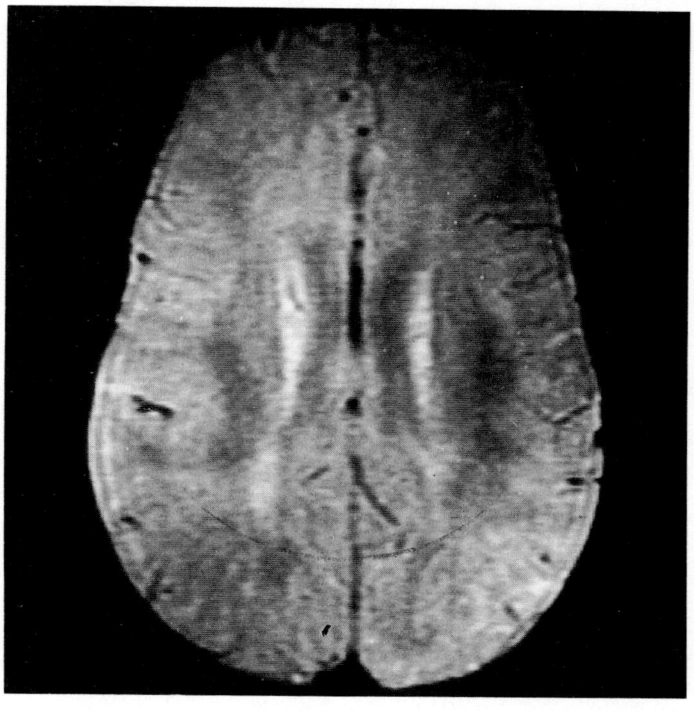

2-72 Axial MR scan of a 9-month-old infant (2000/80). Section 25 in Fig. 2-67.

2/Head, Angiography

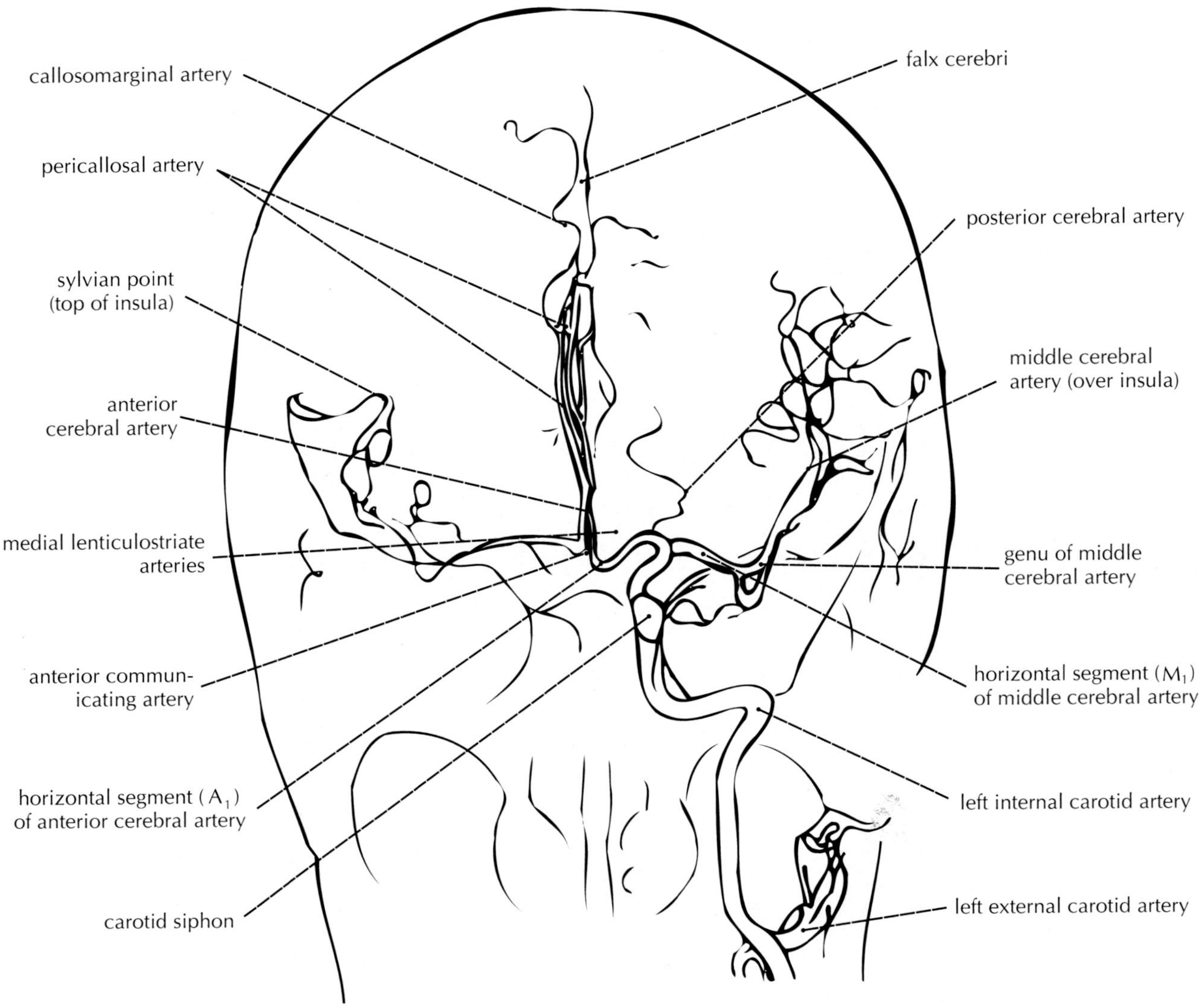

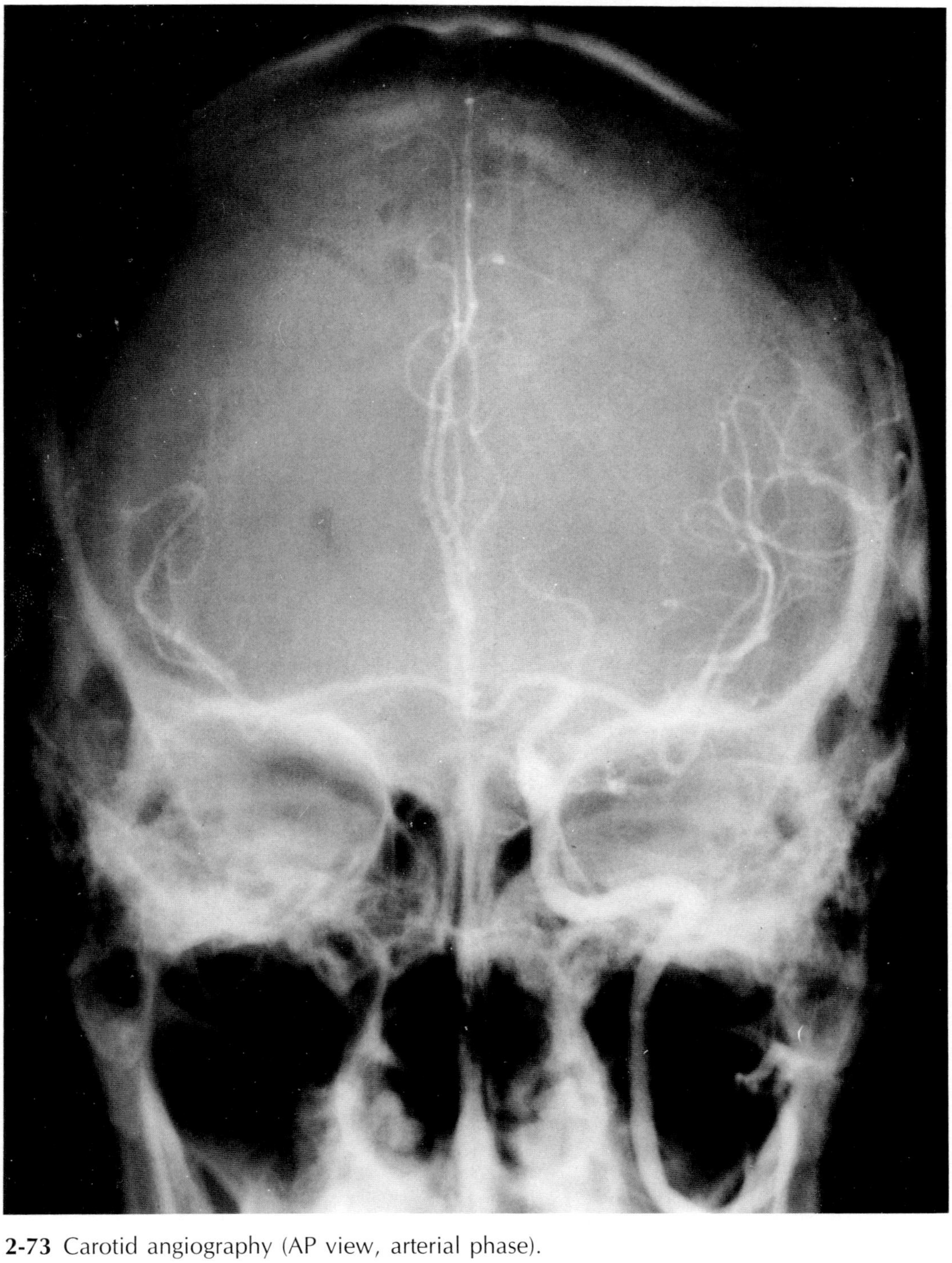

2-73 Carotid angiography (AP view, arterial phase).

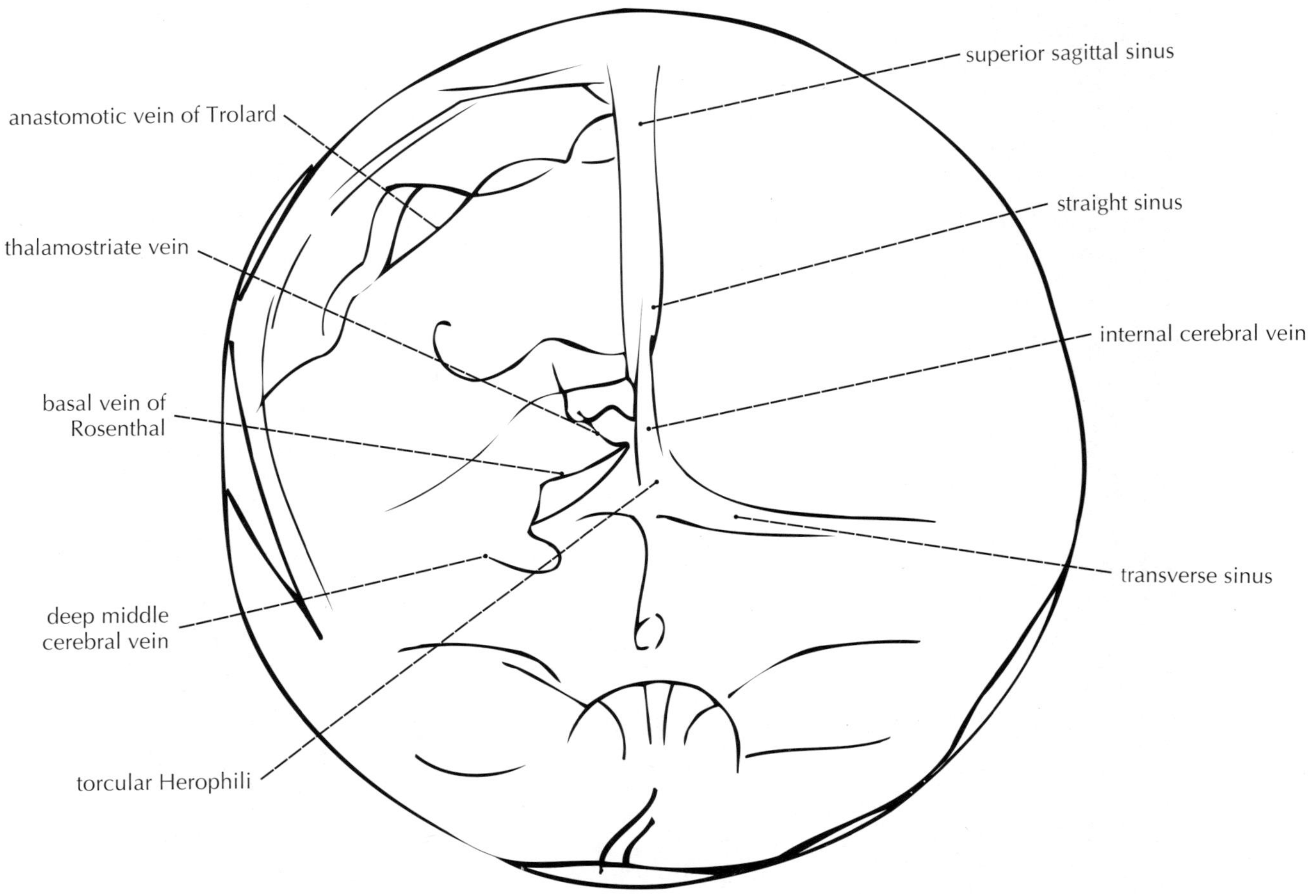
superior sagittal sinus
anastomotic vein of Trolard
straight sinus
thalamostriate vein
internal cerebral vein
basal vein of
Rosenthal
transverse sinus
deep middle
cerebral vein
torcular Herophili

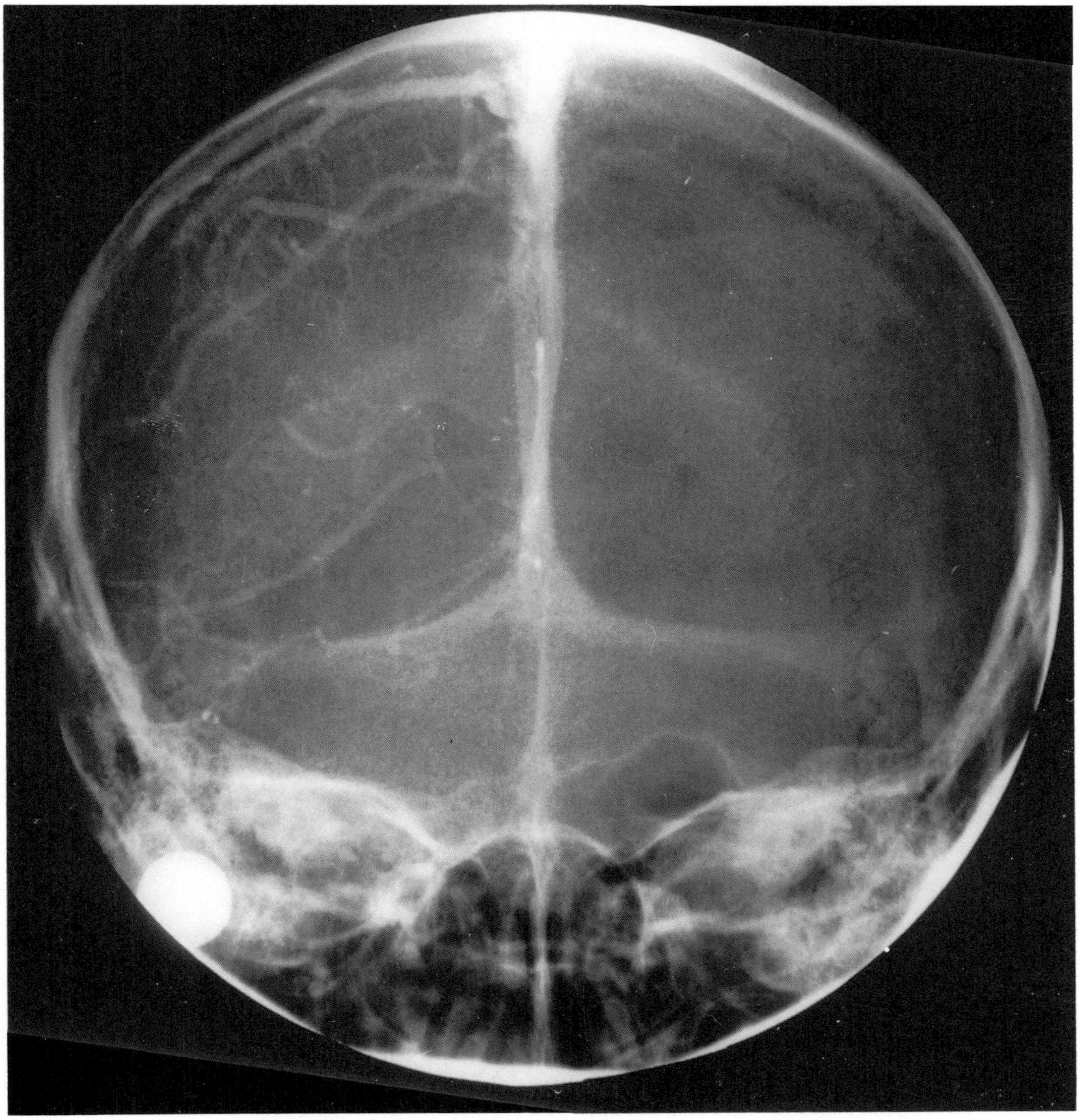

2-74 Carotid angiography (AP view, venous phase).

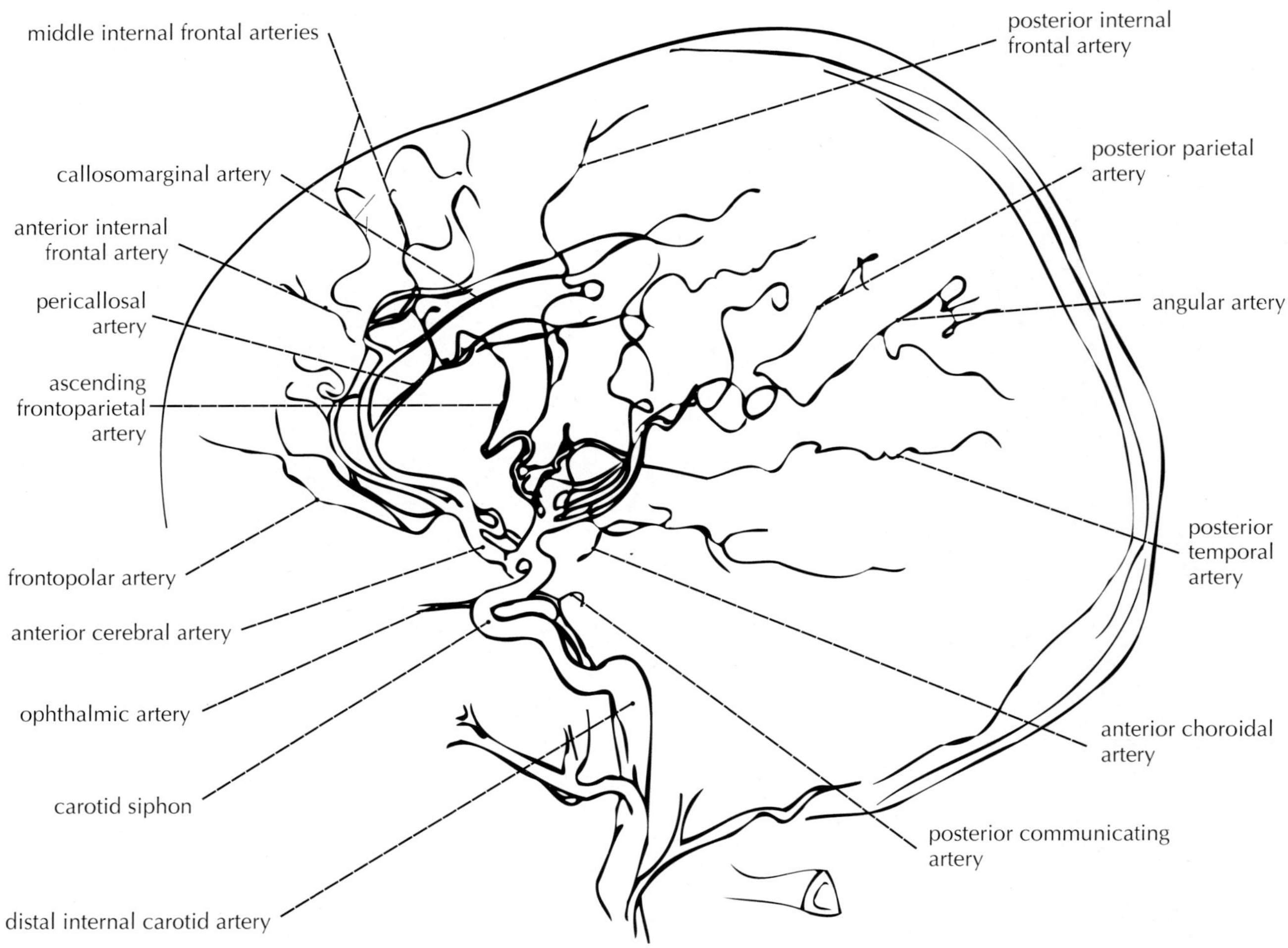
middle internal frontal arteries
callosomarginal artery
anterior internal frontal artery
pericallosal artery
ascending frontoparietal artery
frontopolar artery
anterior cerebral artery
ophthalmic artery
carotid siphon
distal internal carotid artery
posterior internal frontal artery
posterior parietal artery
angular artery
posterior temporal artery
anterior choroidal artery
posterior communicating artery

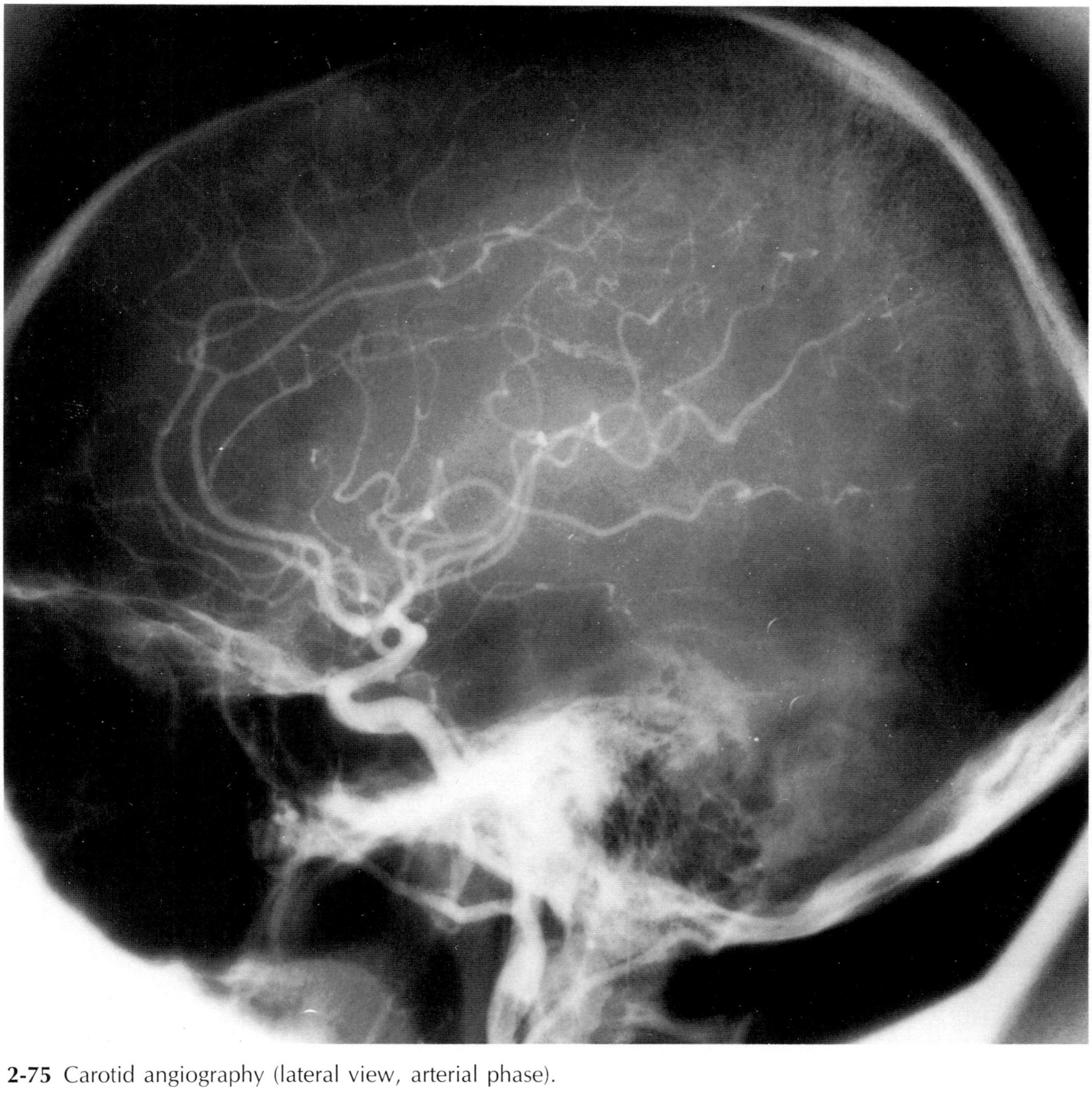

2-75 Carotid angiography (lateral view, arterial phase).

2/Head, Angiography

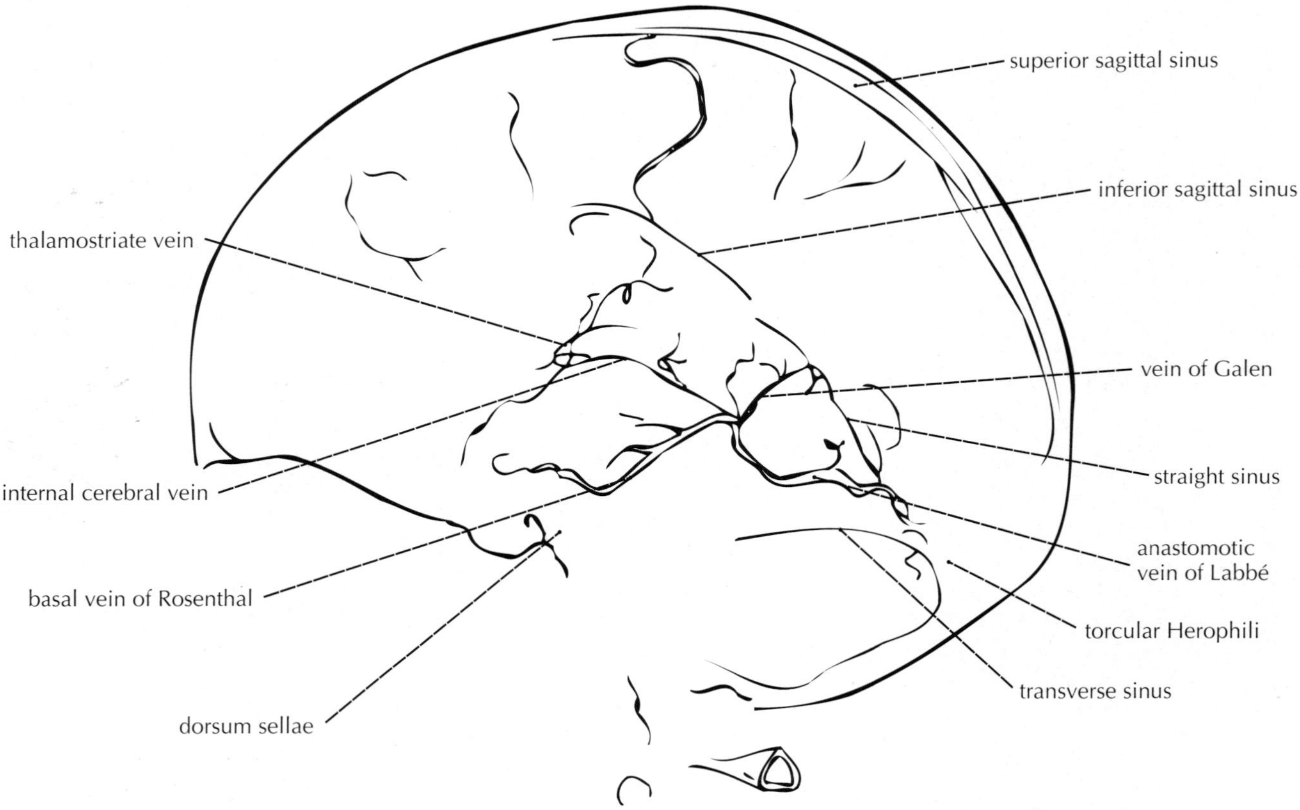

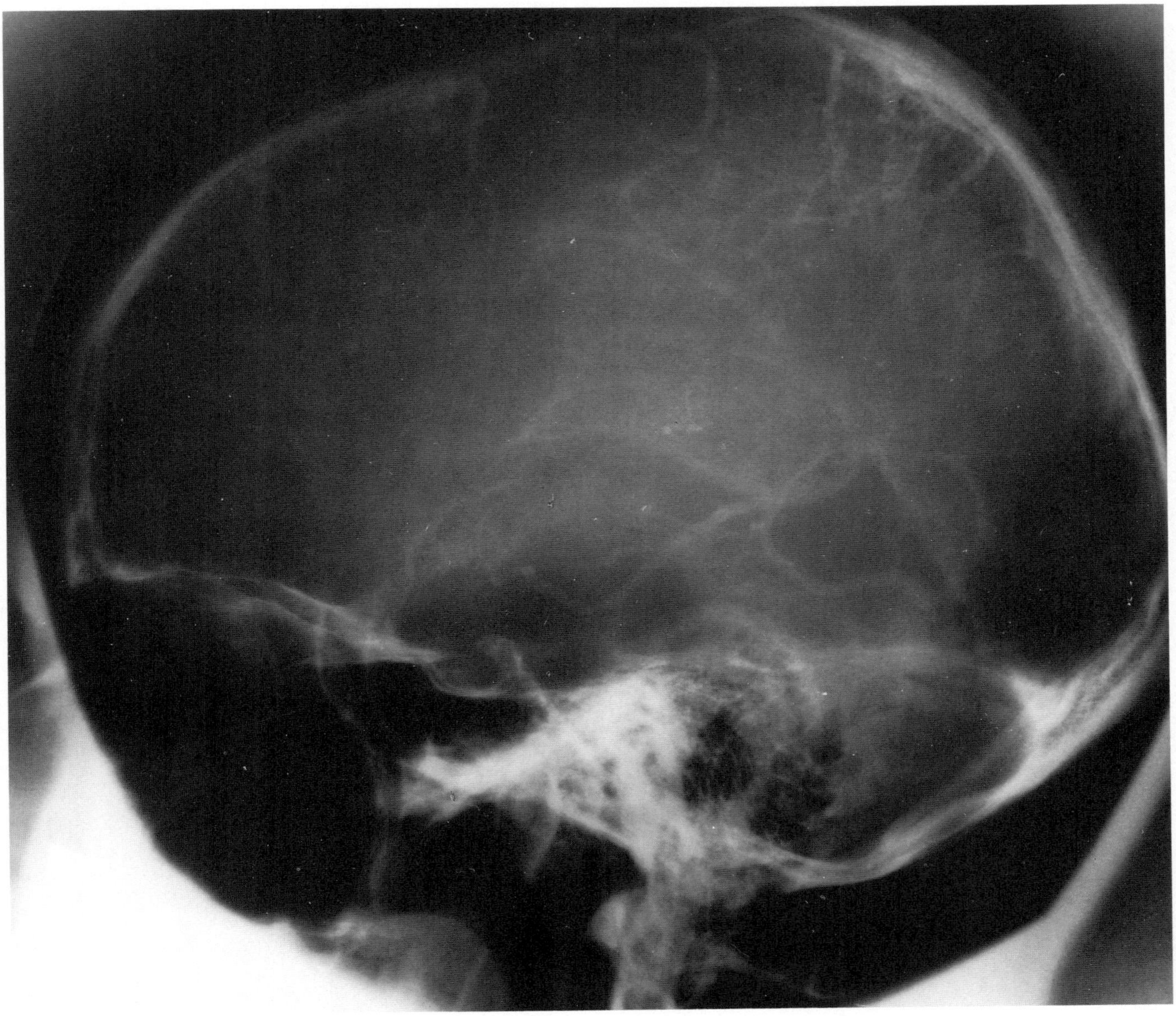

2-76 Carotid arteriography (lateral view, venous phase).

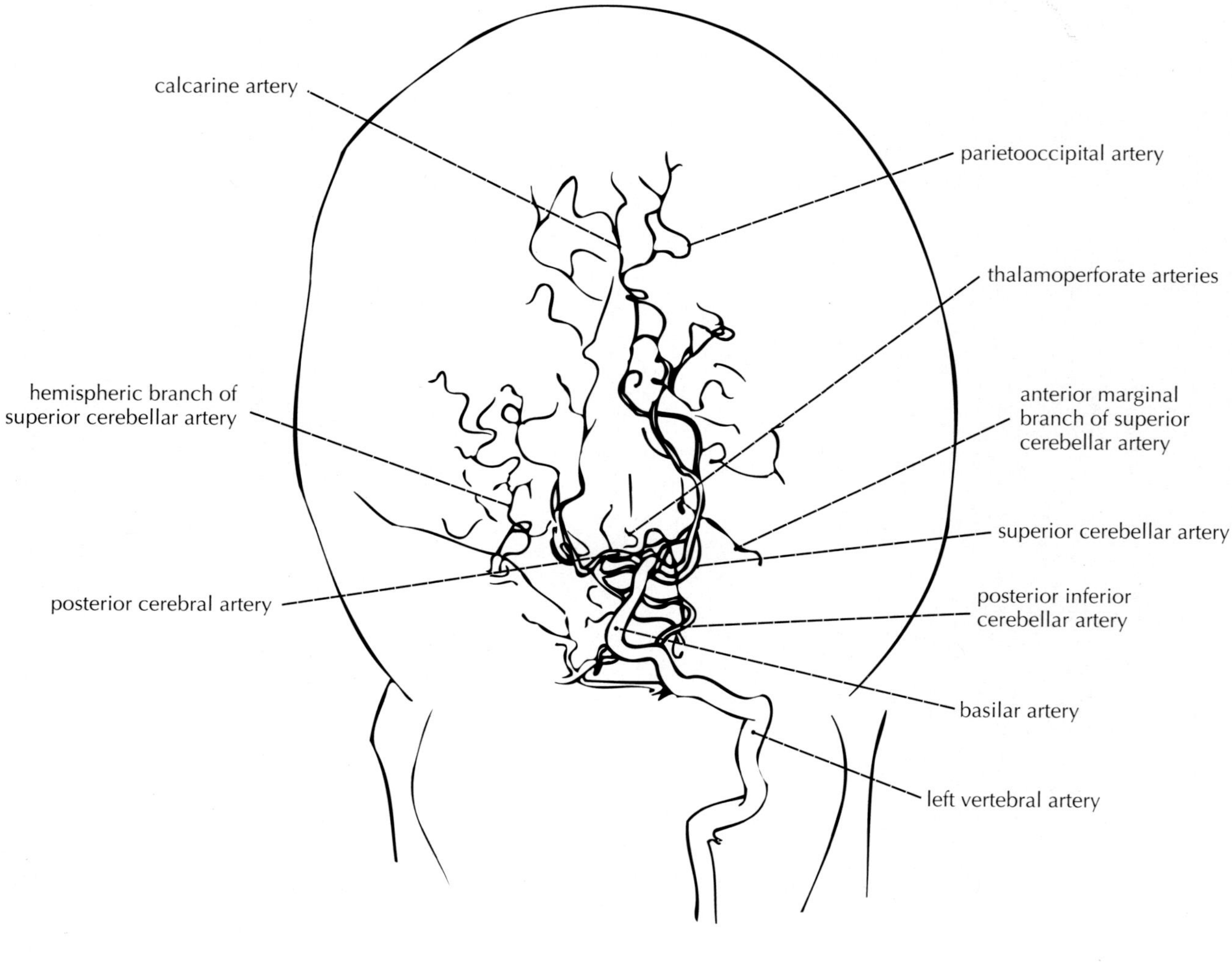
calcarine artery
parietooccipital artery
thalamoperforate arteries
hemispheric branch of superior cerebellar artery
anterior marginal branch of superior cerebellar artery
superior cerebellar artery
posterior cerebral artery
posterior inferior cerebellar artery
basilar artery
left vertebral artery

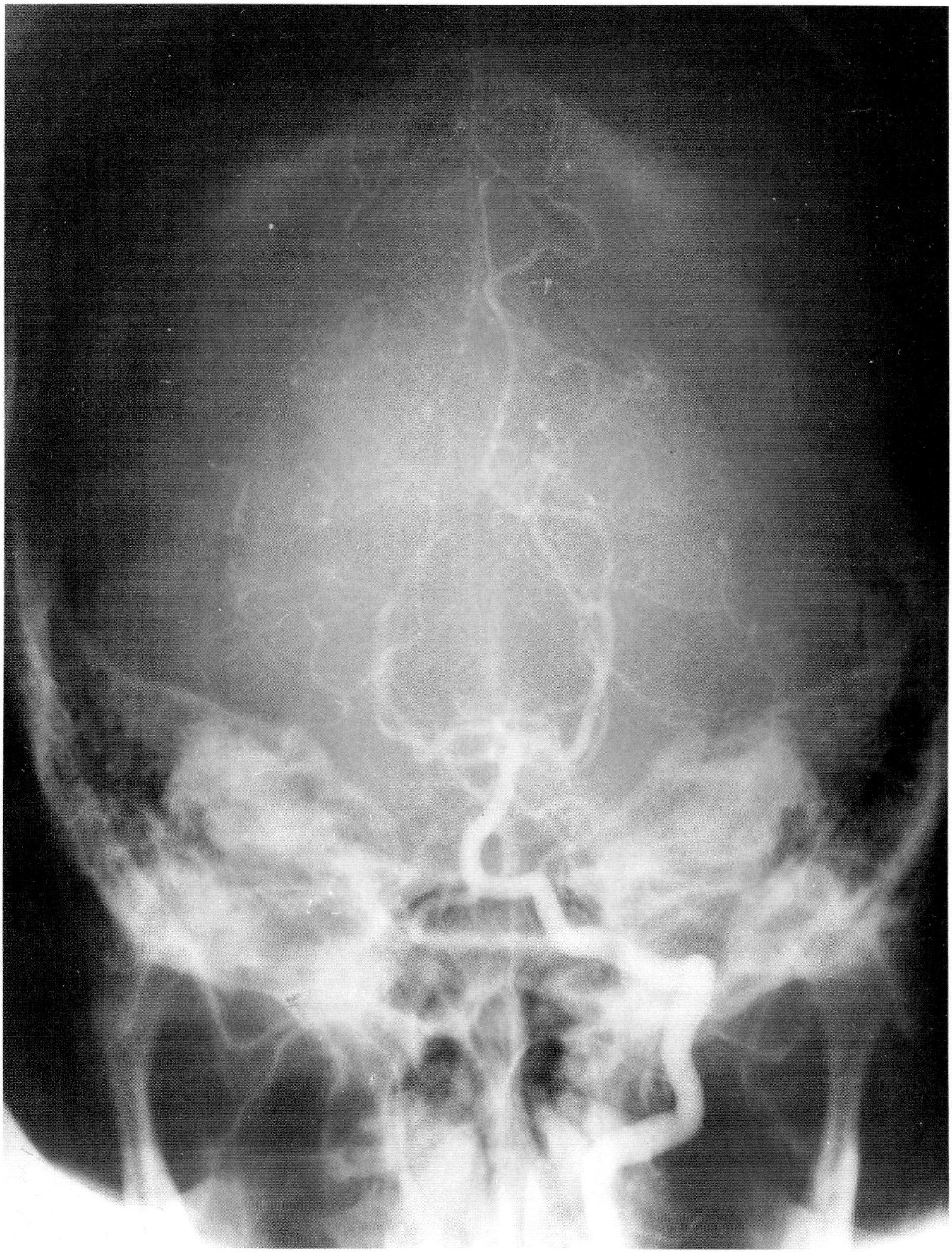

2-77 Vertebral angiography (AP view, arterial phase).

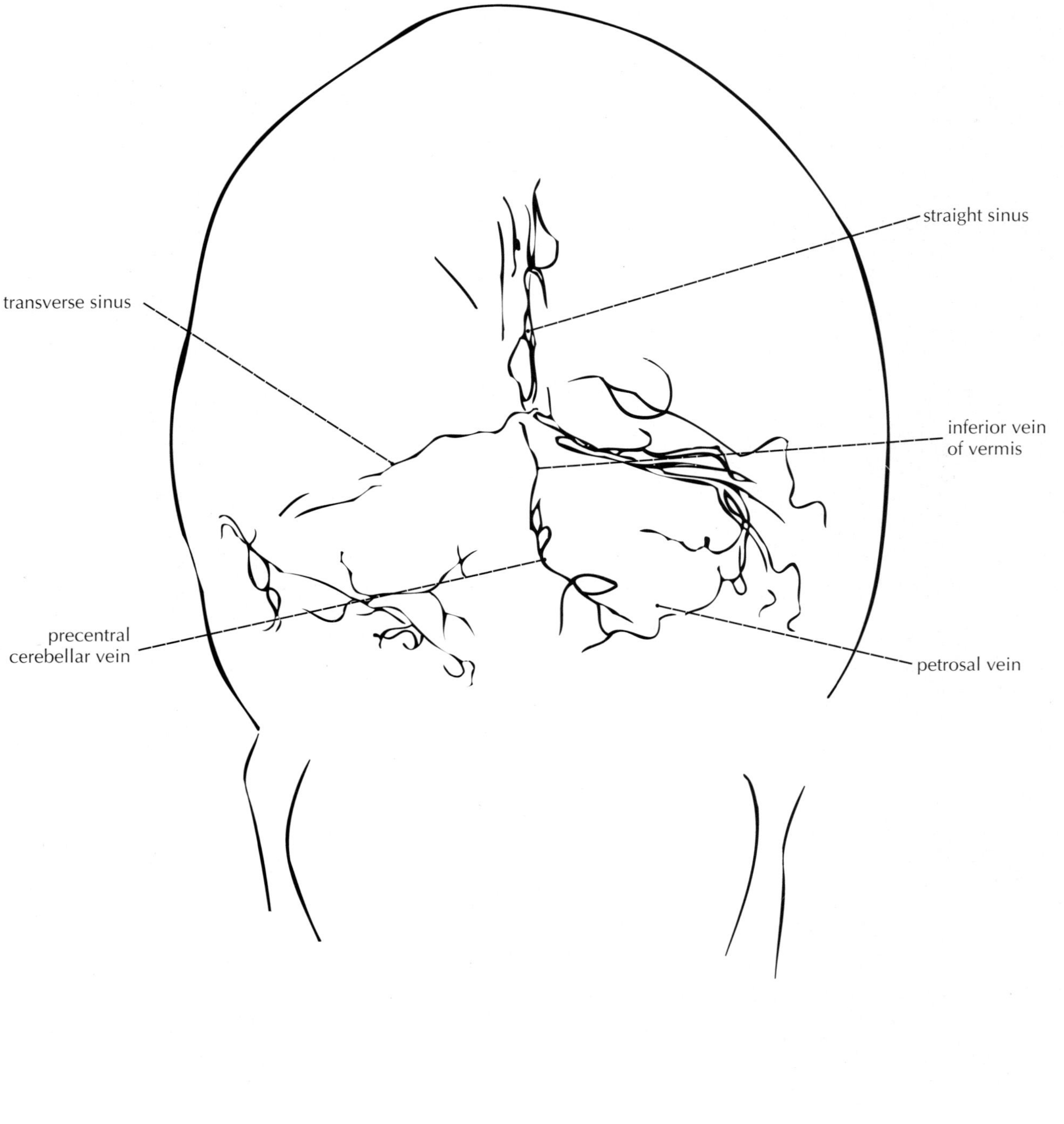
straight sinus
transverse sinus
inferior vein
of vermis
precentral
cerebellar vein
petrosal vein

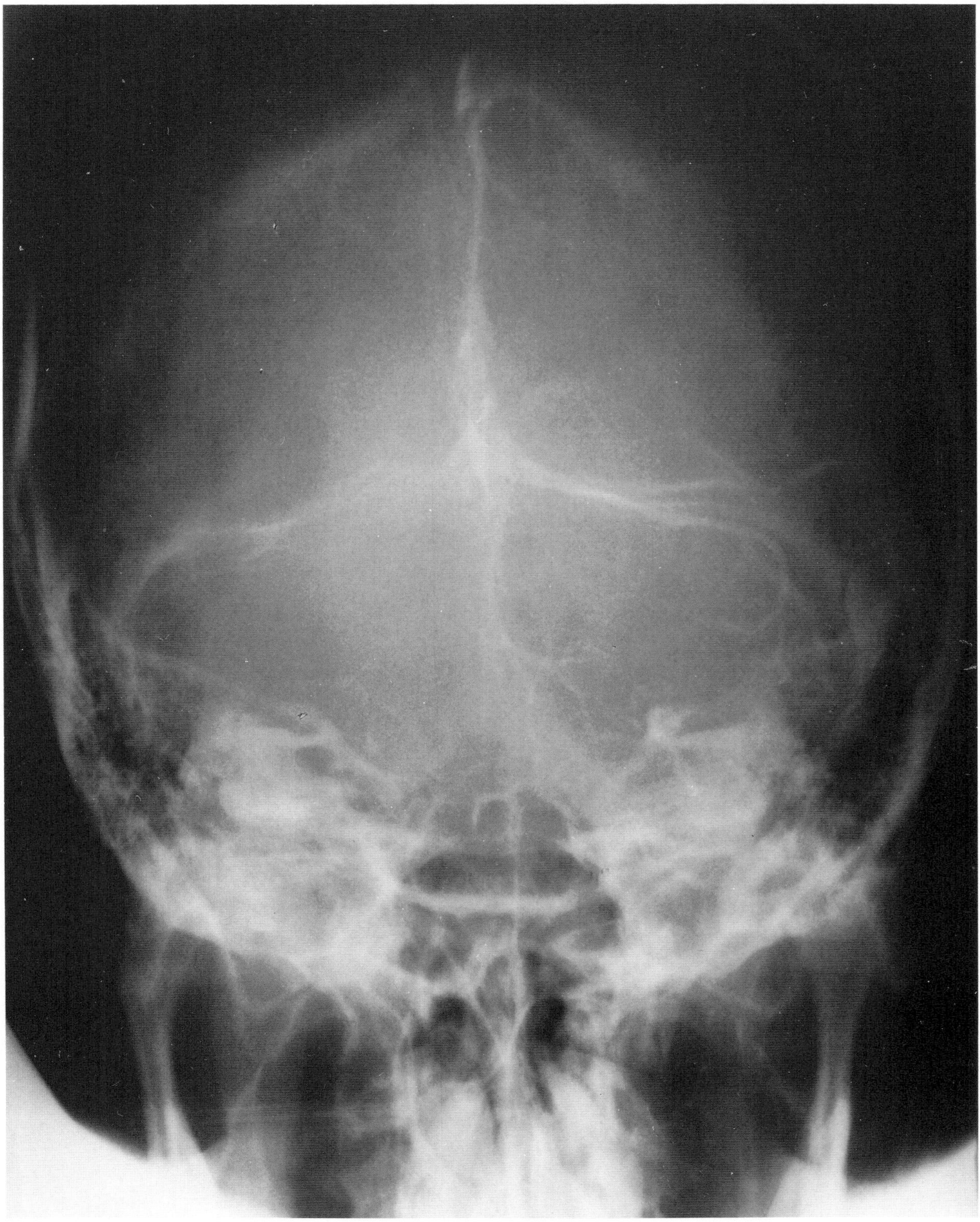

2-78 Vertebral angiography (AP view, venous phase).

2/Head, Angiography

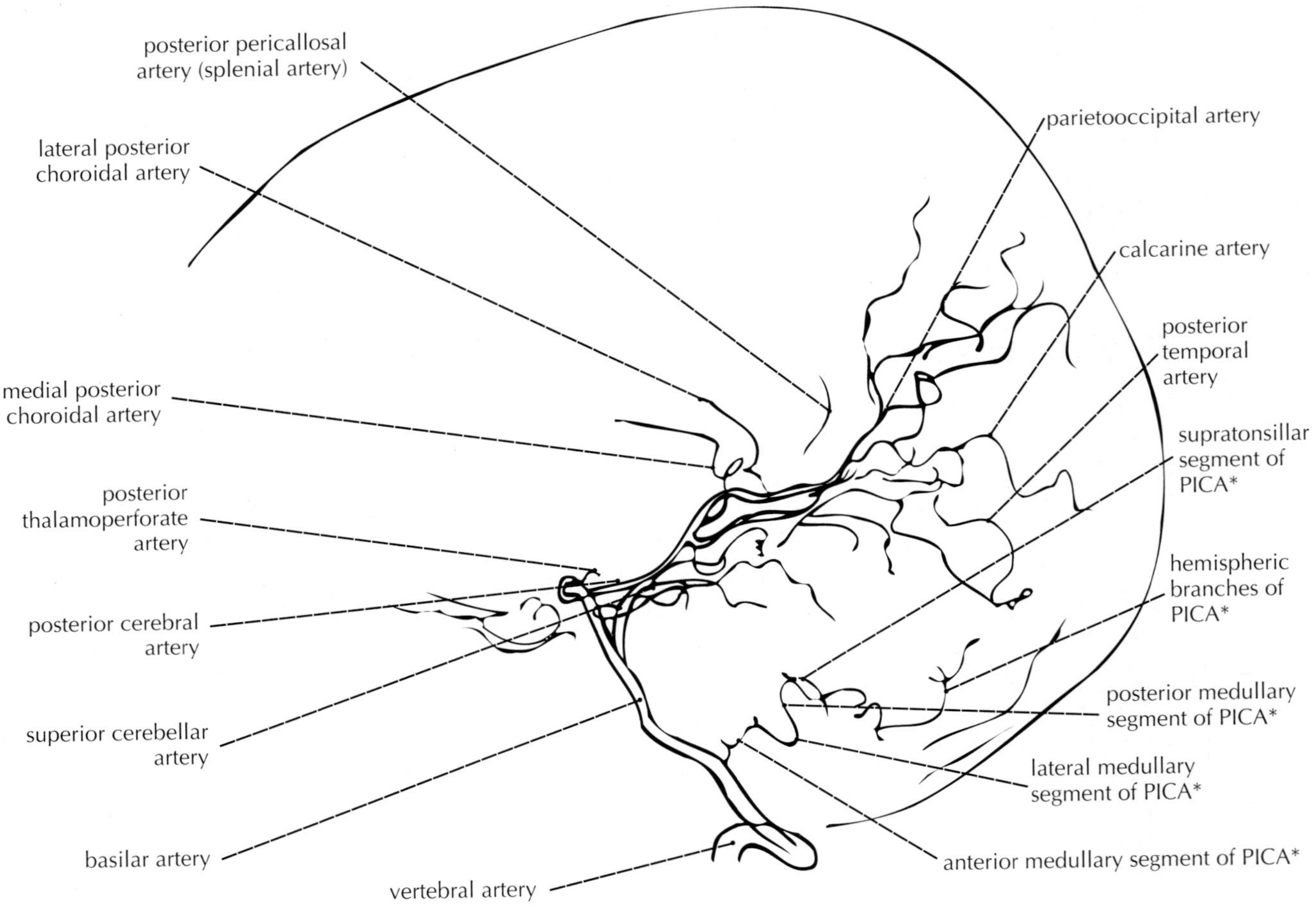

*PICA = posterior inferior cerebellar artery

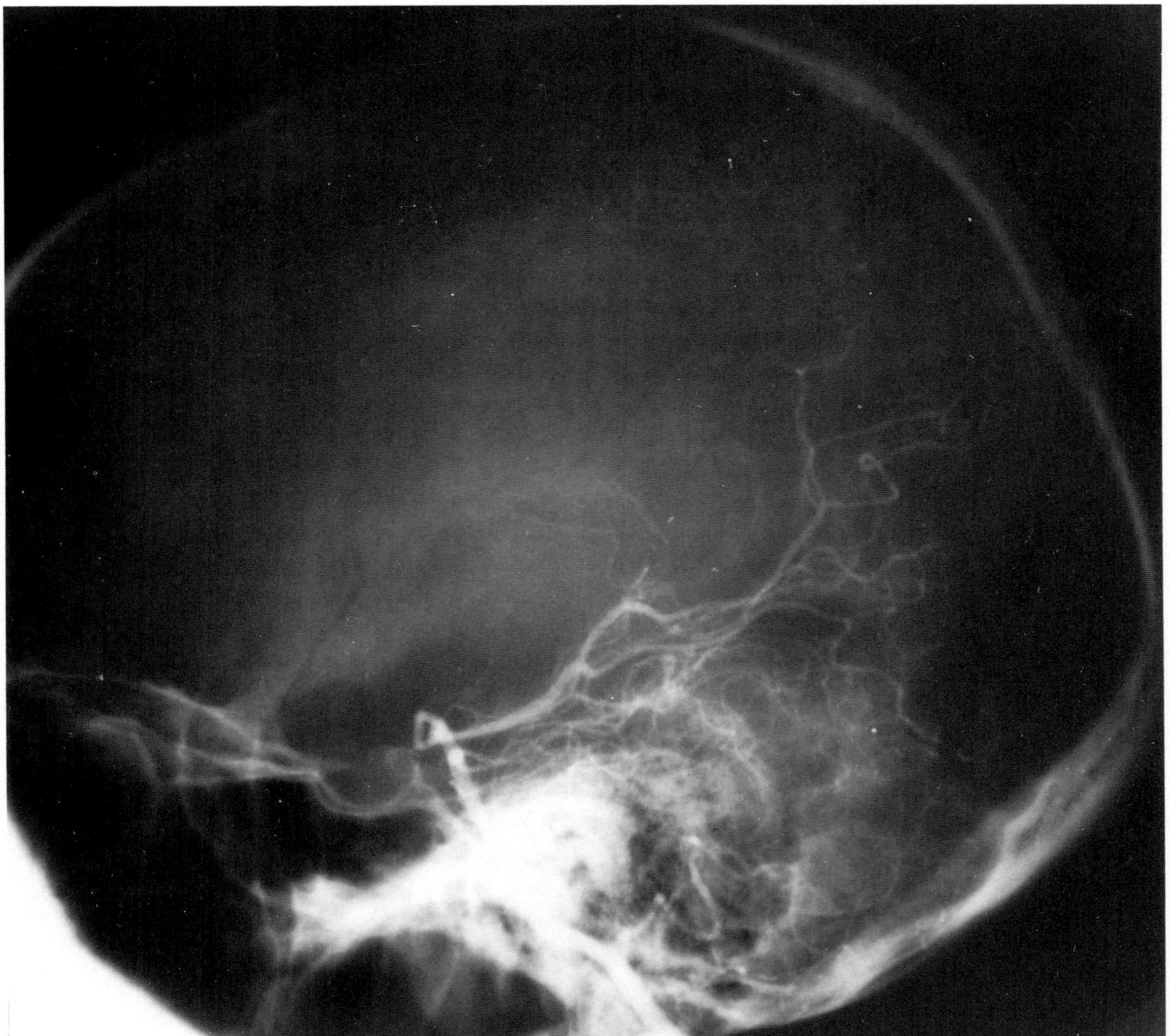

2-79 Vertebral angiography (lateral view, arterial phase).

2/Head, Angiography

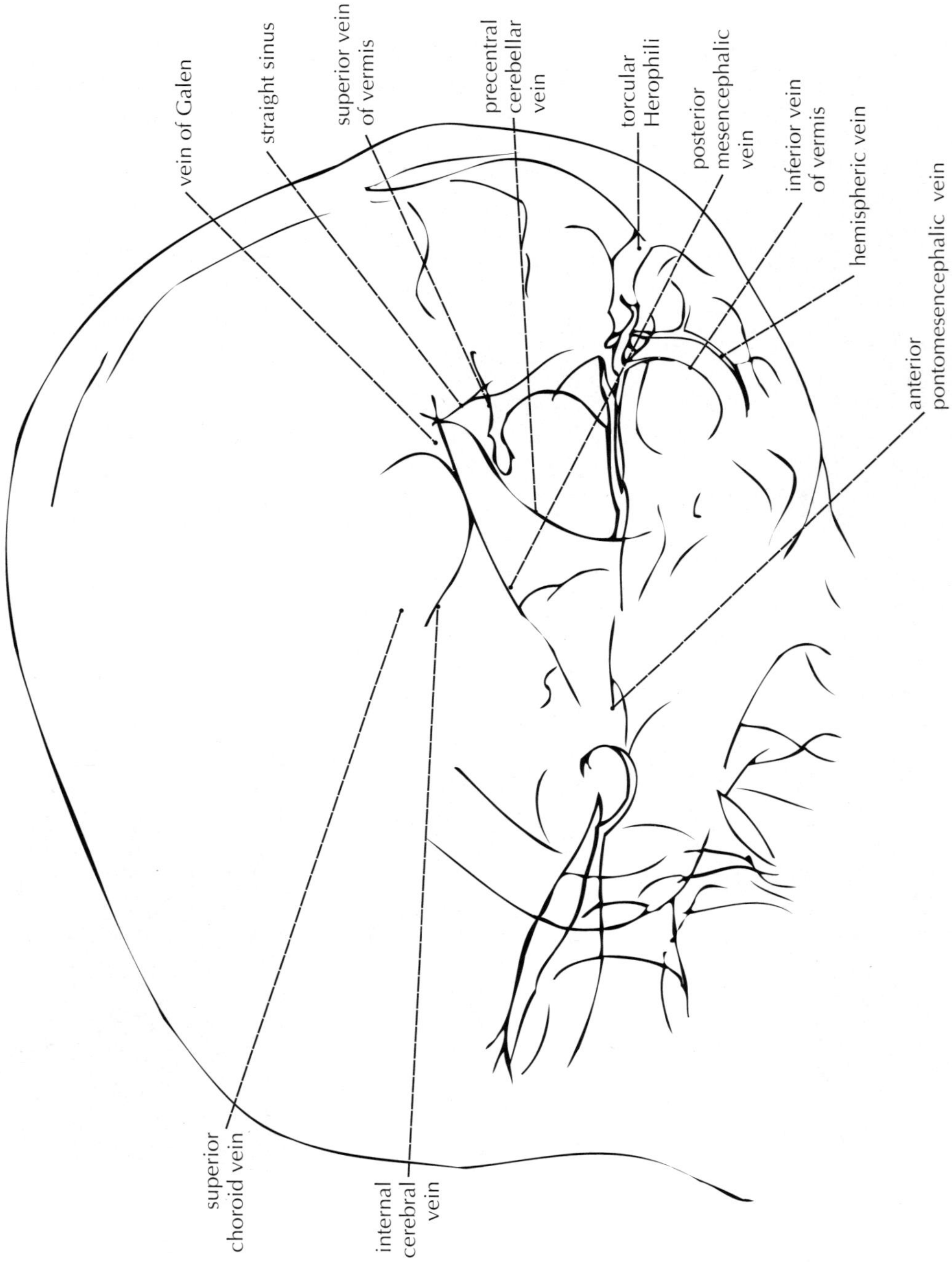

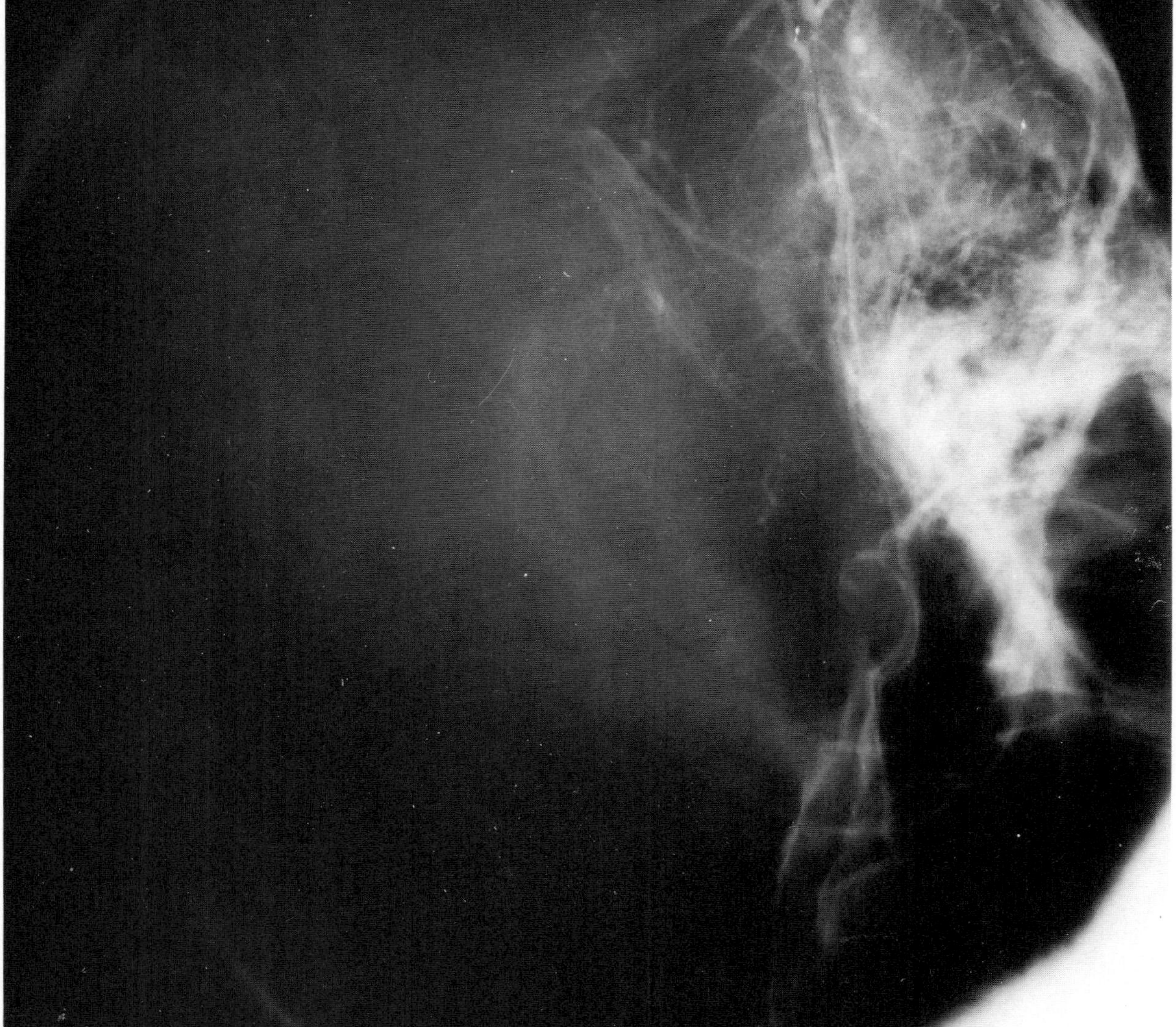

2-80 Vertebral angiography (lateral view, venous phase).

2/Head, MR Angiography

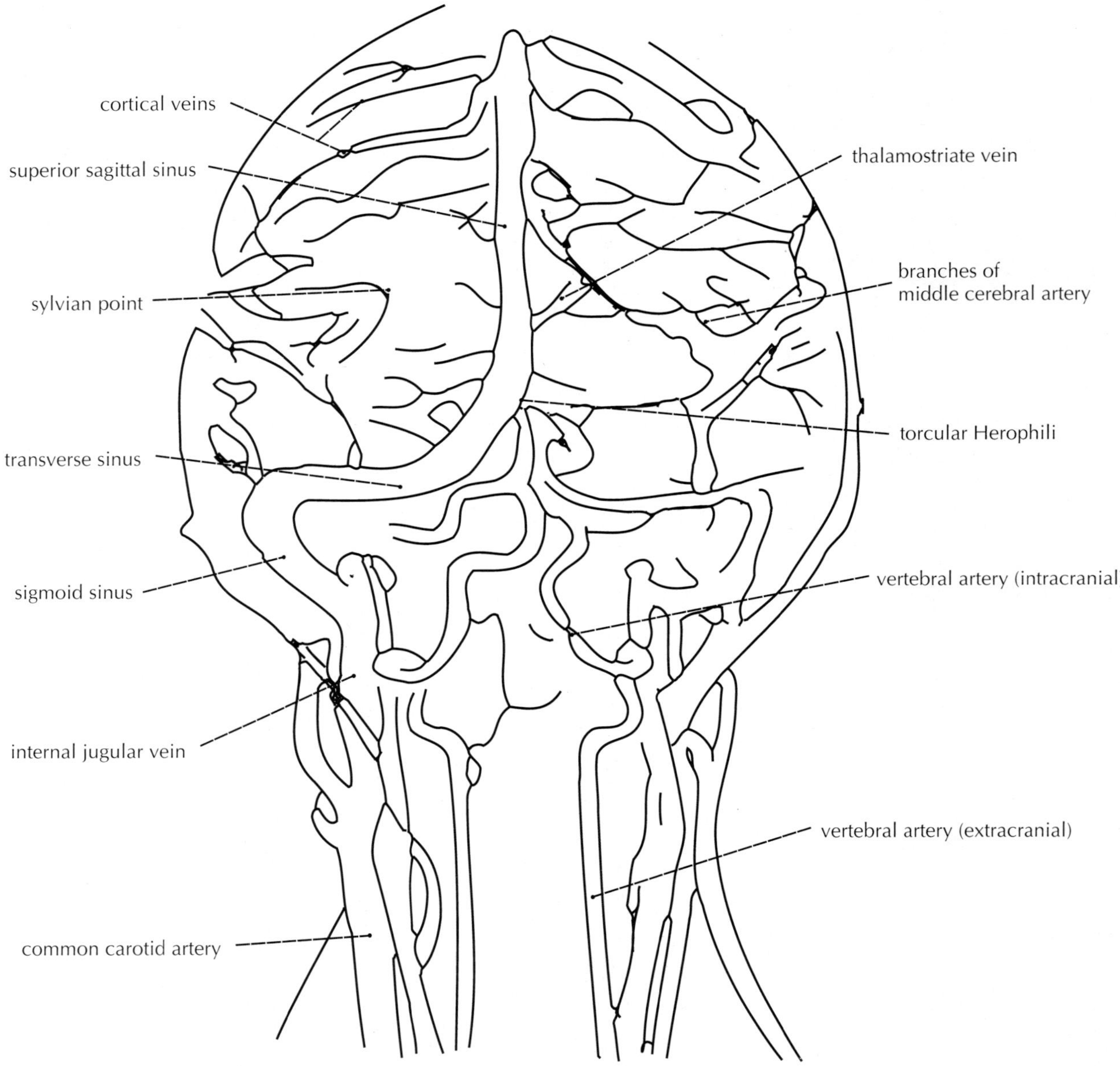

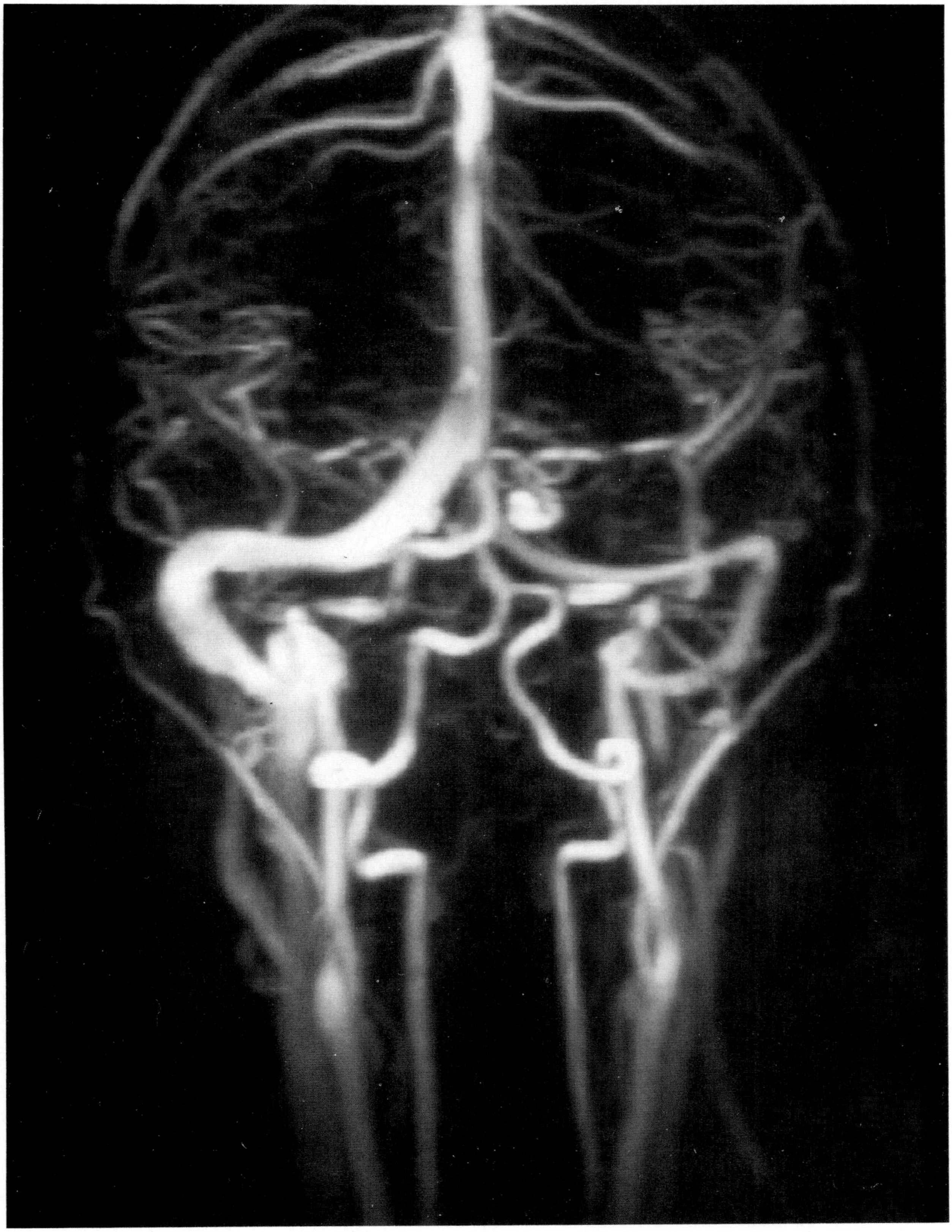

2-81 Intracranial angiography (noncontrast MR scan, frontal view).

2/Head, MR Angiography

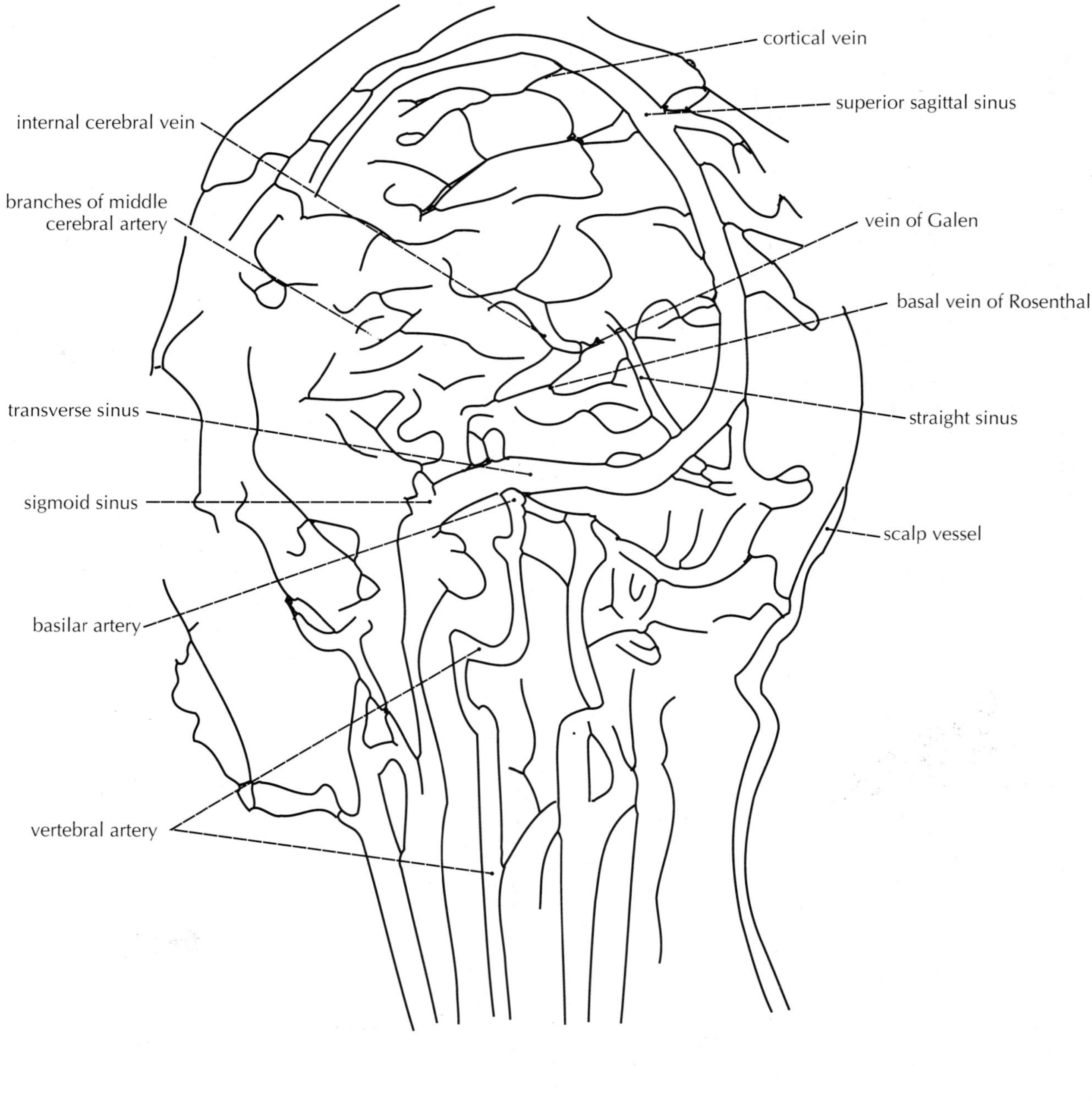

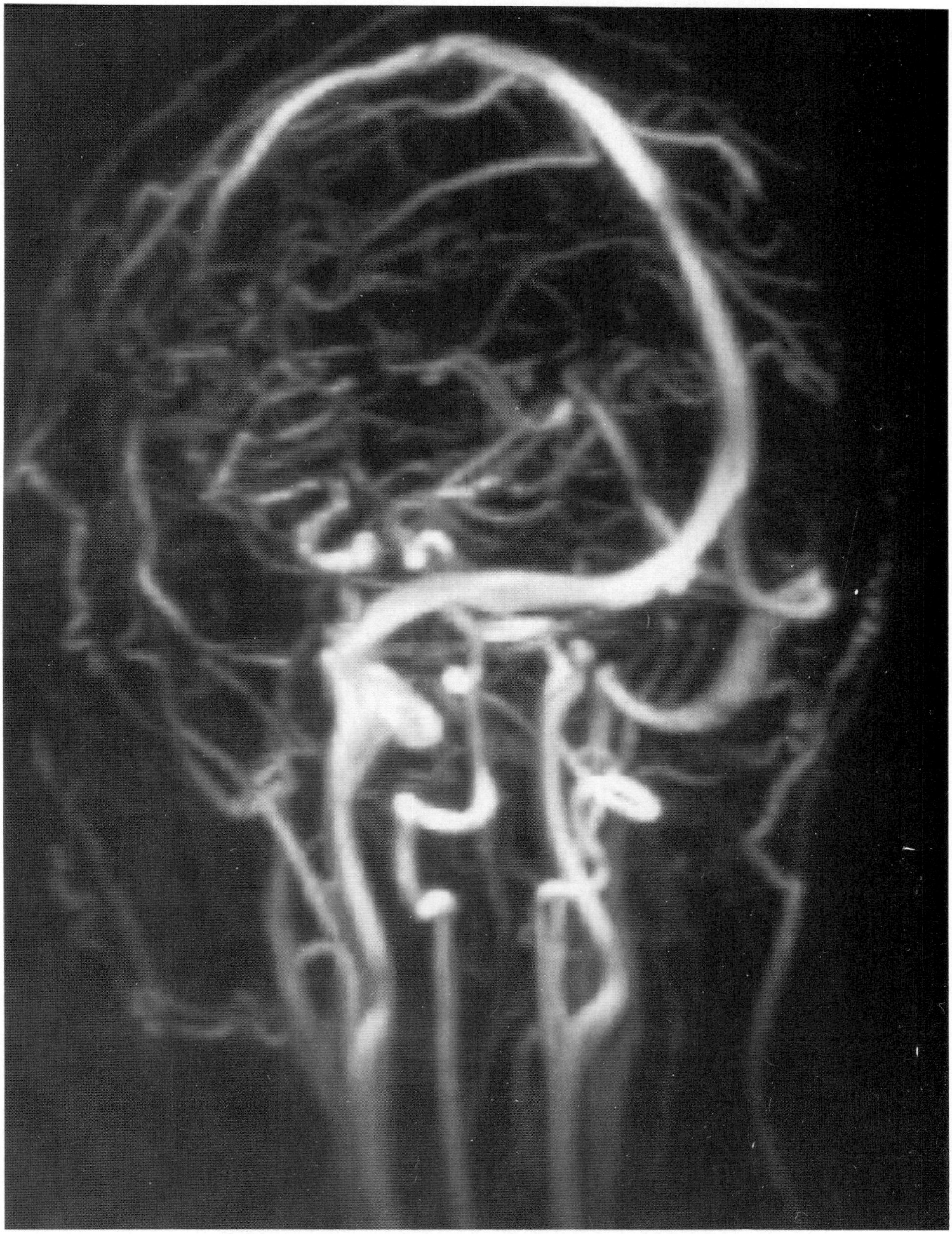

2-82 Intracranial angiography (noncontrast MR scan, oblique view).

2/Sella Turcica, X-Ray

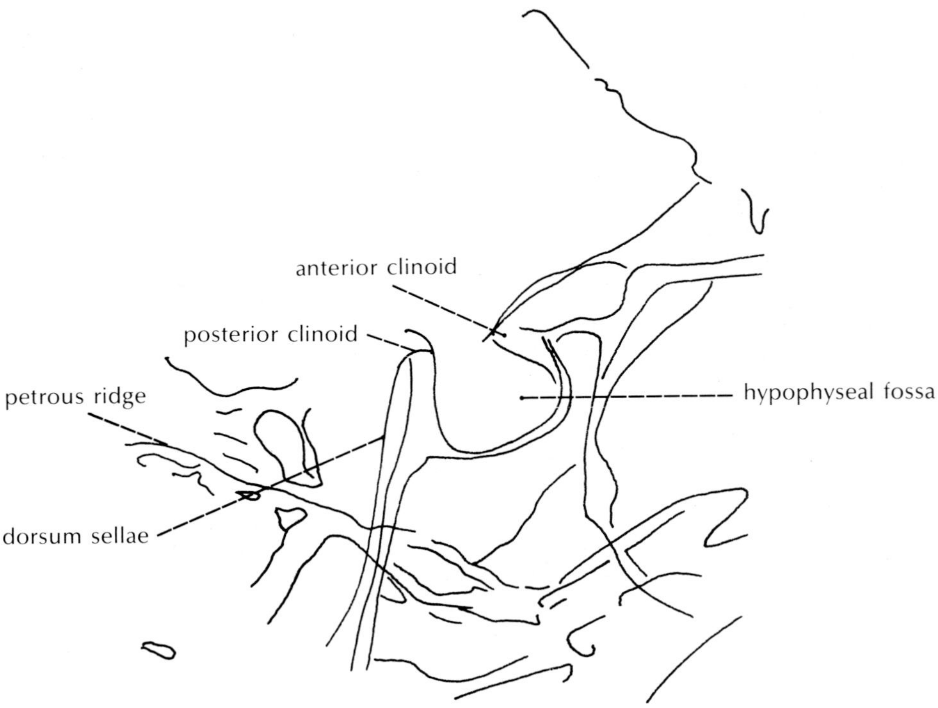

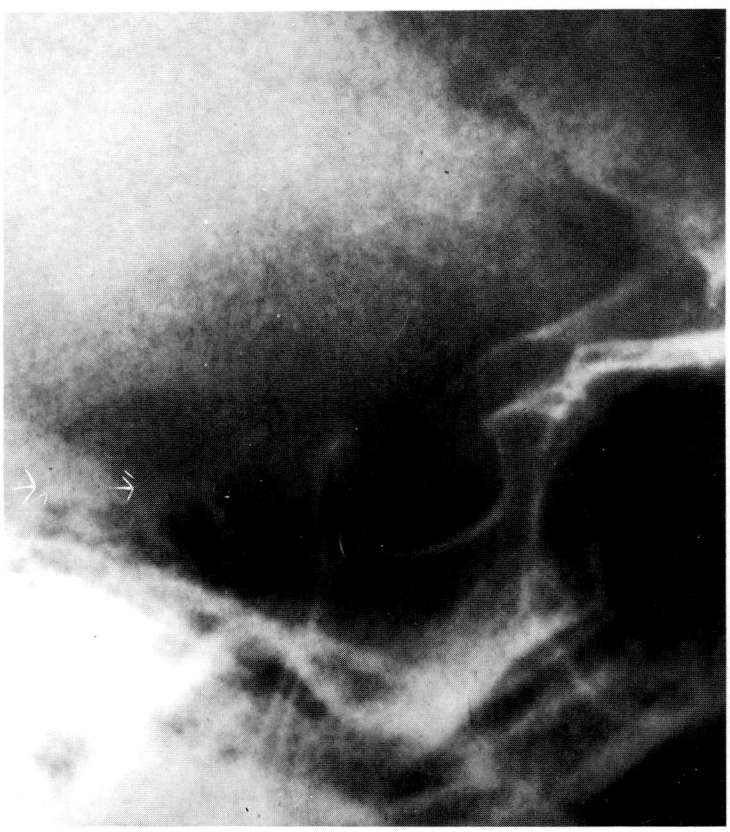

2-83 Sella turcica, lateral view.

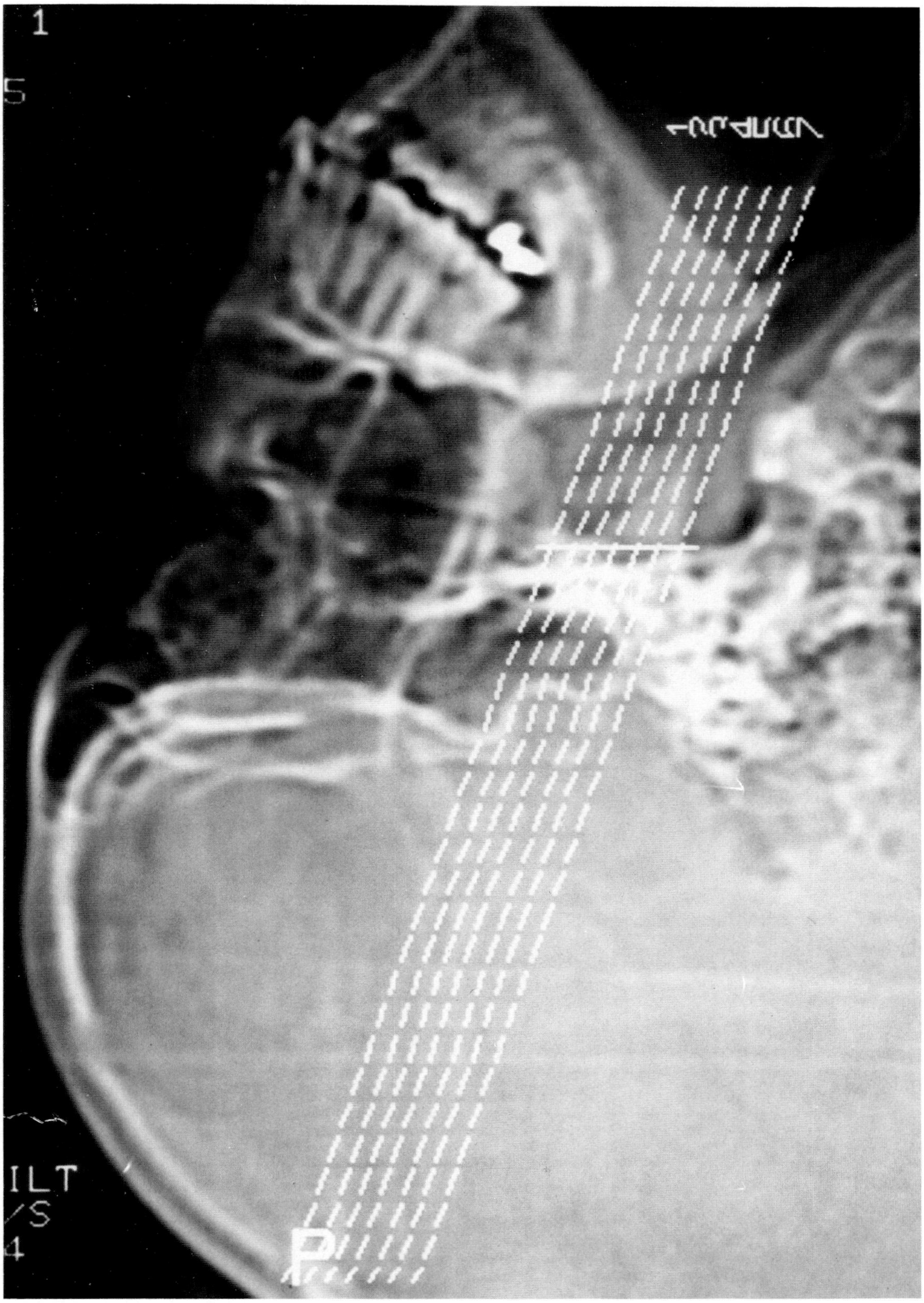

2-84 This sagittal scout CT scan is used to demonstrate the sellar sections. (Section 3 is used in Figs. 2-85 and 2-86.)

2/Sella Turcica, Coronal CT

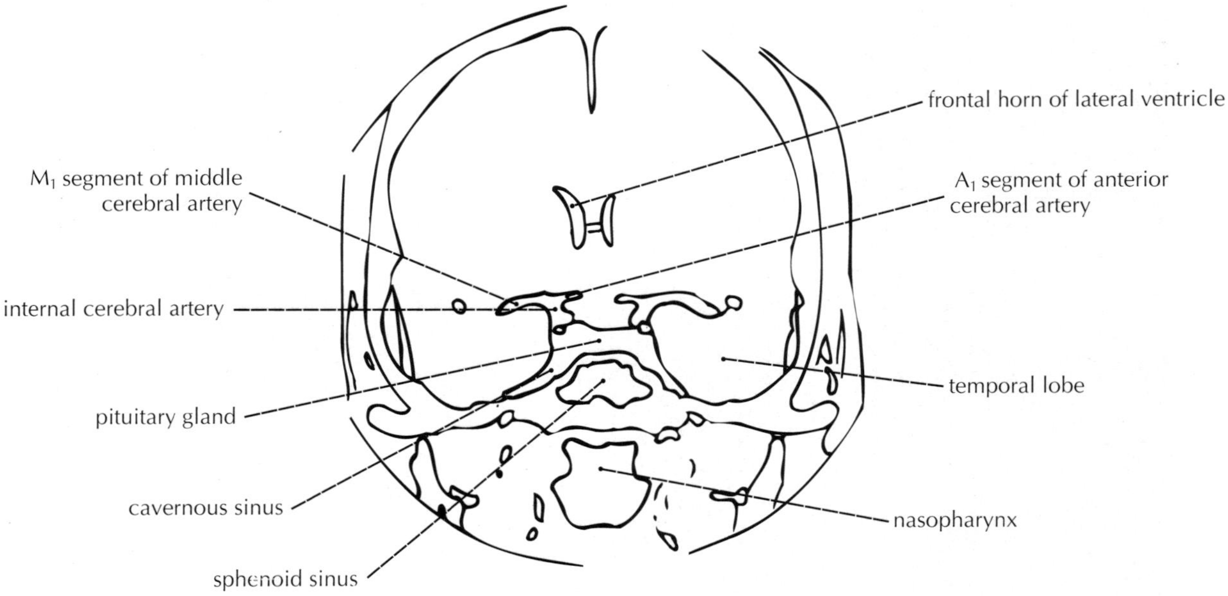

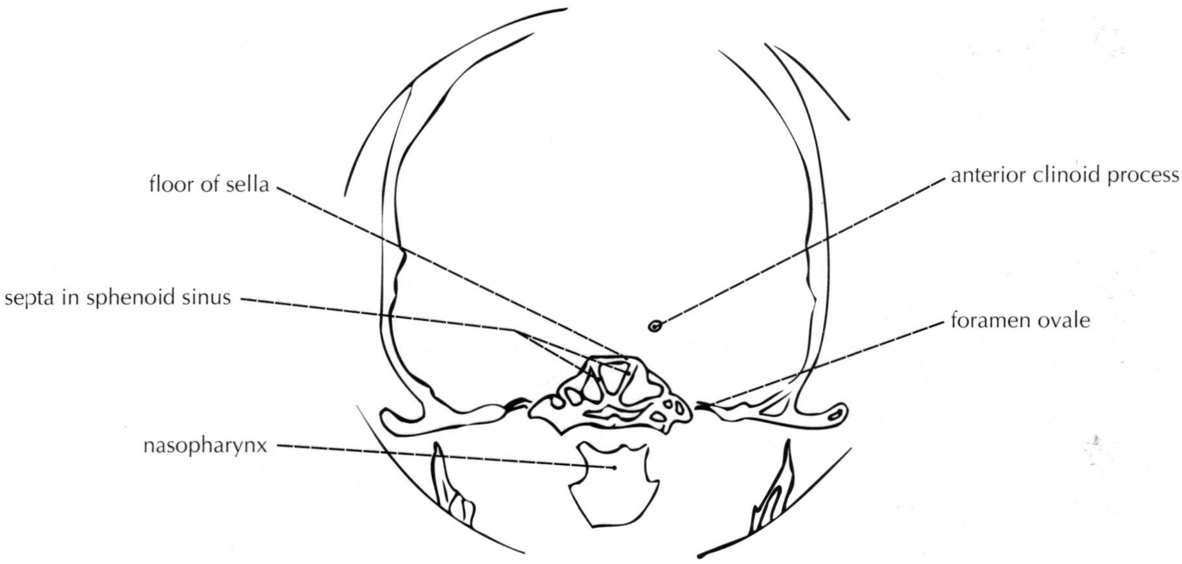

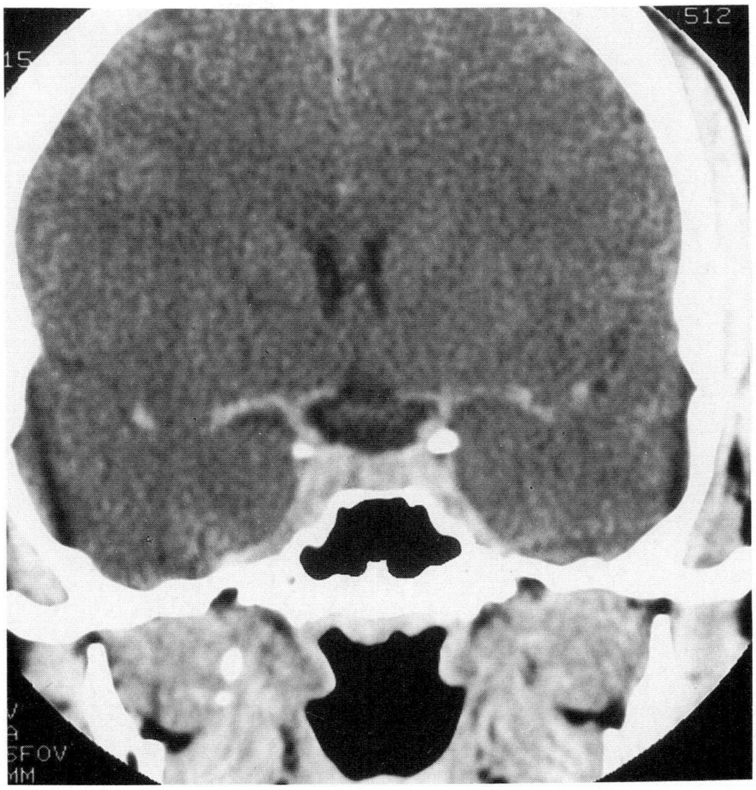

2-85 Coronal CT scan of pituitary gland with intravenous contrast enhancement.

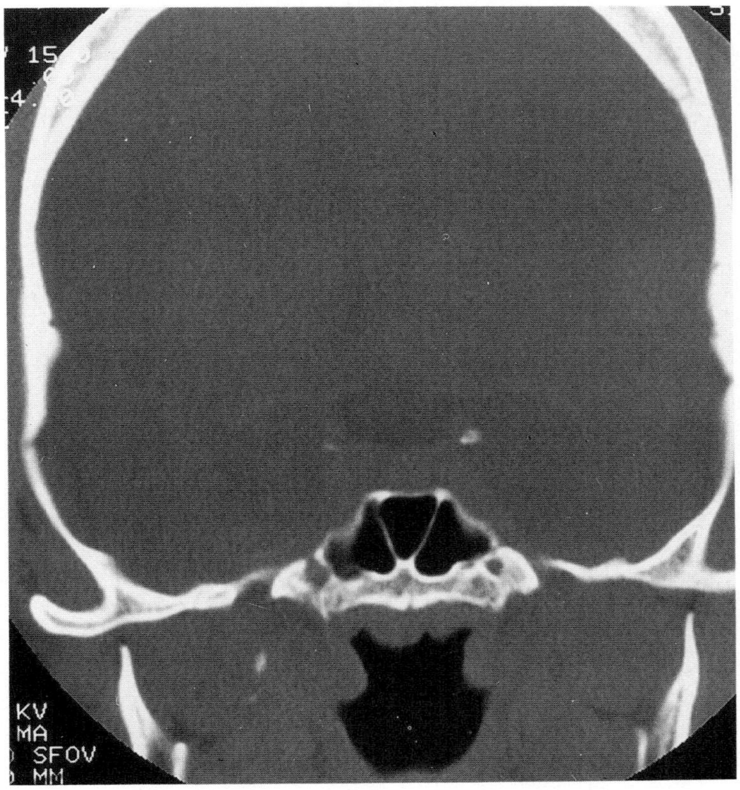

2-86 Coronal CT scan of pituitary area (same image as Fig. 2-85, but with bone window).

2/Sella Turcica, Axial MRI

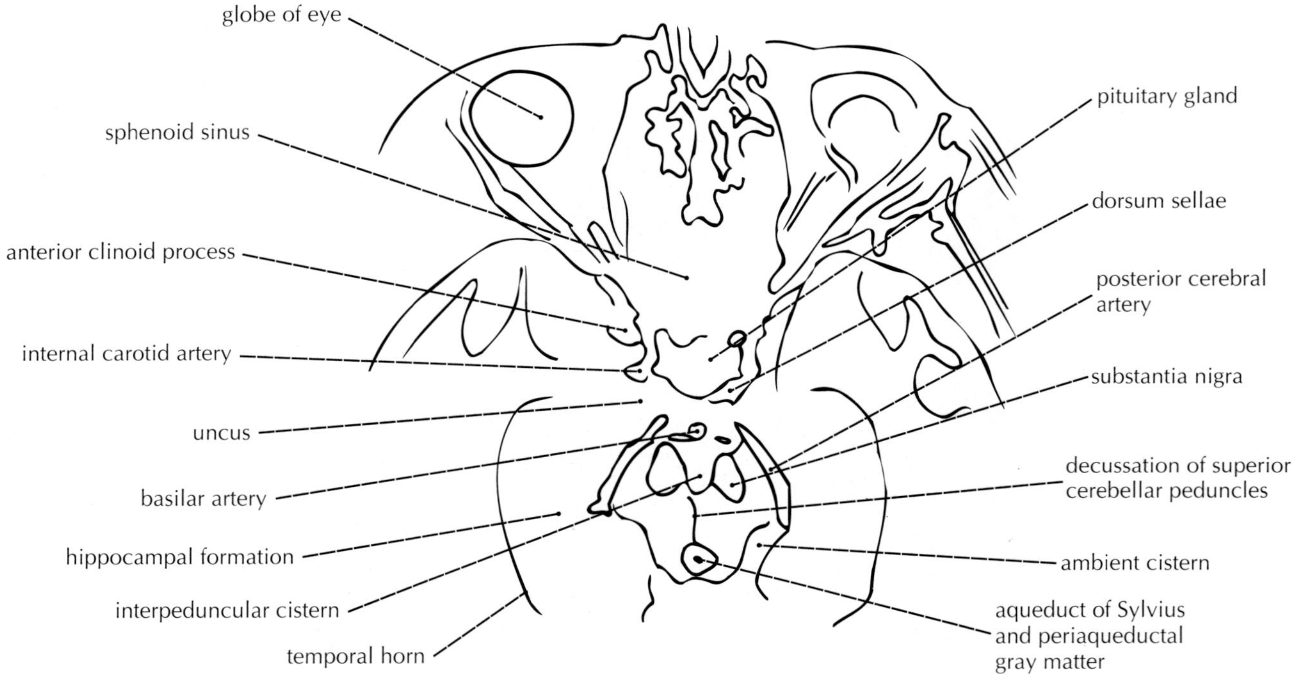

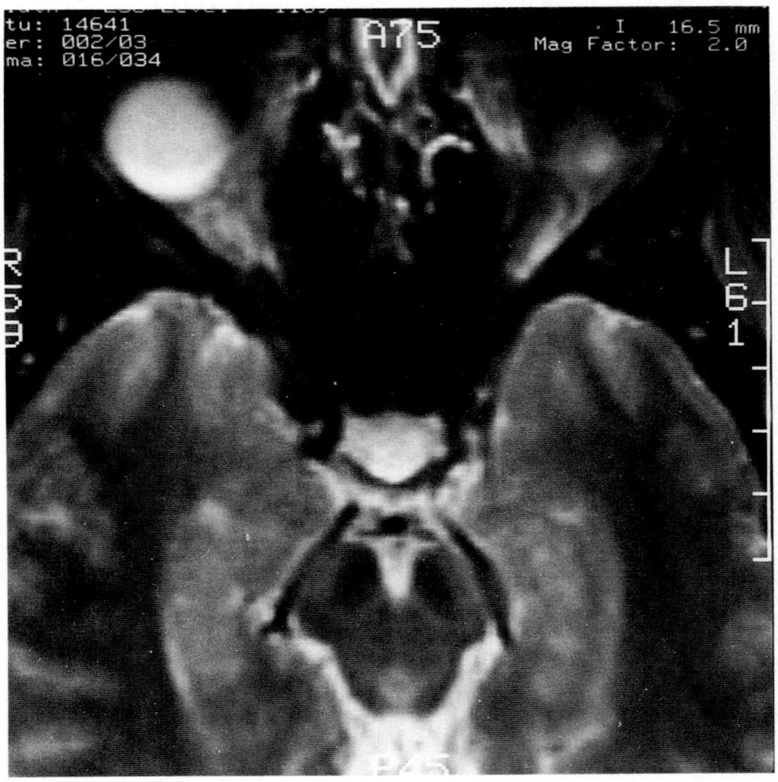

2-87 Axial MR scan of pituitary gland (2000/90).

2/Sella Turcica, Sagittal Scout MRI and Coronal MRI

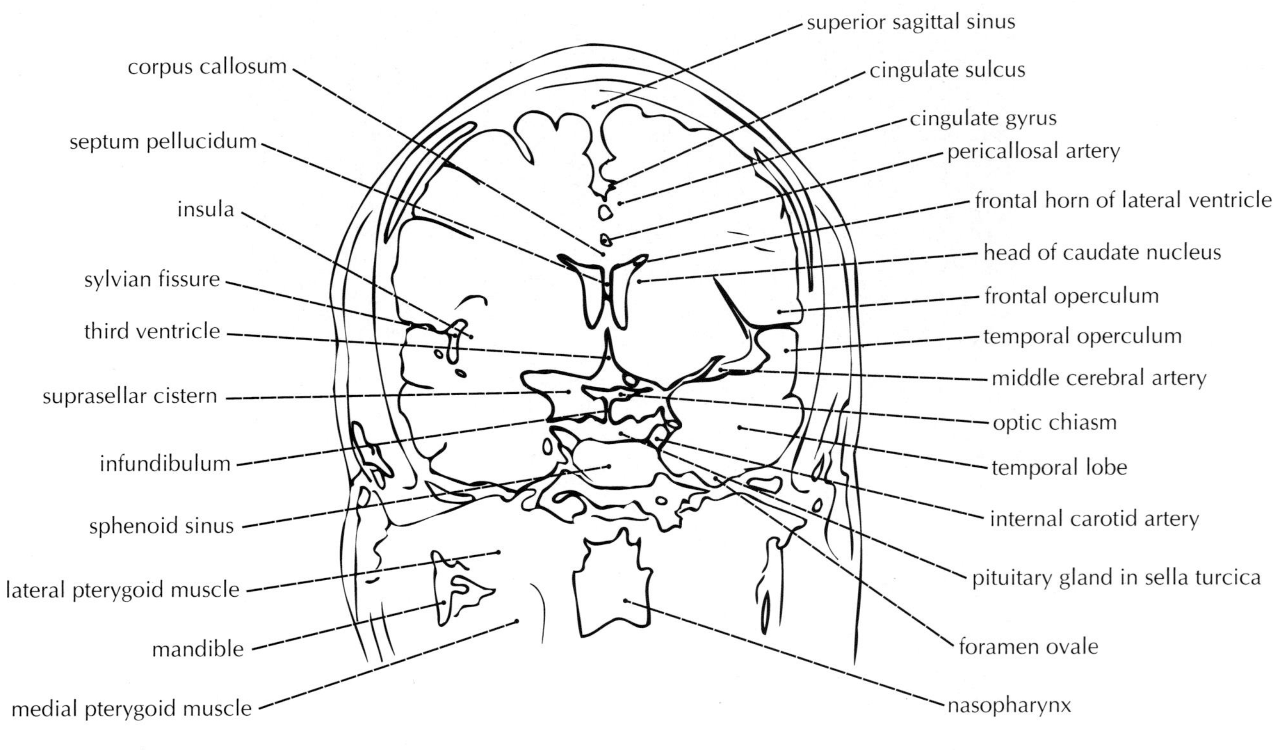

2/Sella Turcica, Sagittal Scout MRI and Coronal MRI

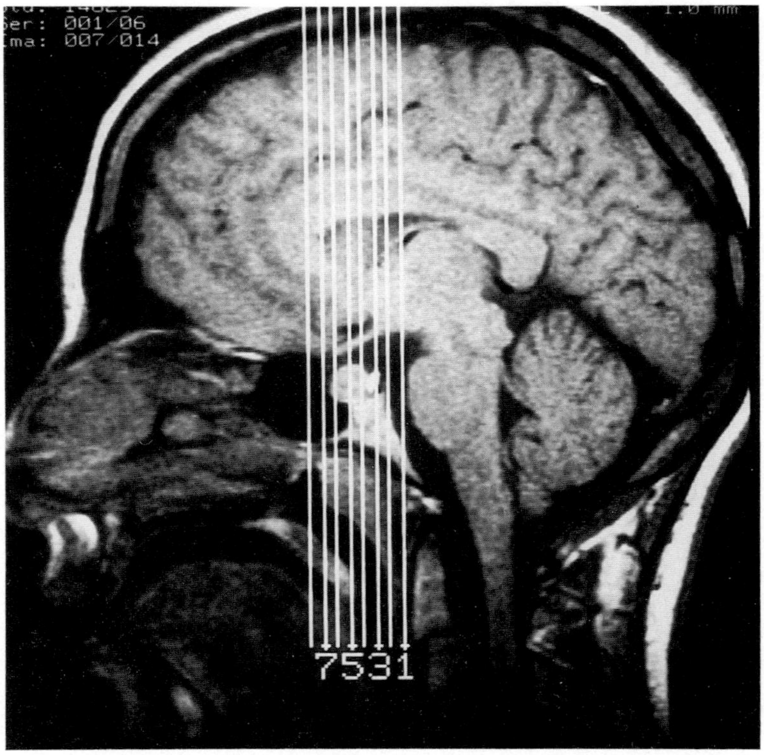

2-88 This sagittal scout MR scan is used to demonstrate the coronal sections of the pituitary and parapituitary areas. (Sections 6, 5, and 4 are used in Figs. 2-89, 2-90, and 2-91, respectively.)

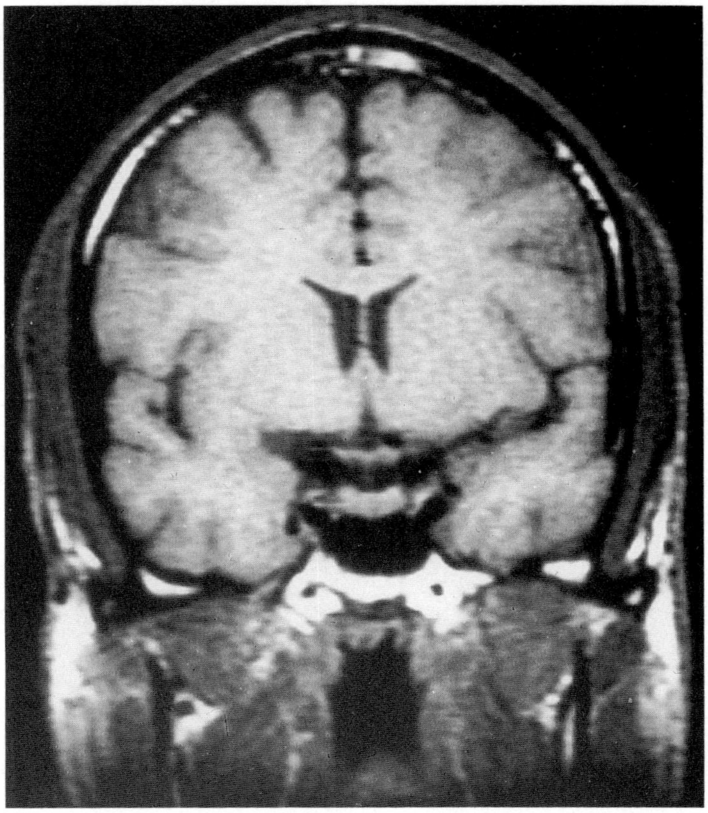

2-89 Coronal noncontrast MR scan through pituitary gland (section 6 in Fig. 2-88) (600/20).

2/Sella Turcica, Coronal MRI

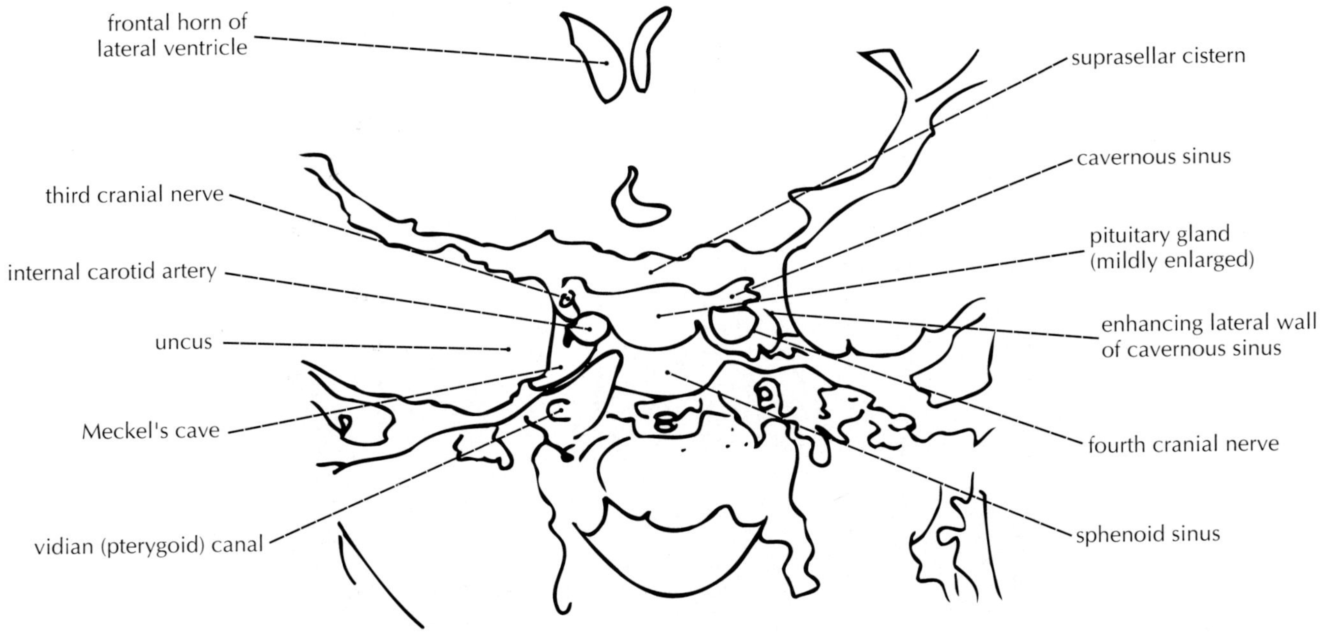

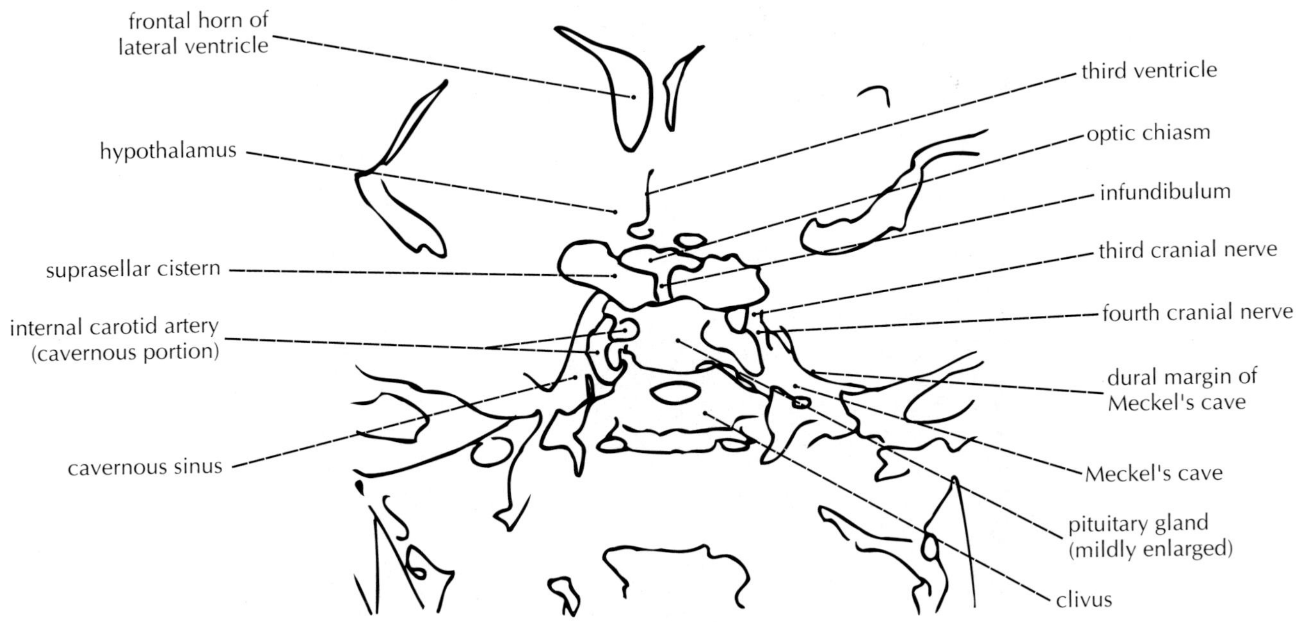

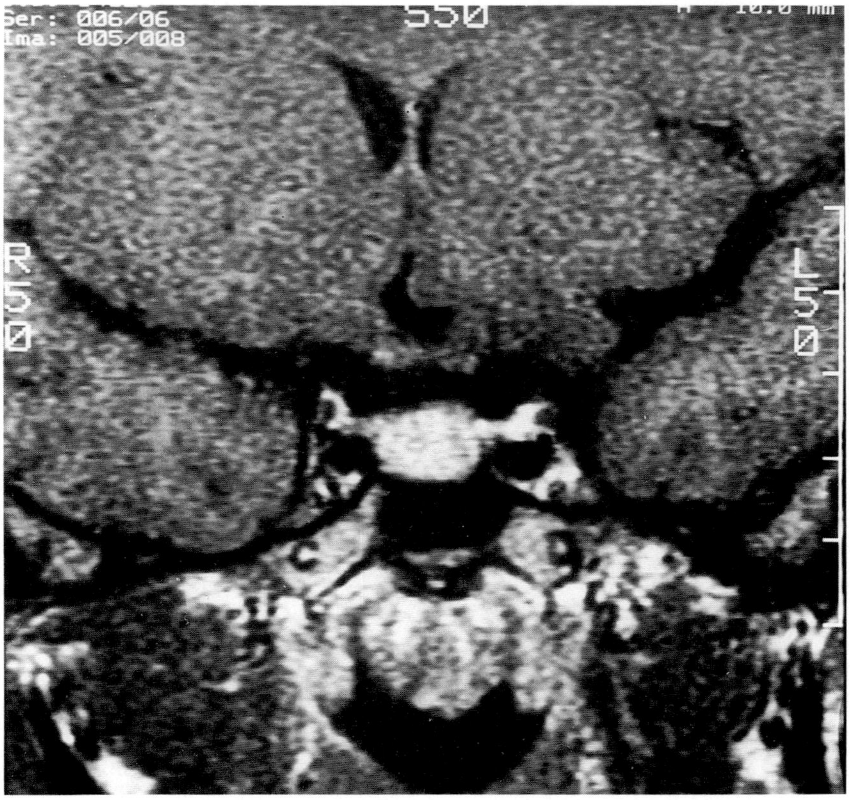

2-90 Coronal MR scan through pituitary gland with intravenous contrast enhancement (gadolinium-DTPA) (section 5 in Fig. 2-88).

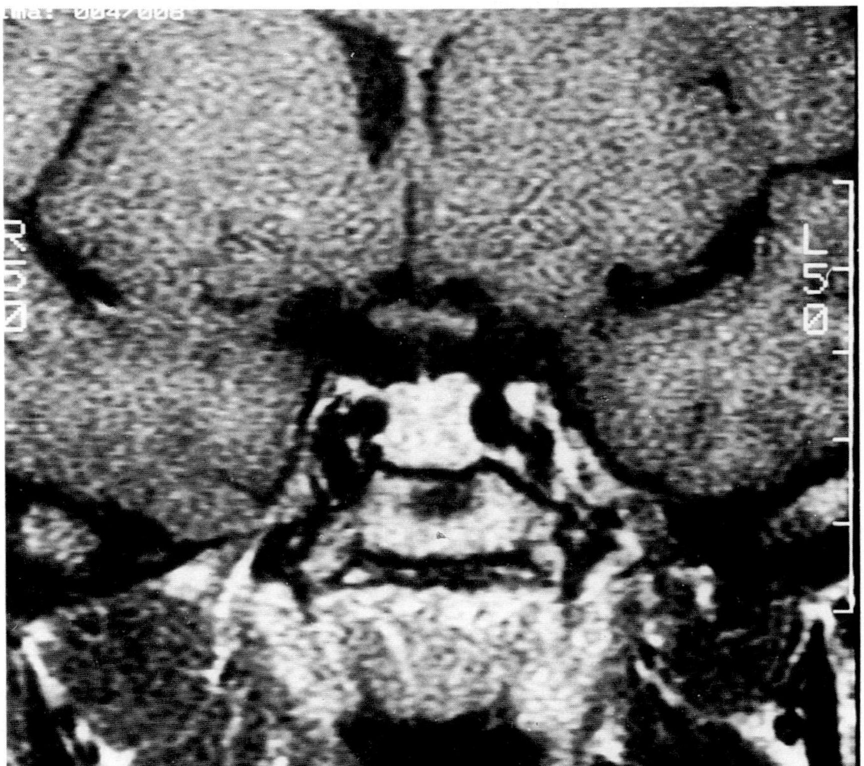

2-91 Coronal MR scan through pituitary gland with intravenous contrast enhancement (gadolinium-DTPA) (section 4 in Fig. 2-88).

2/Mastoid, X-Ray

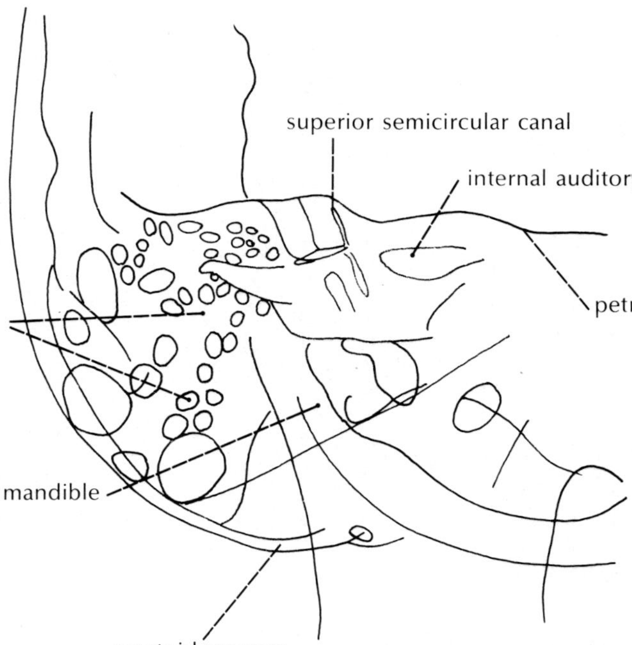

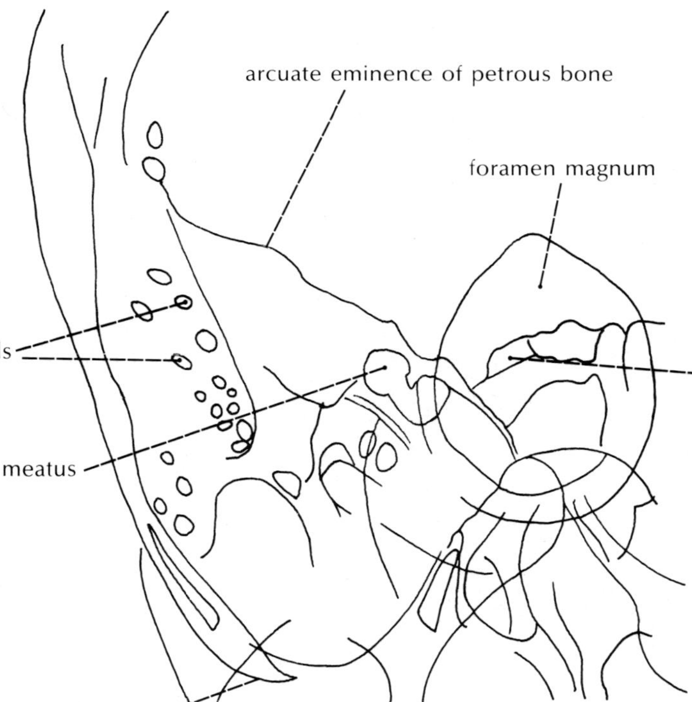

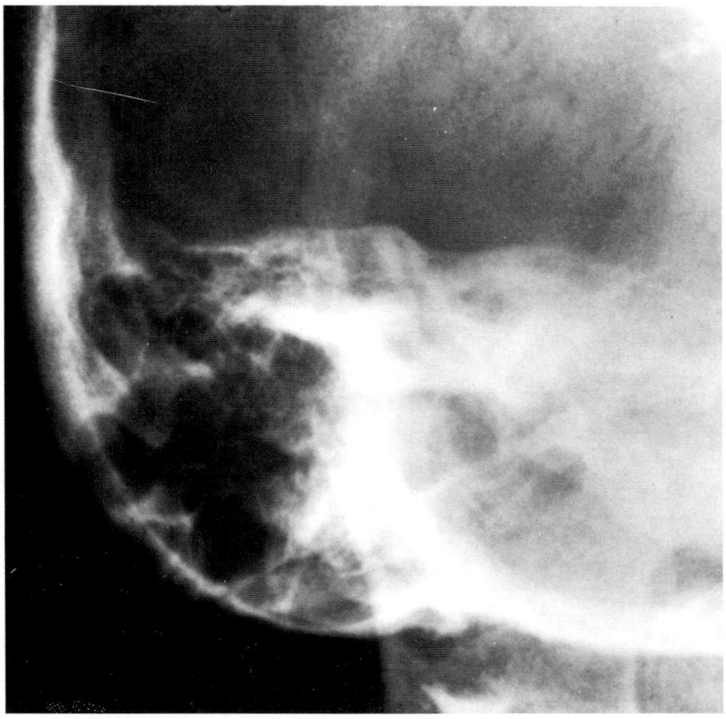

2-92 Mastoid, Stenvers view.

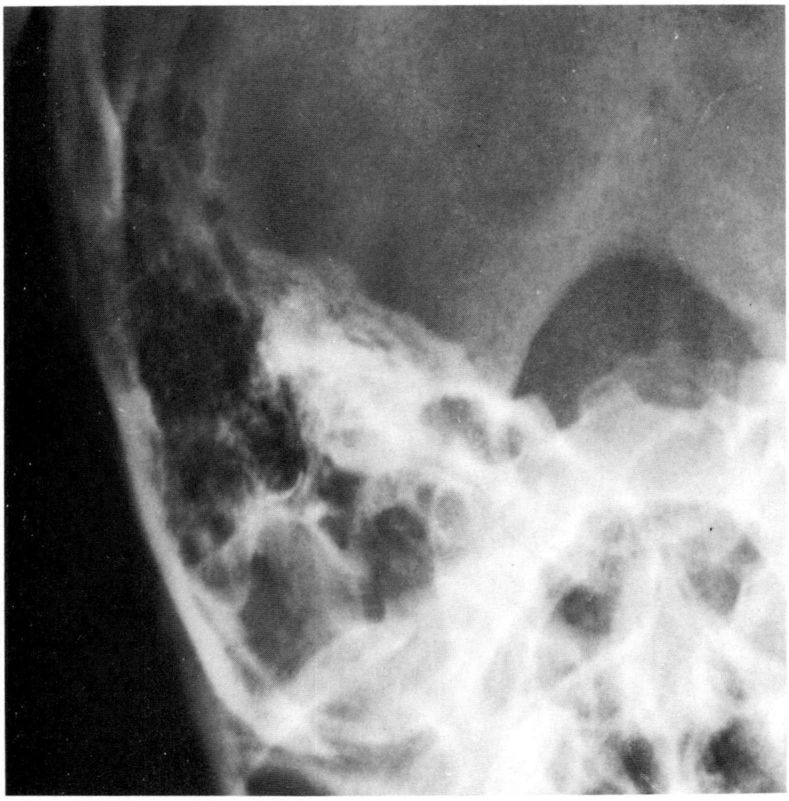

2-93 Mastoid, Towne view.

2/Temporal Bone, Axial CT

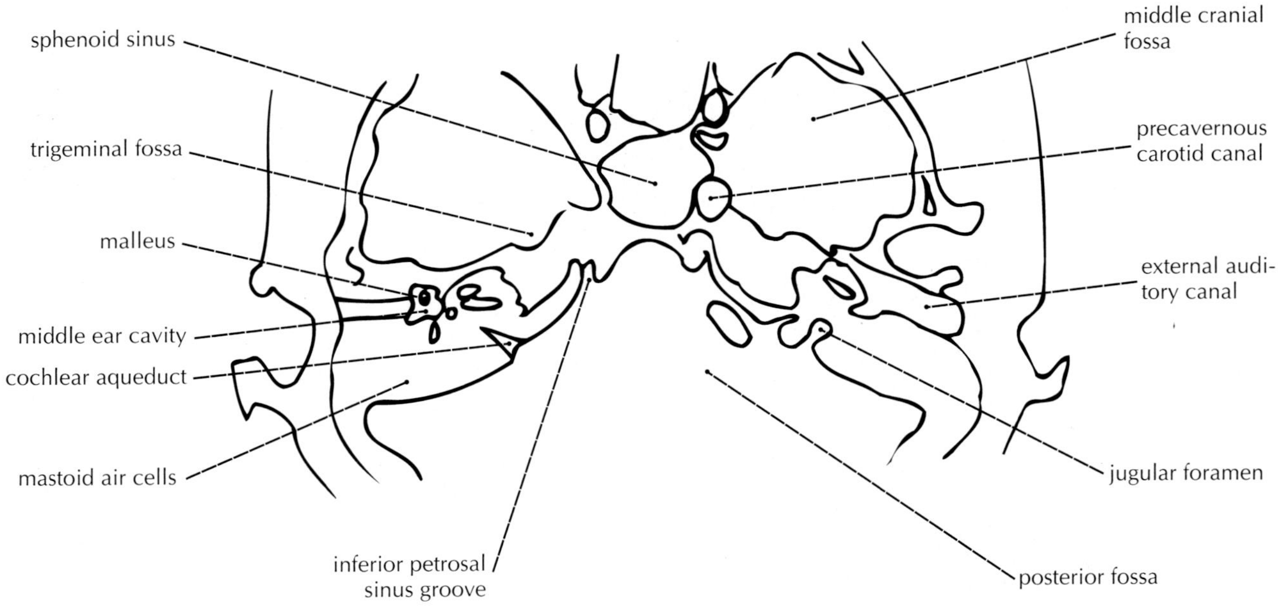

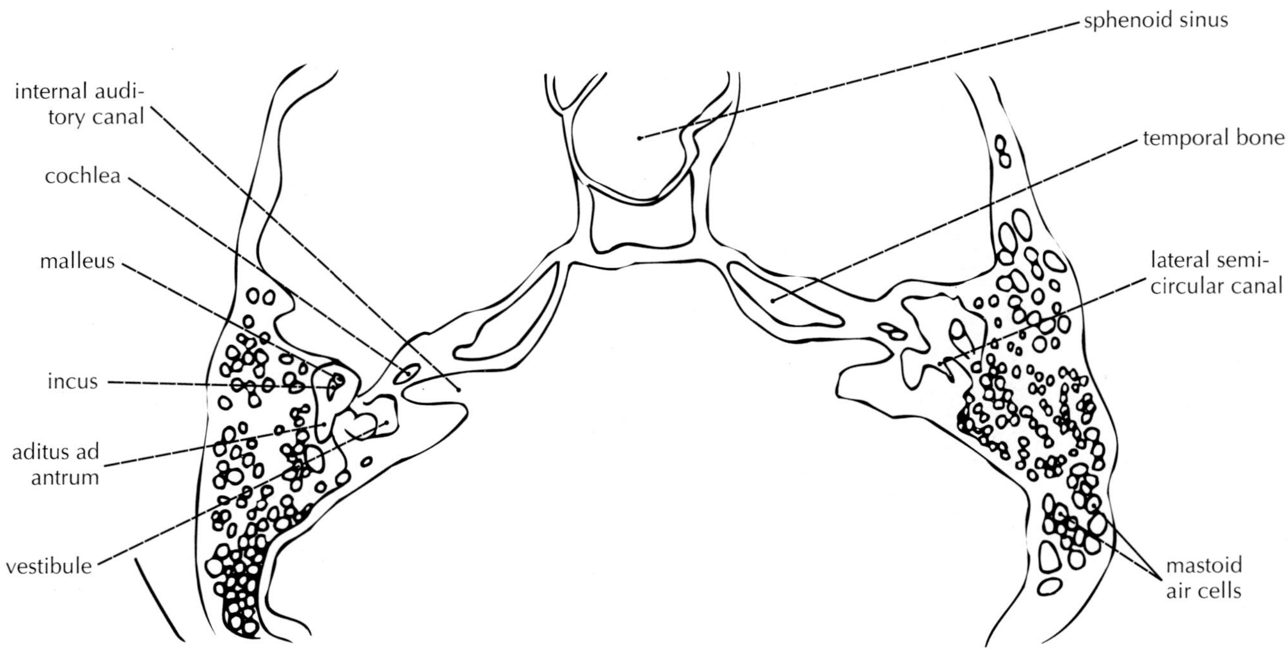

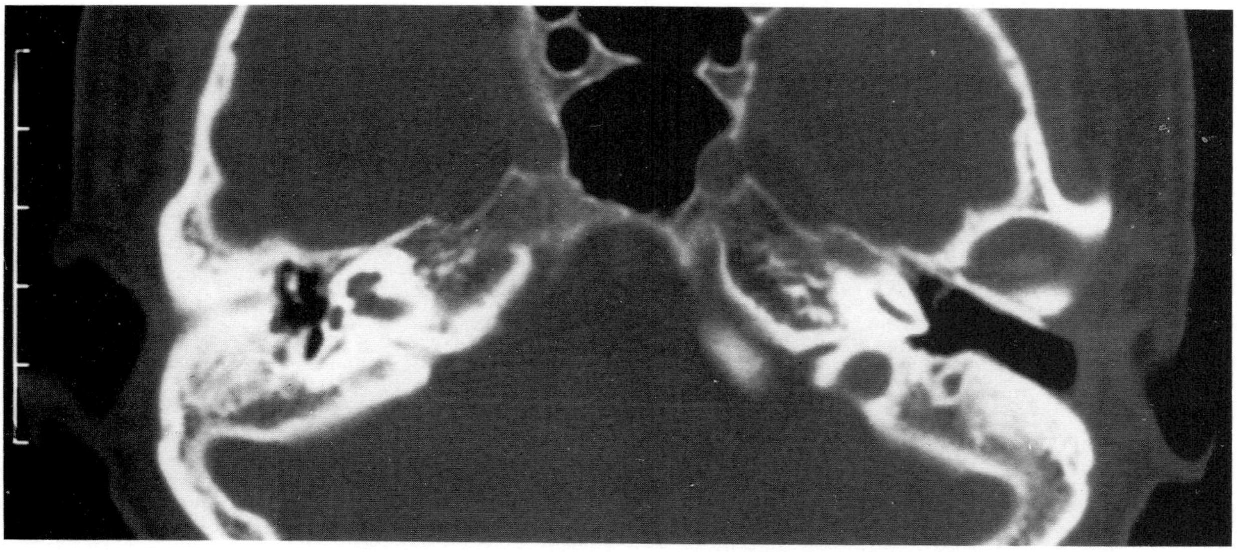

2-94 Axial CT scan through temporal bone. Section 11 in Fig. 1-6 (p. 13).

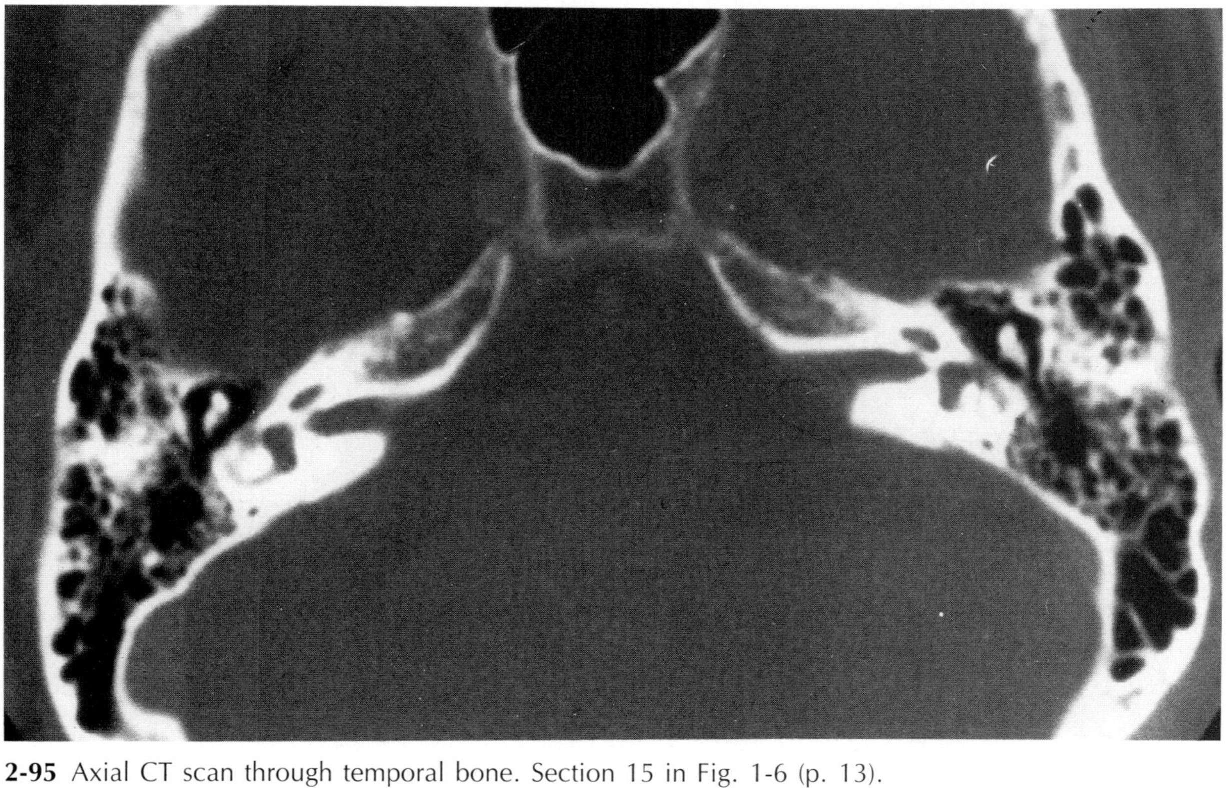

2-95 Axial CT scan through temporal bone. Section 15 in Fig. 1-6 (p. 13).

2/Temporal Bone, Coronal CT

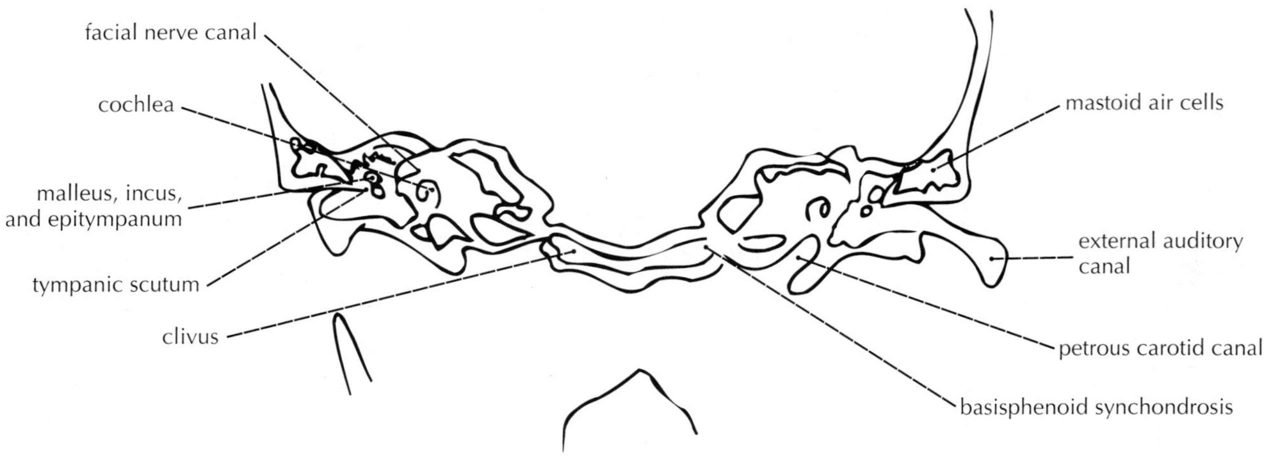

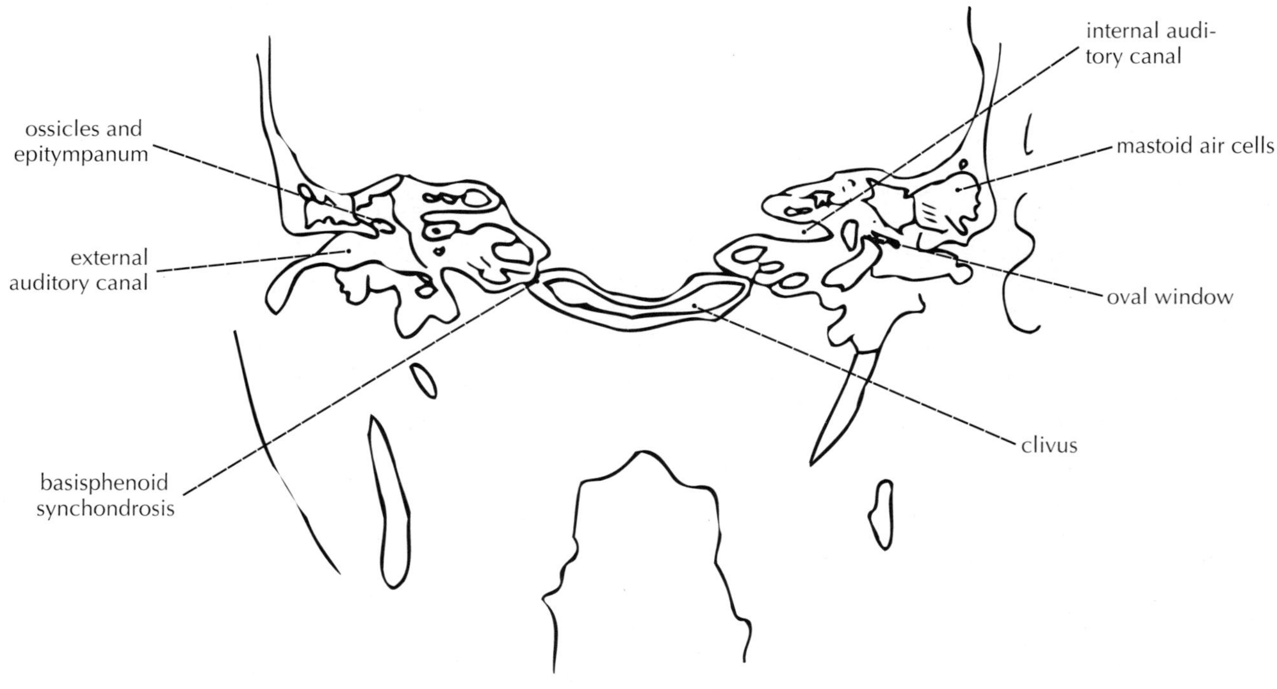

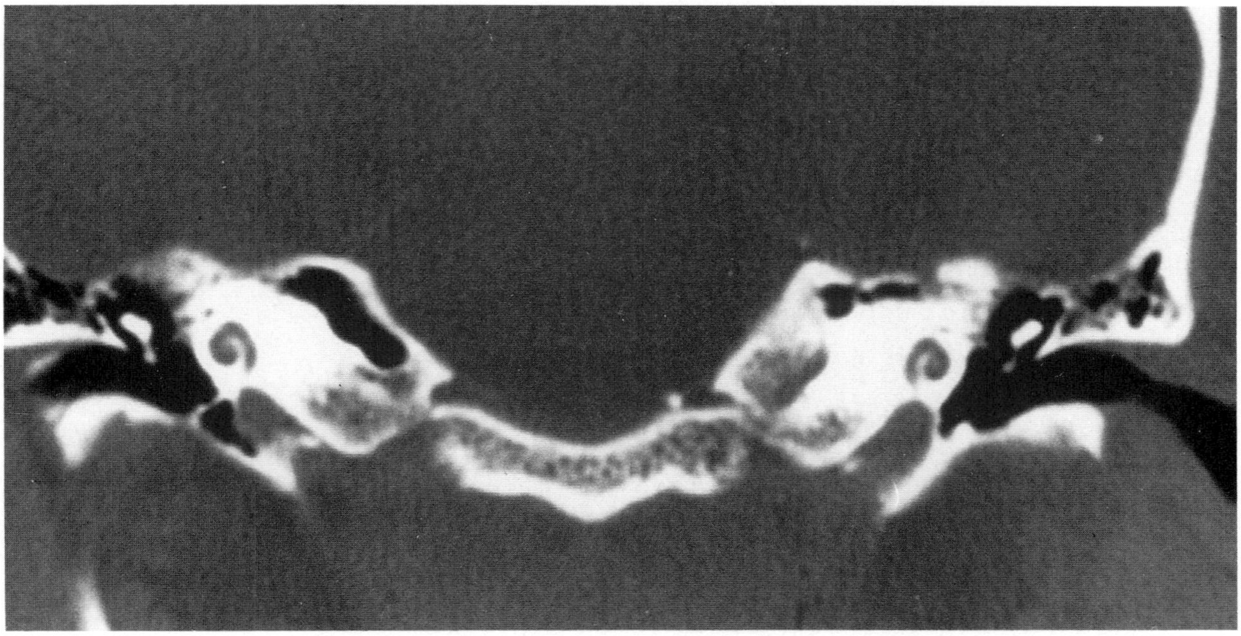

2-96 Coronal CT scan through skull base. Section 27 in Fig. 1-11 (p. 19).

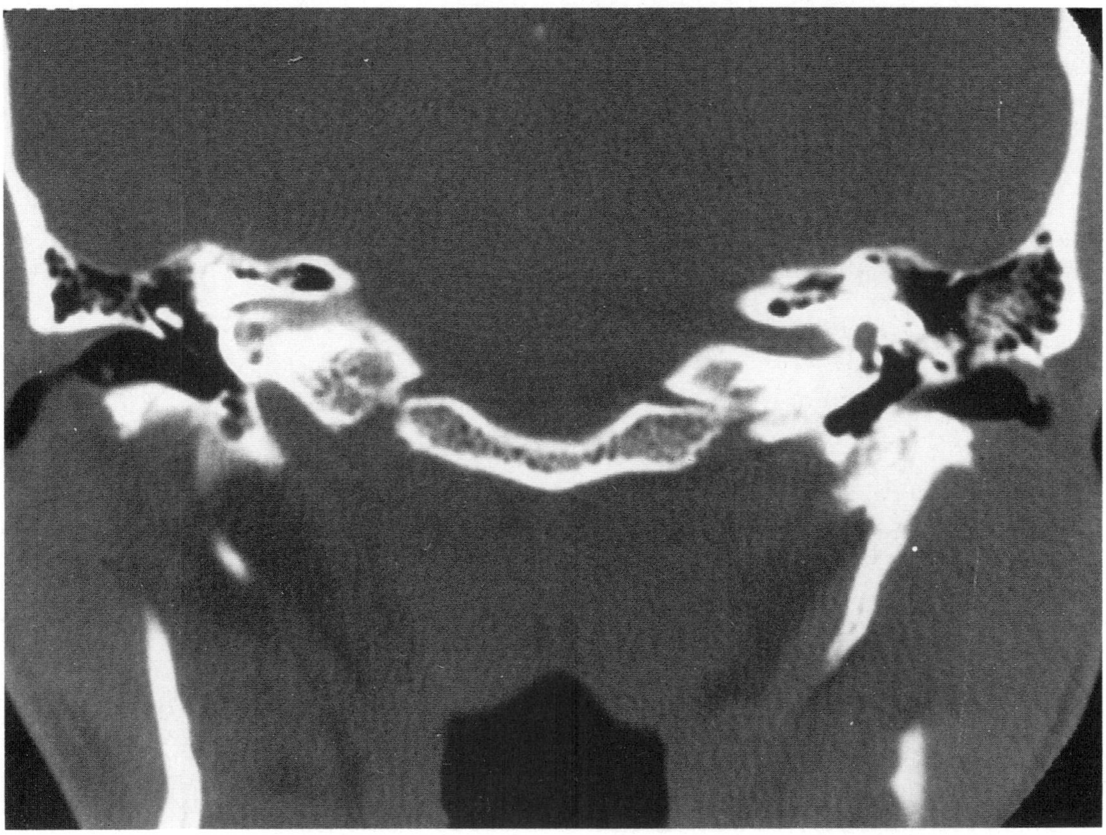

2-97 Coronal CT scan through skull base and internal auditory canals. Section 7 in Fig. 1-11 (p. 19).

2/Temporal Bone, Axial MRI

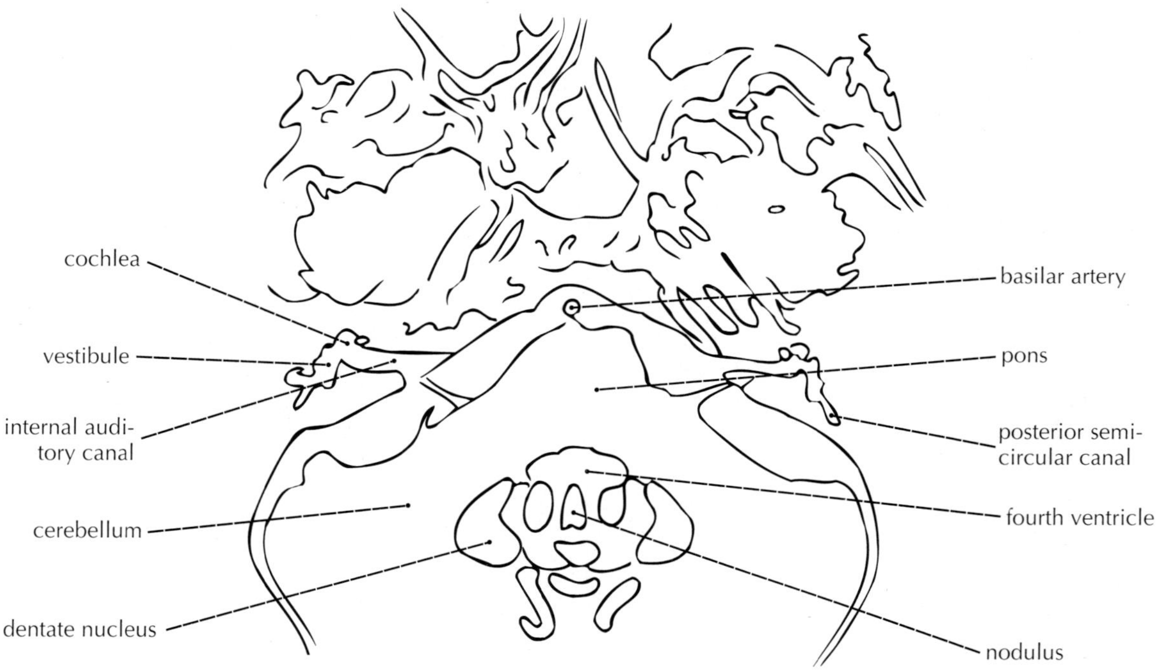

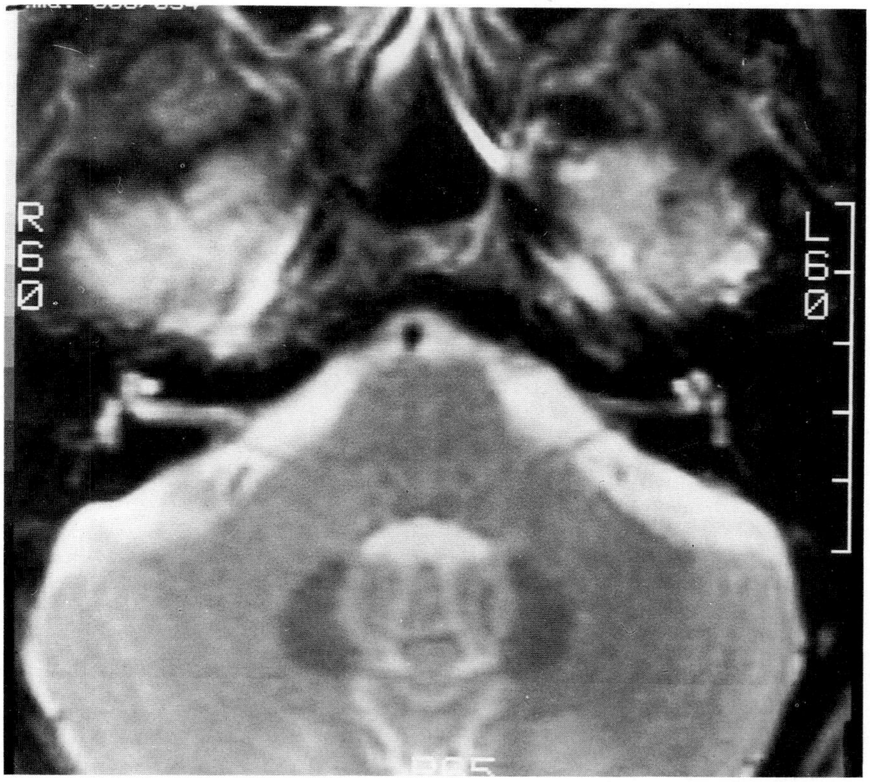

2-98 Axial MR scan through internal auditory canal (2000/90).

2/Temporal Bone, Axial Scout MRI and Coronal MRI

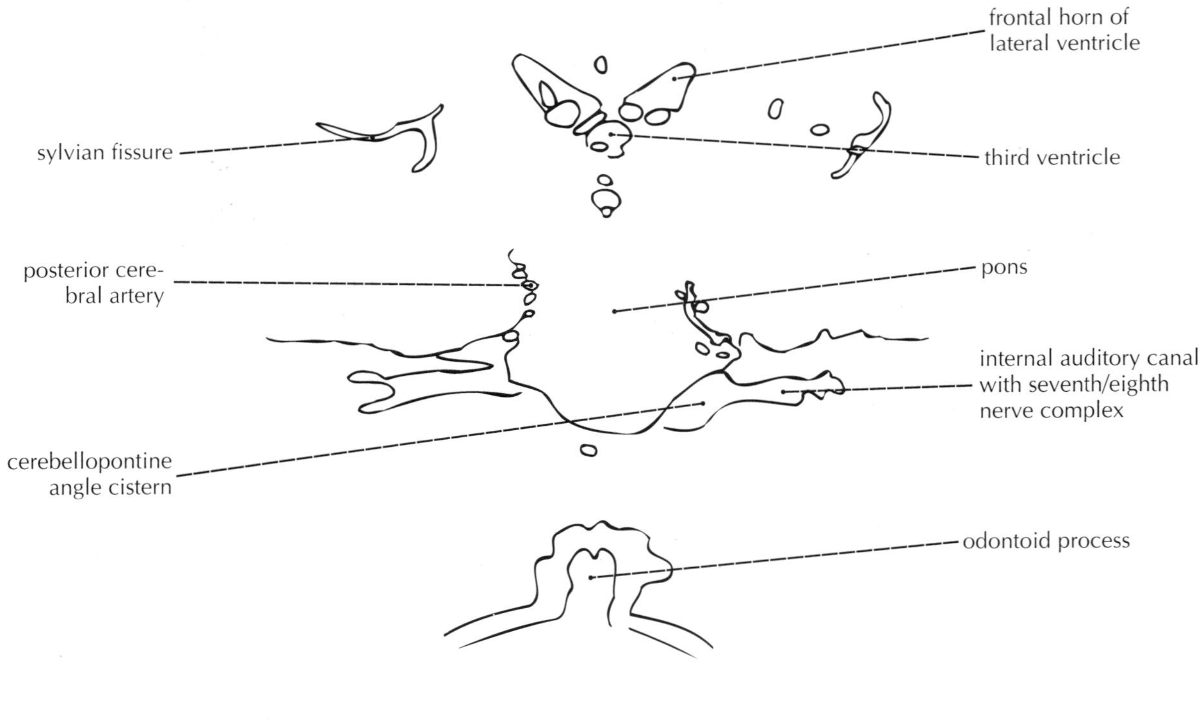

2/Temporal Bone, Axial Scout MRI and Coronal MRI

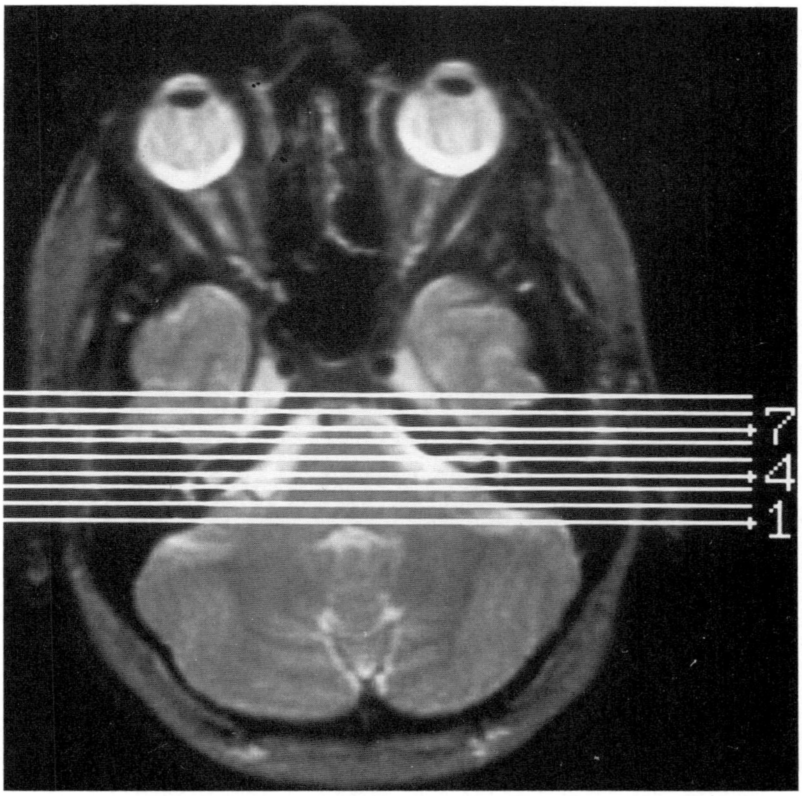

2-99 Axial scout MRI for the coronal MRI.

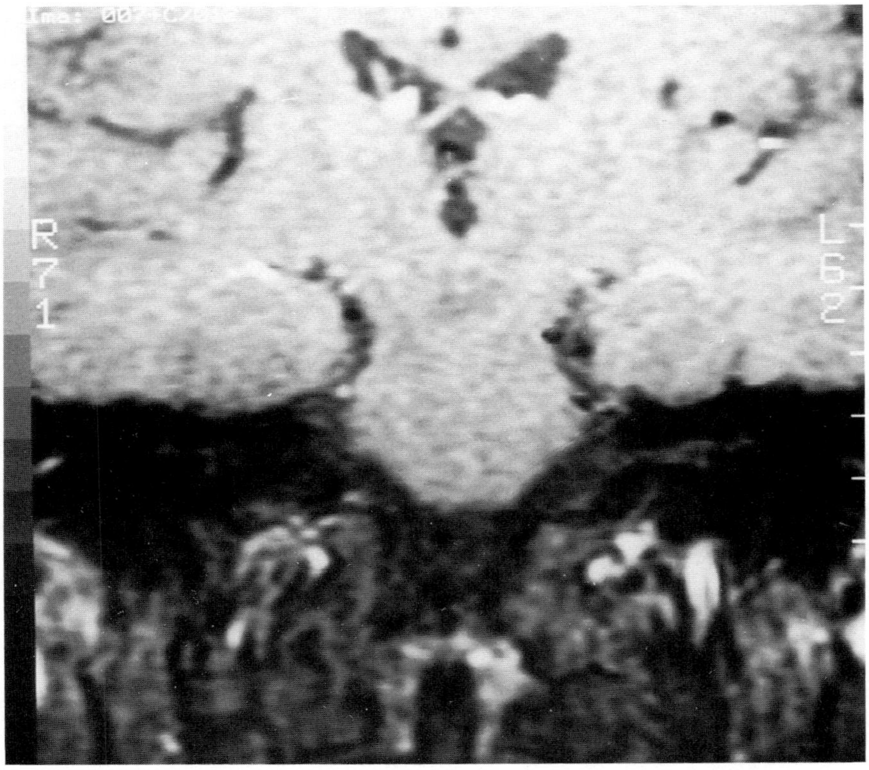

2-100 Coronal MR scan through internal auditory canal (gadolinium-DTPA–enhanced study) (600/20). Section 5 in Fig. 2-99.

PART 2

THE NECK AND SPINE

3/Cervical Spine □ Cervical Spine, X-Ray

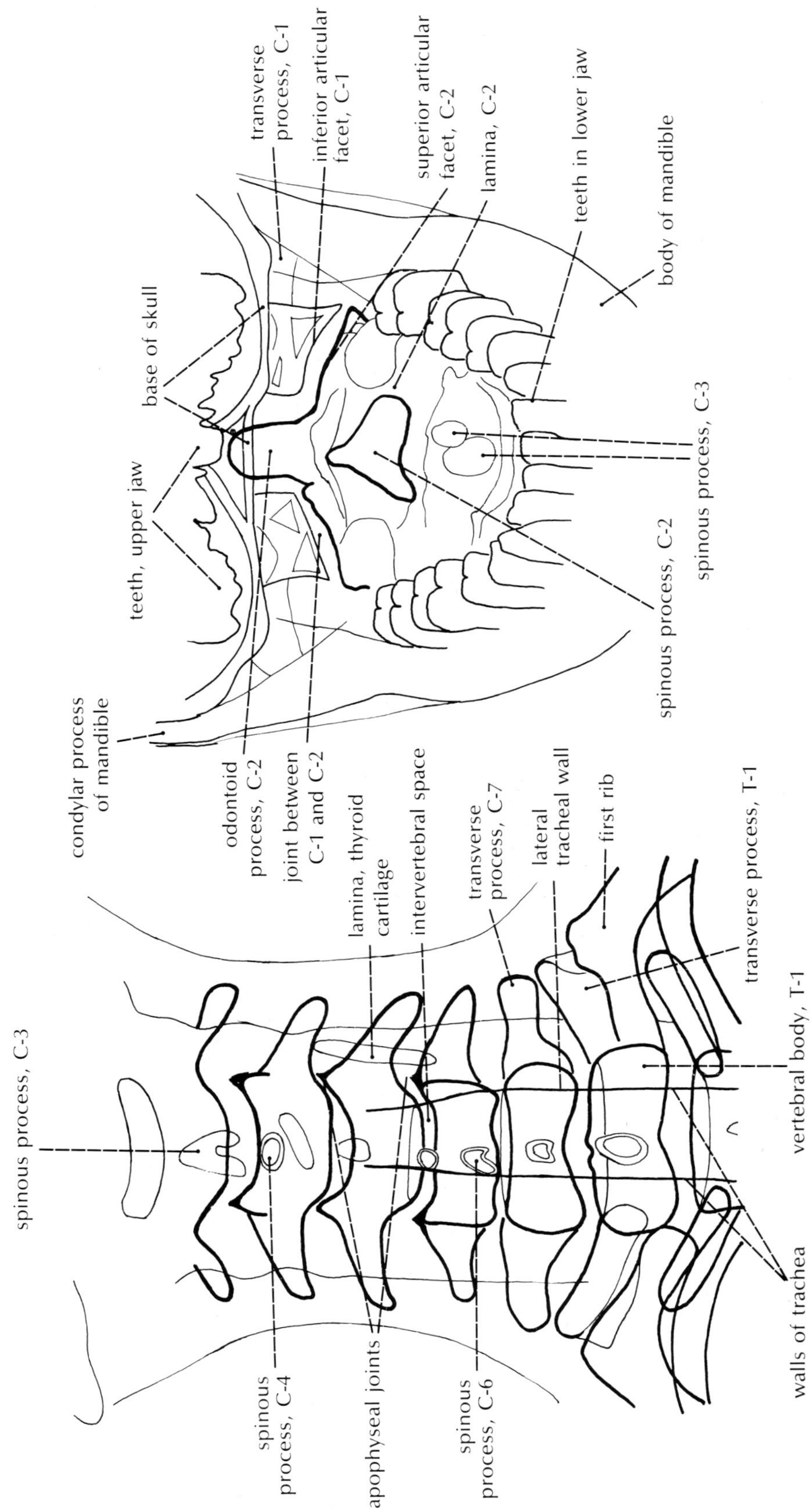

3/Cervical Spine, X-Ray

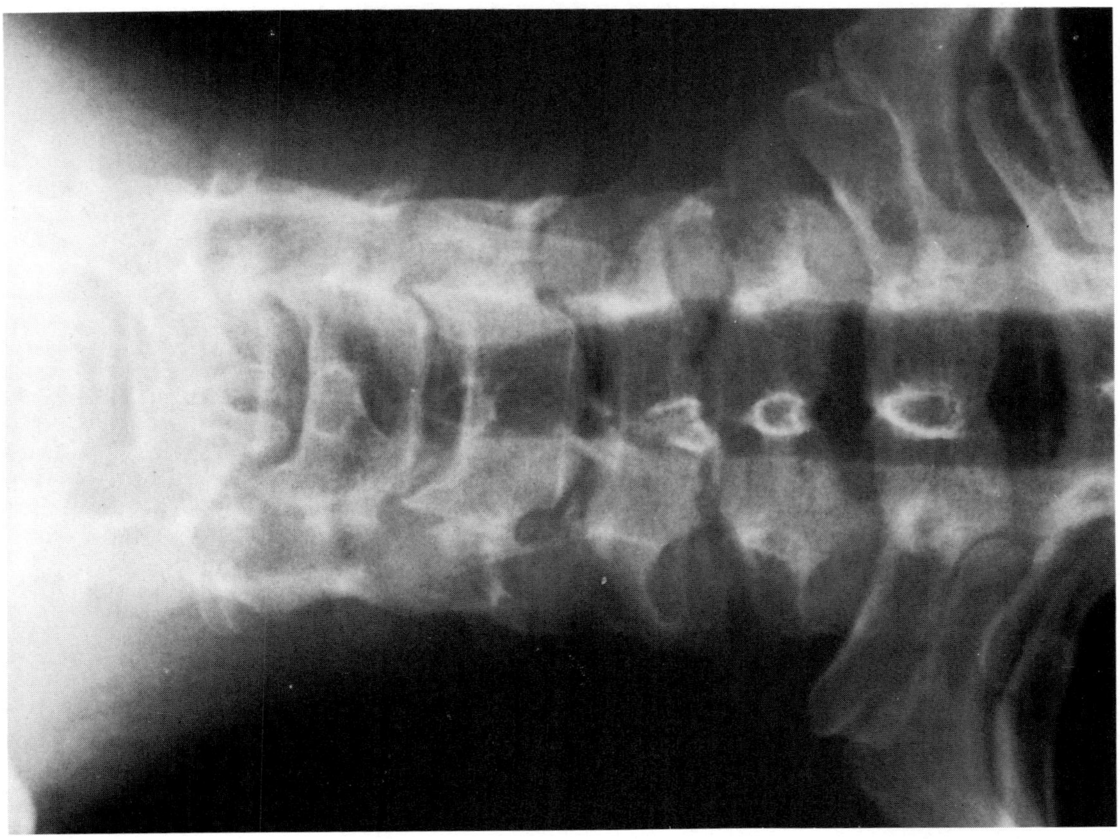

3-1 Cervical spine, AP view.

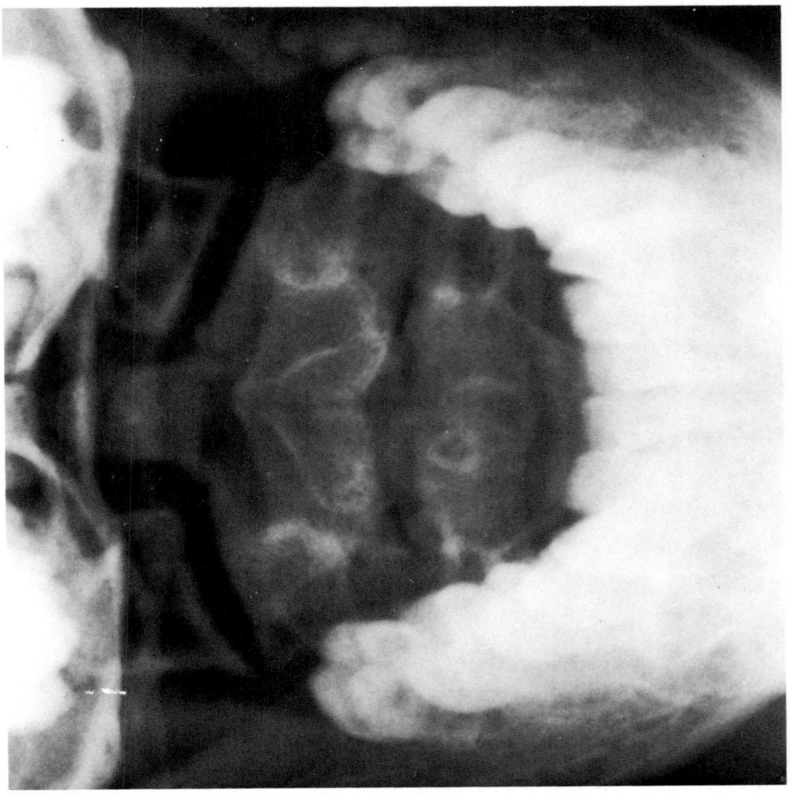

3-2 Cervical spine, open-mouth view.

3/Cervical Spine, X-Ray

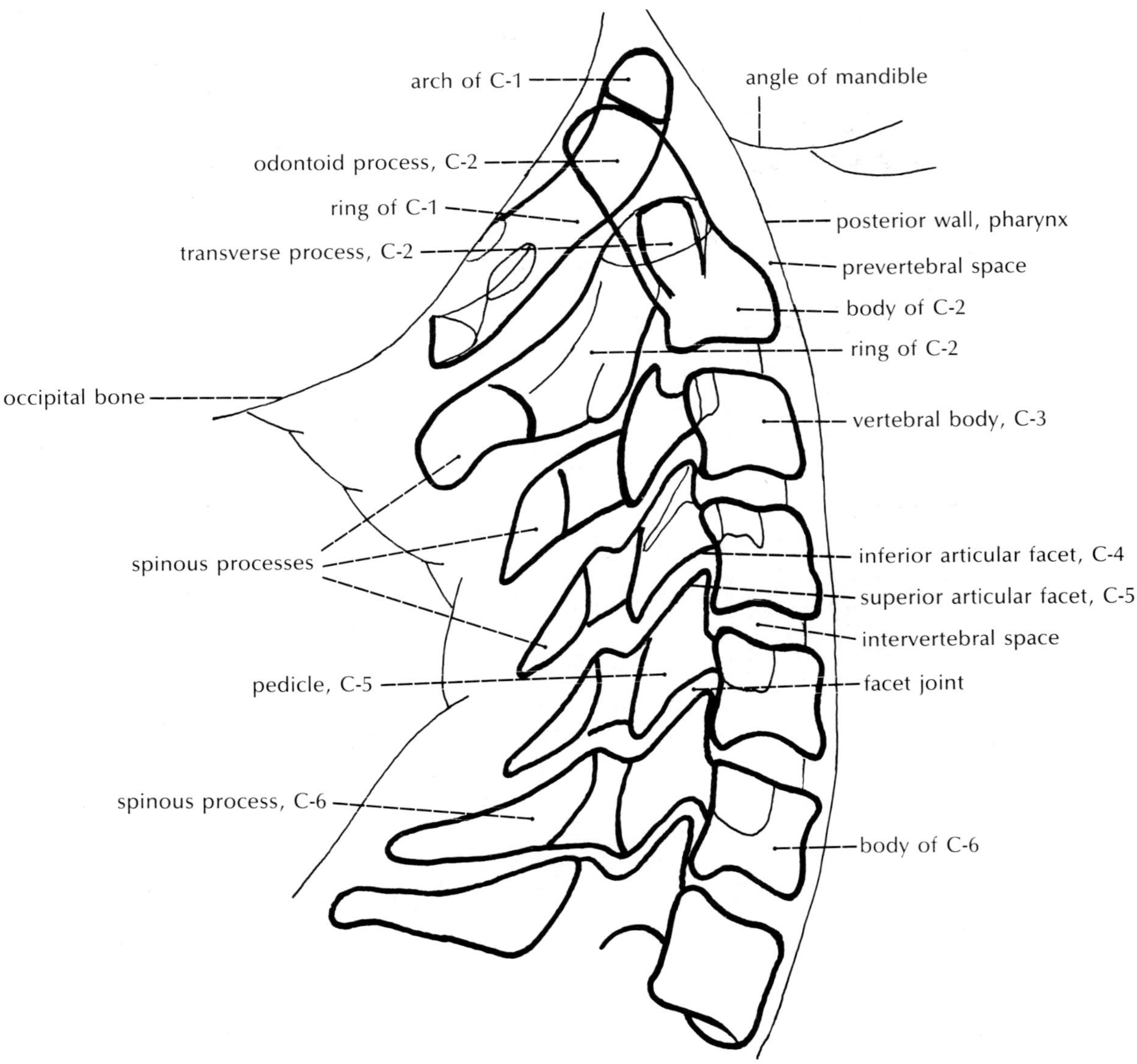

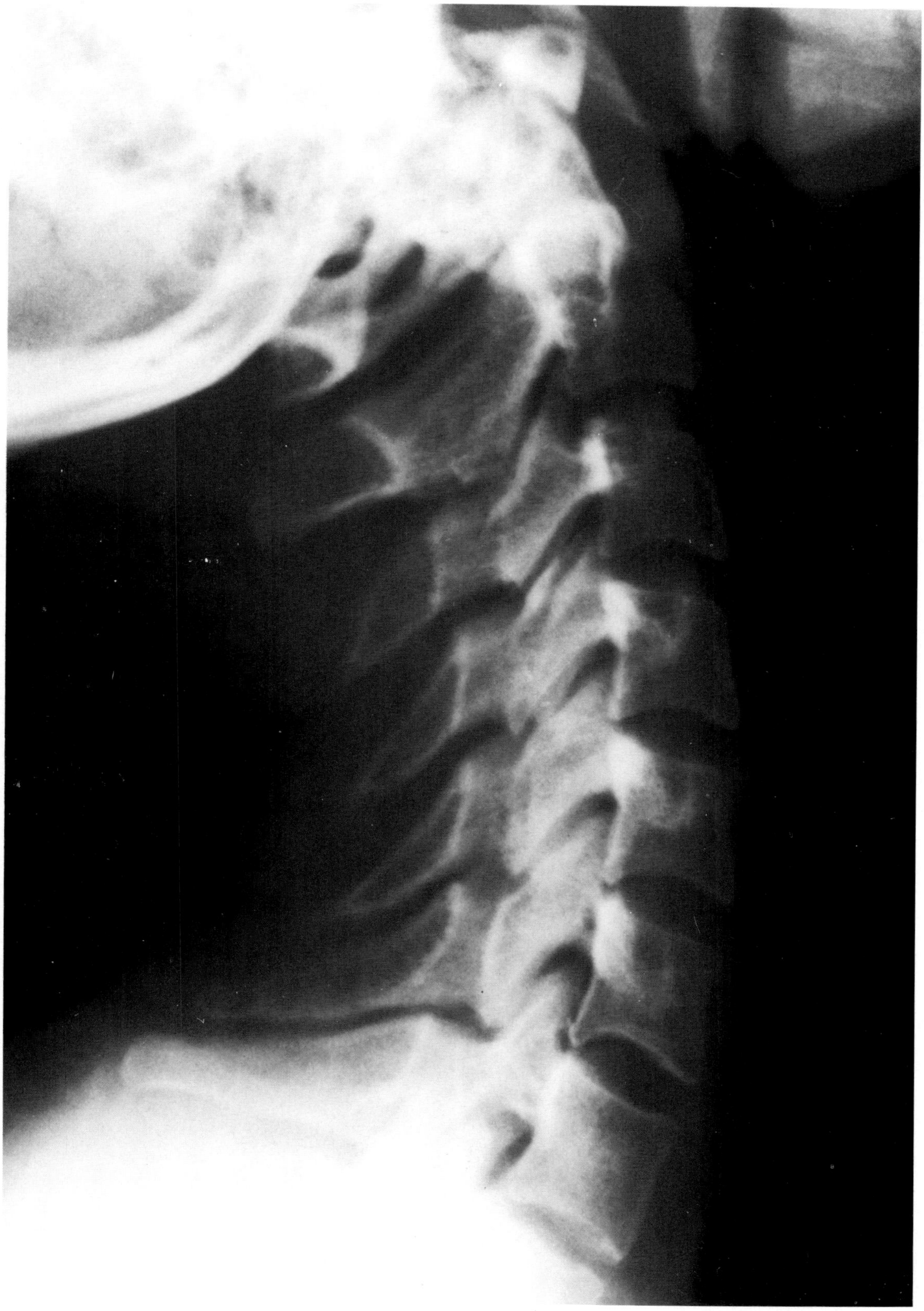

3-3 Cervical spine, lateral view.

3/Cervical Spine, X-Ray

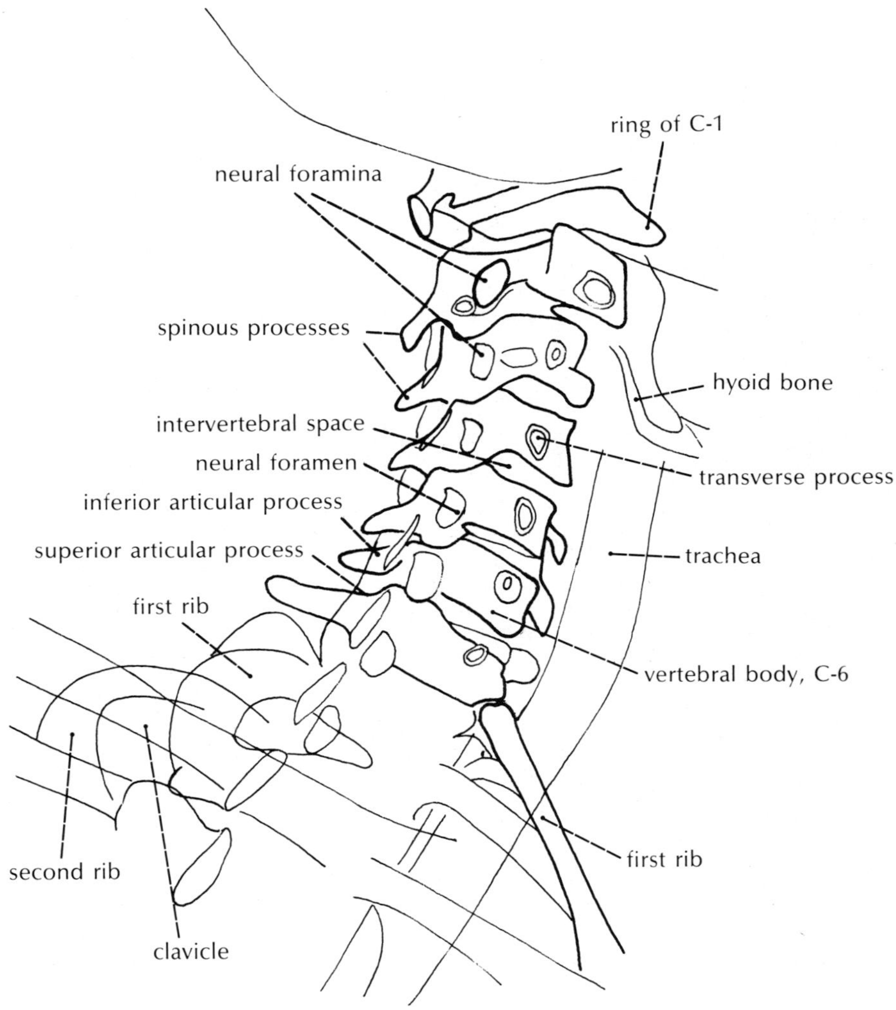

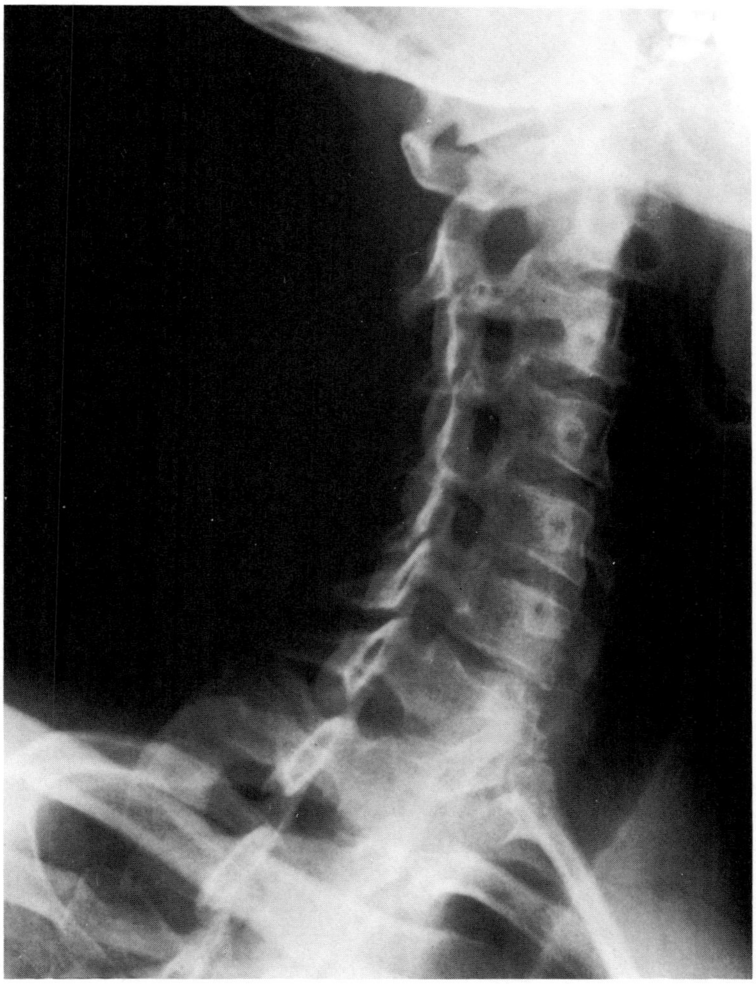

3-4 Cervical spine, oblique view.

3/Cervical Spine, Sagittal Scout CT and Axial CT

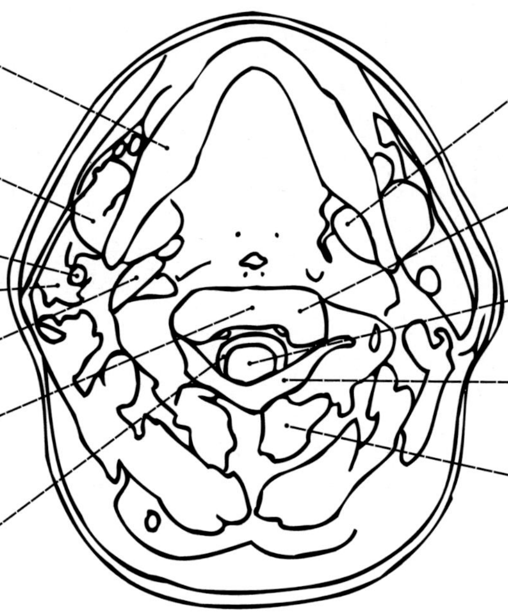

3/Cervical Spine, Sagittal Scout CT and Axial CT

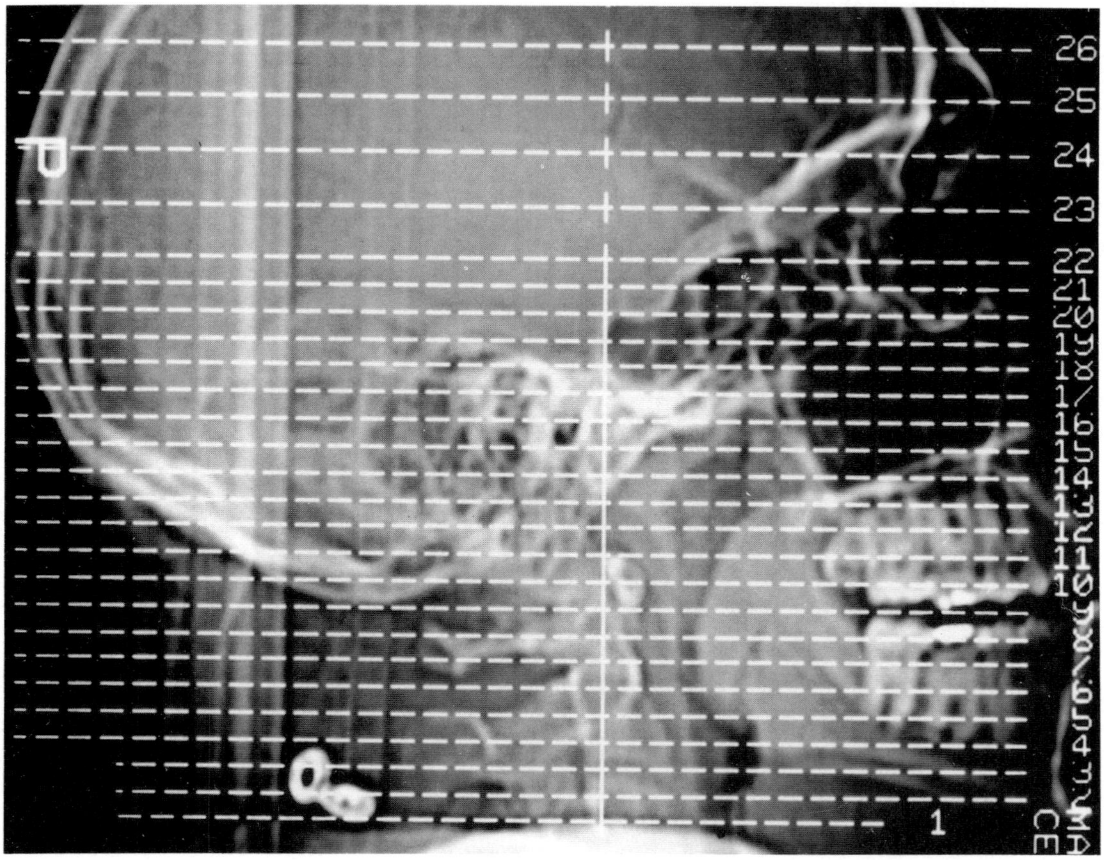

3-5 This sagittal scout CT scan illustrates the location of selected axial CT scans. Sections 7, 2, 9, and 3 are shown.

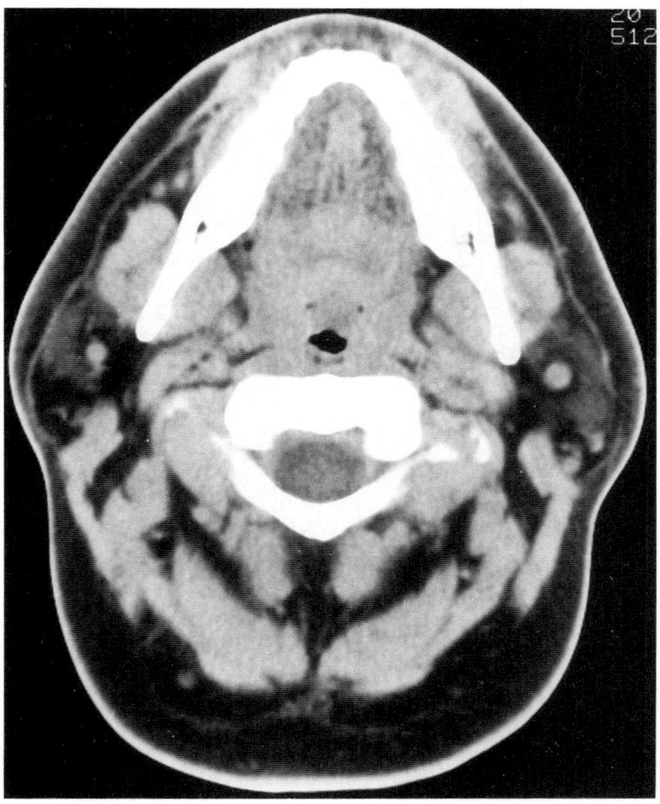

3-6 Axial CT scan through body of C-2. Section 7 in Fig. 3-5.

3/Cervical Spine, Axial CT

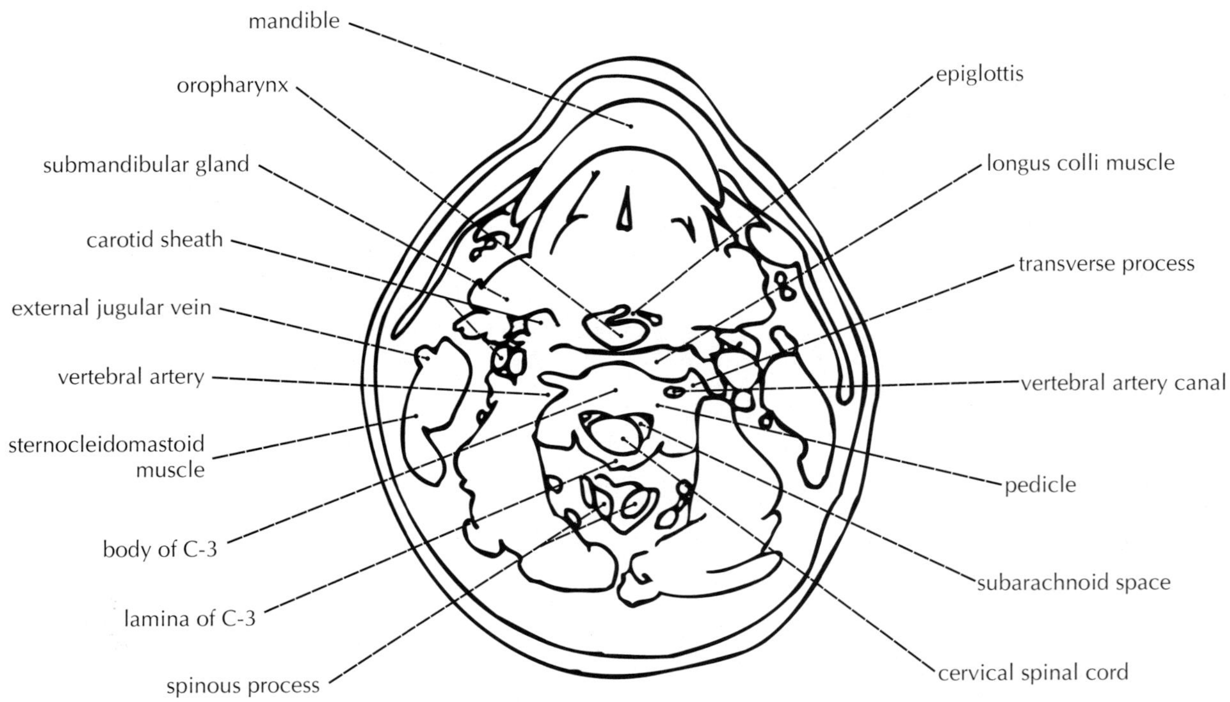

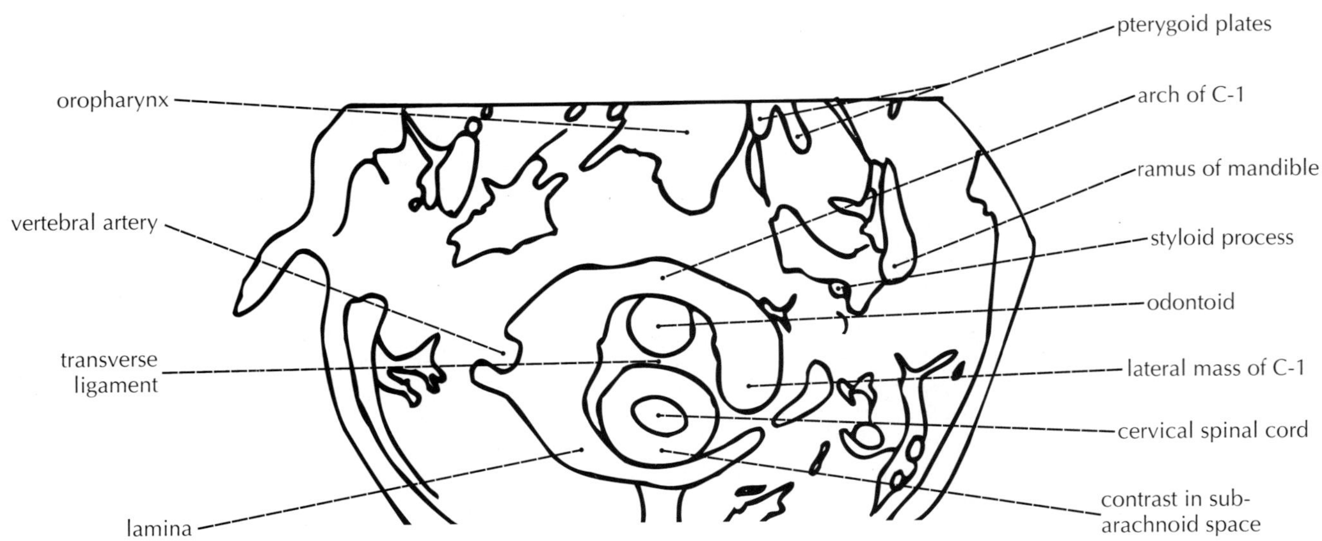

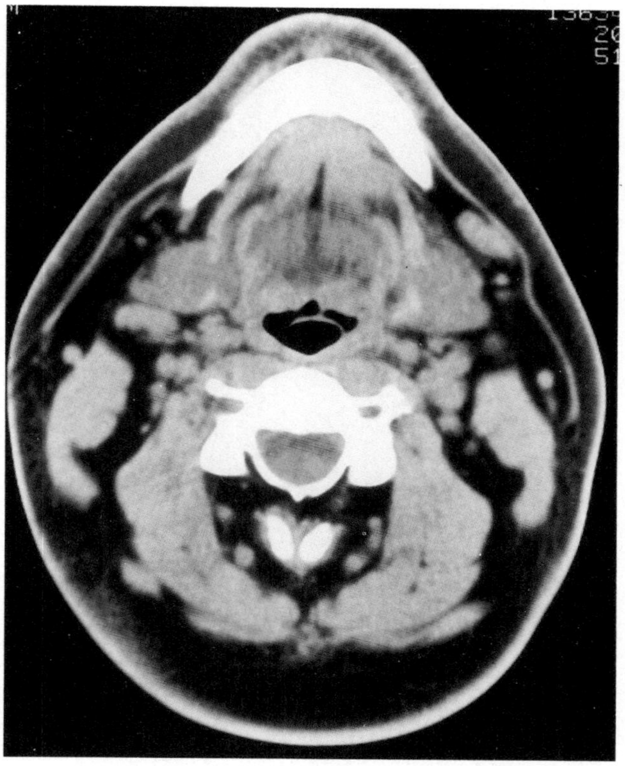

3-7 Axial CT scan through body of C-3. Section 2 in Fig. 3-5.

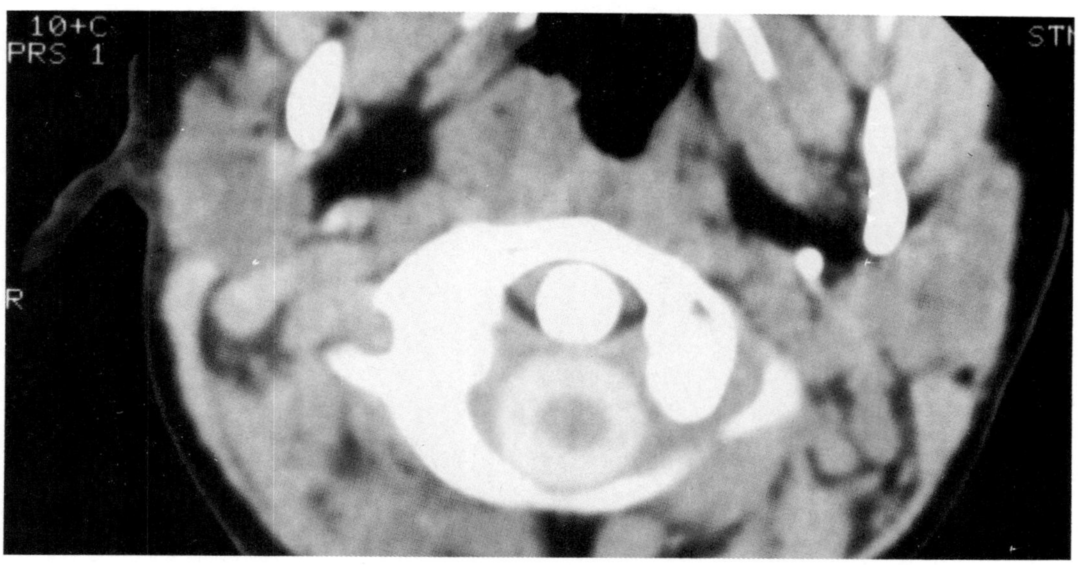

3-8 Axial CT scan through cervical spine (with intrathecal contrast) at C-1–C-2 level. Section 9 in Fig. 3-5.

3/Cervical Spine, Axial CT

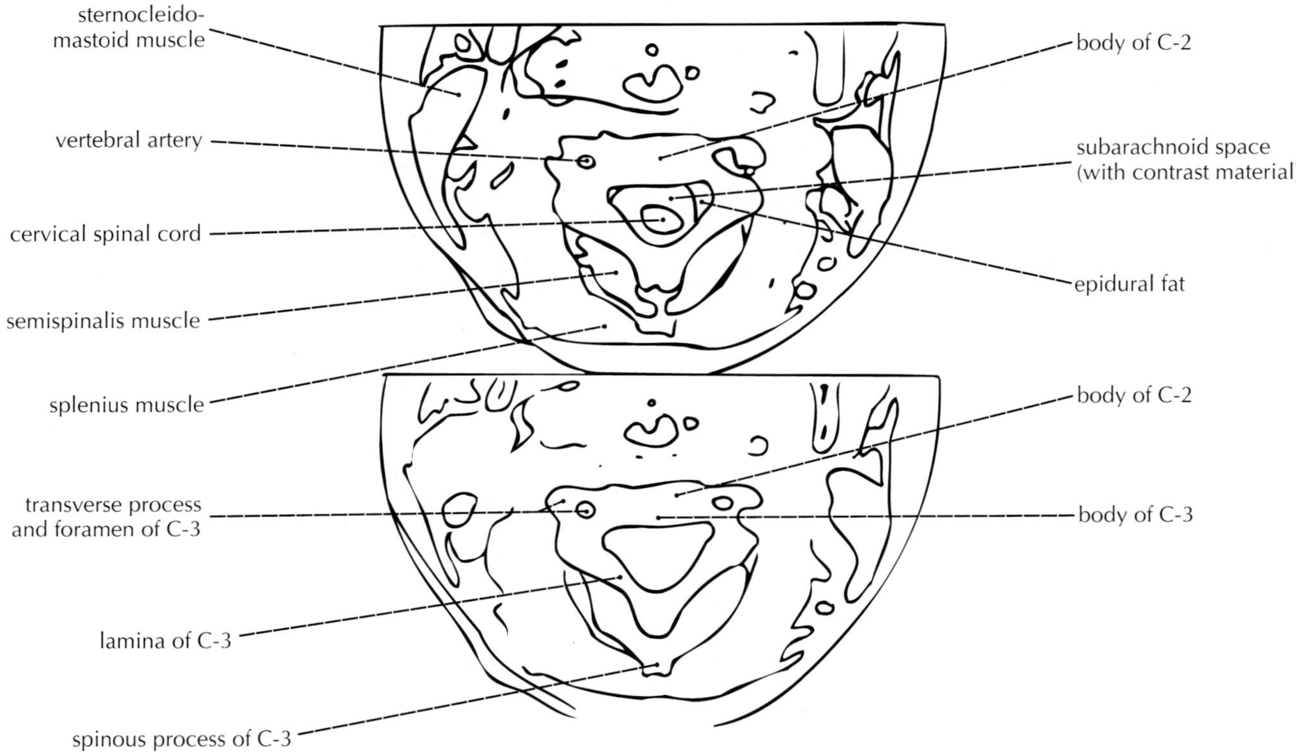

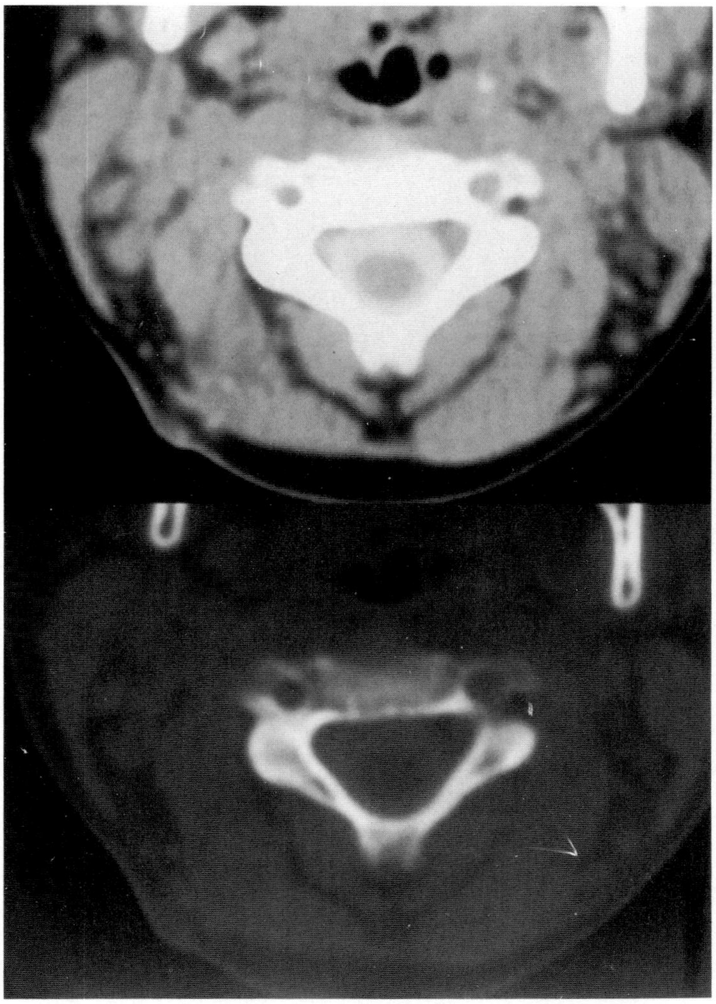

3-9 Axial CT scans through C-2 and C-3 with intrathecal contrast (soft tissue and bone window). Section 3 in Fig. 3-5.

3/Cervical Spine, Sagittal and Parasagittal MRI

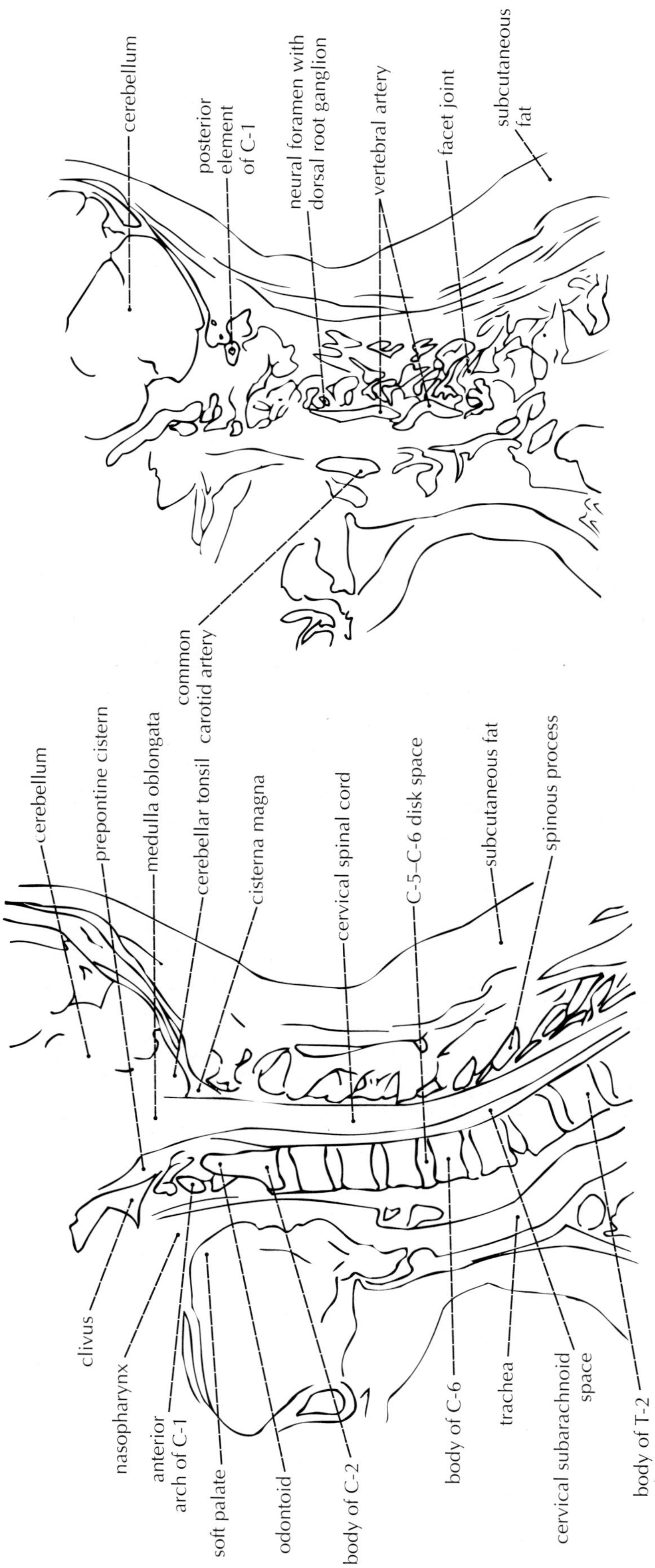

3/Cervical Spine, Sagittal and Parasagittal MRI

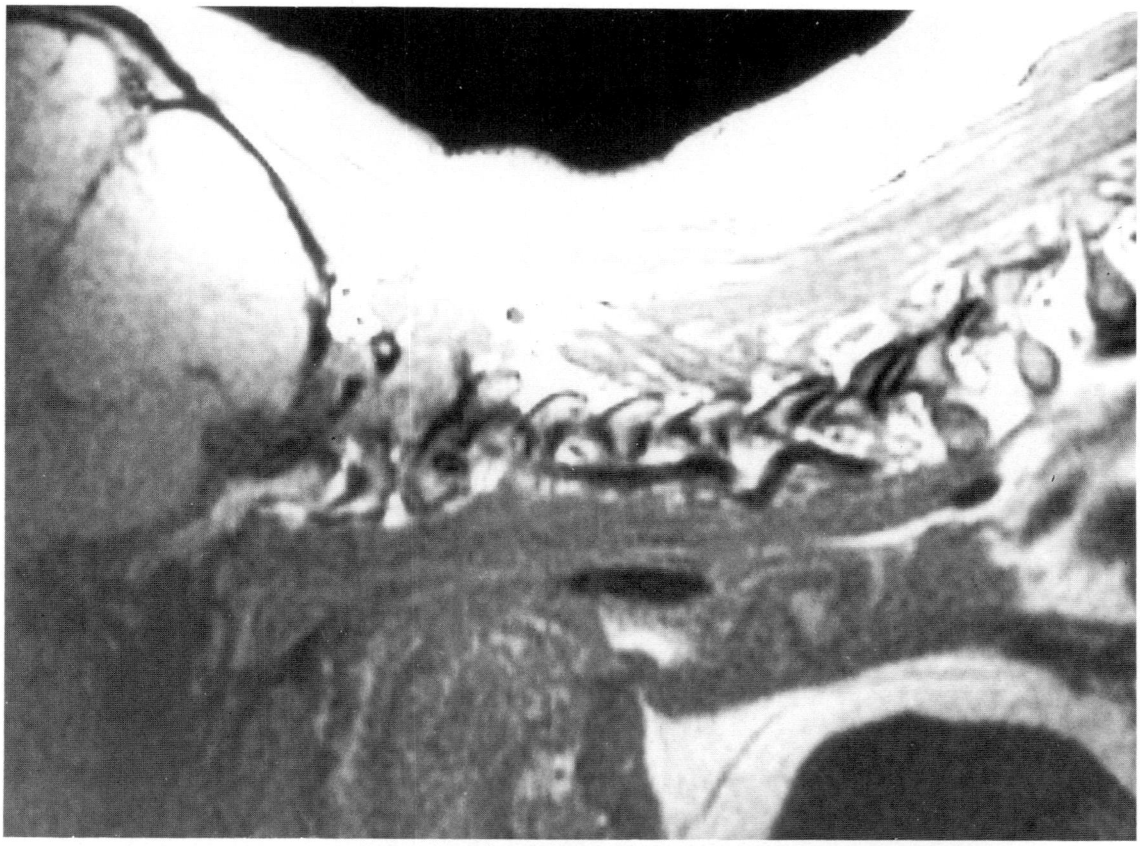

3-11 Parasagittal MR scan through cervical spine (600/20). Section is 1.5 cm lateral to midline.

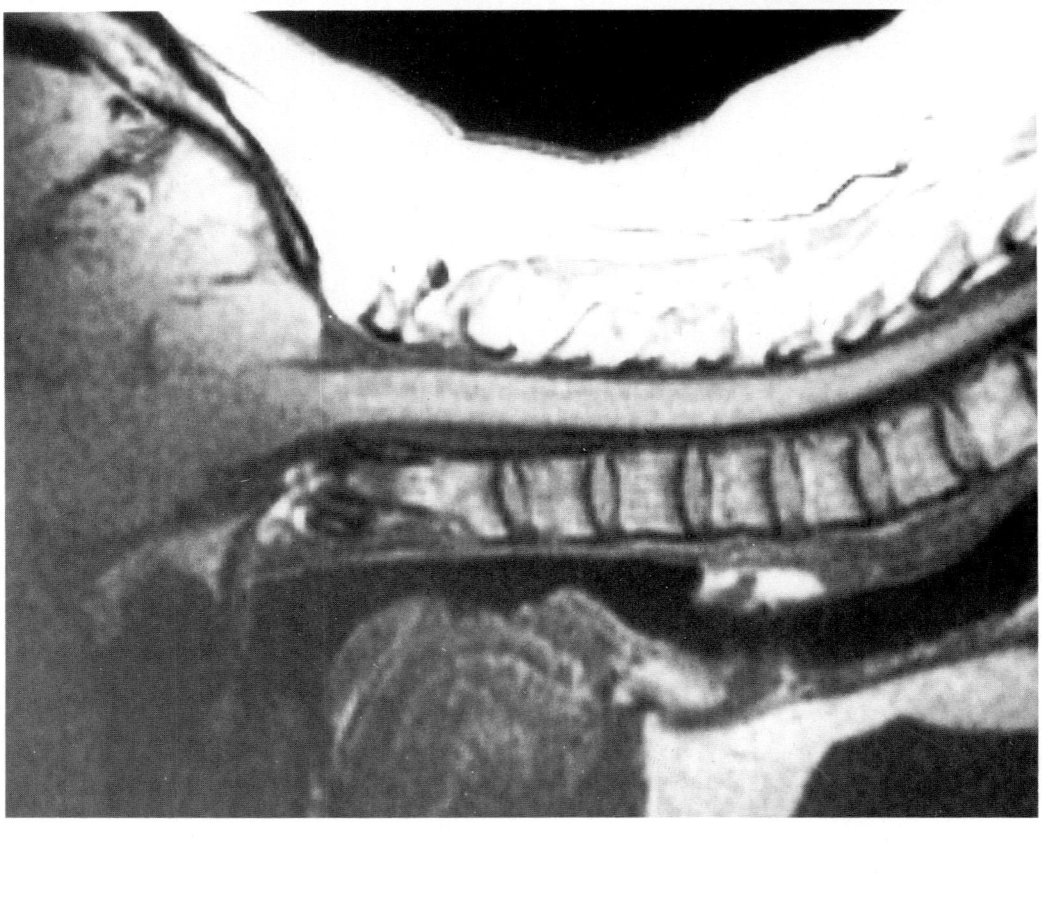

3-10 Sagittal midline MR scan of cervical spine (600/20).

3/Cervical Spine, Sagittal MRI

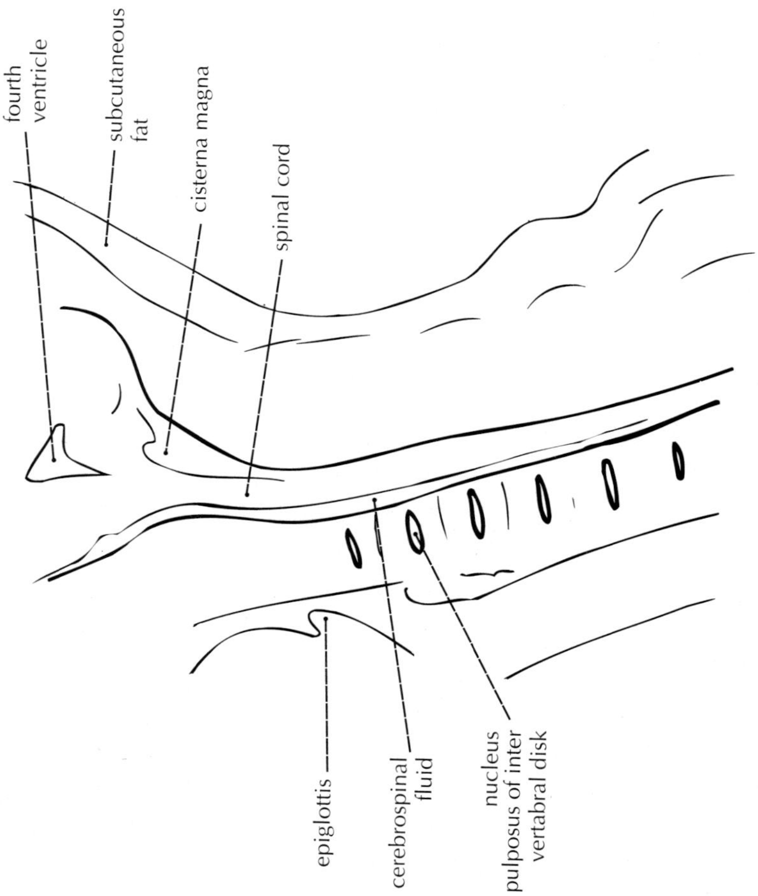

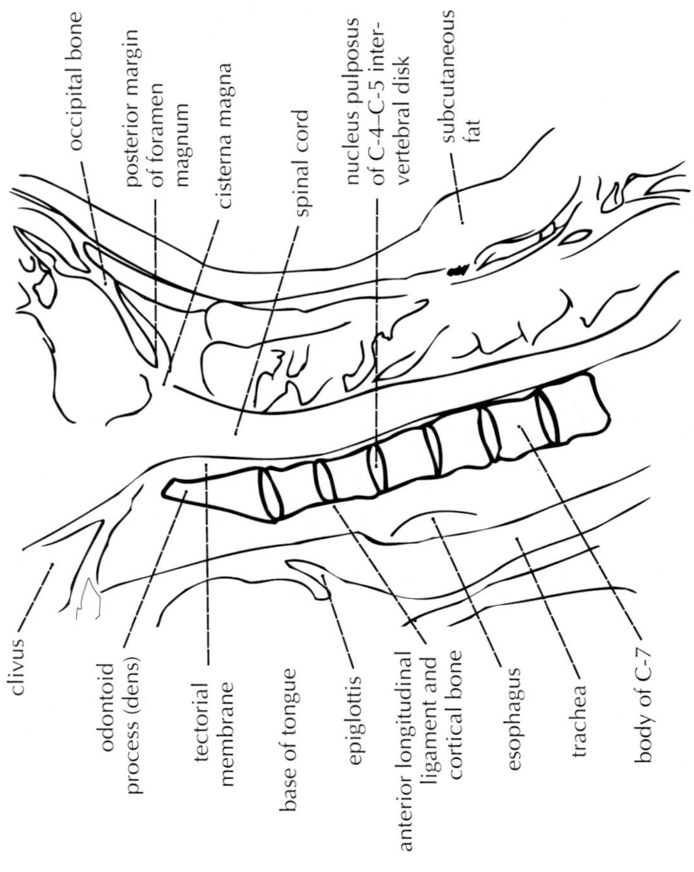

3/Cervical Spine, Sagittal MRI

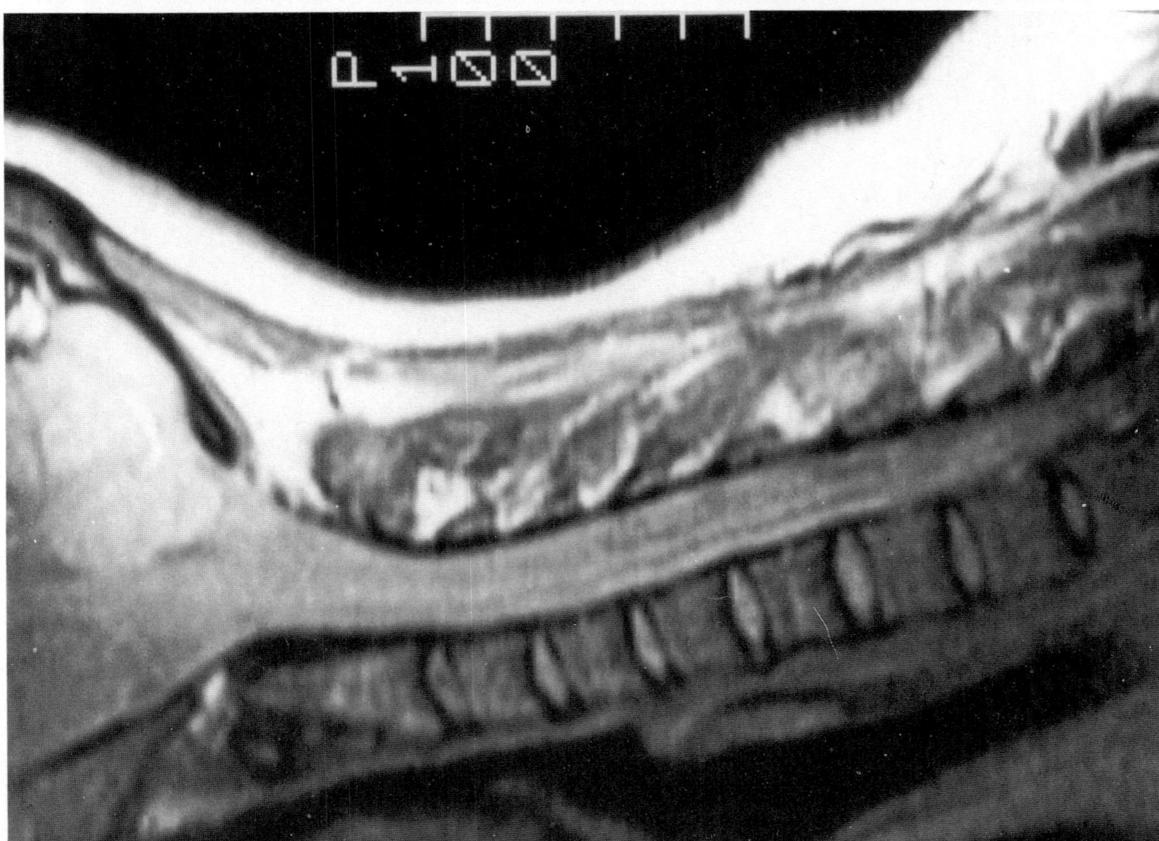

3-12 Sagittal MR scan through cervical spine (2000/30). Midline section.

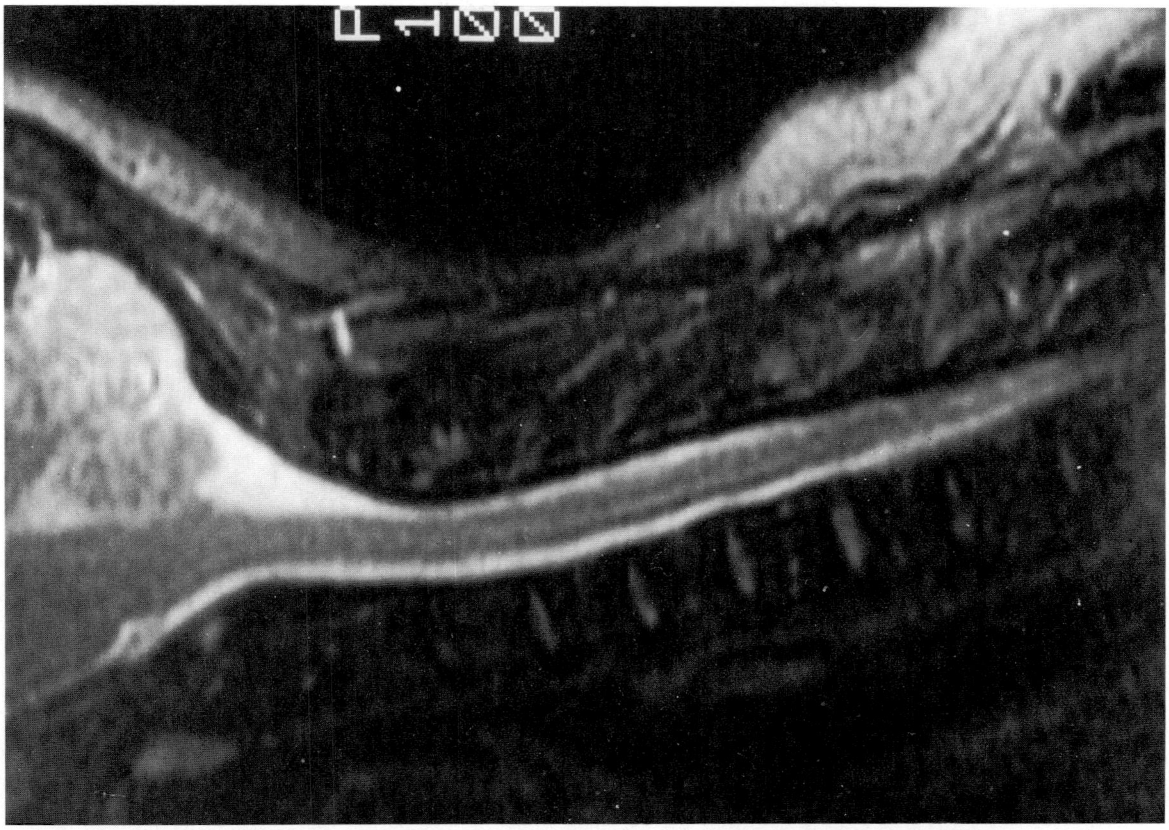

3-13 Sagittal MR scan through cervical spine (2000/90). Midline section.

3/Cervical Spine, Sagittal Scout MRI and Axial MRI

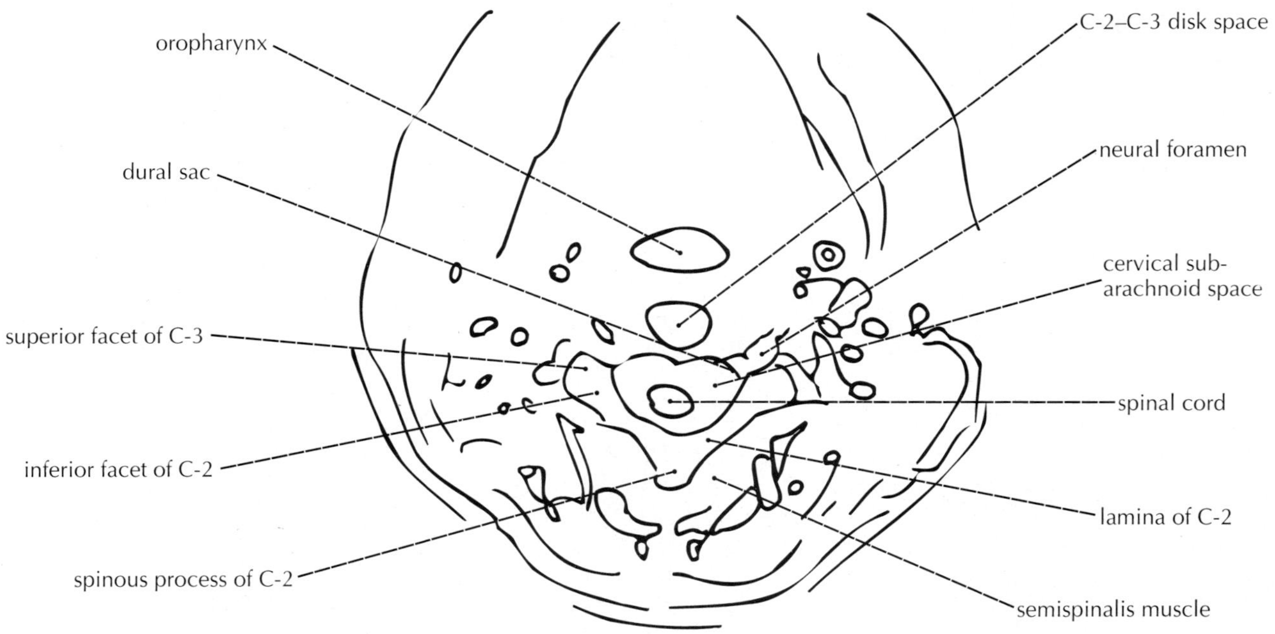

3/Cervical Spine, Sagittal Scout MRI and Axial MRI

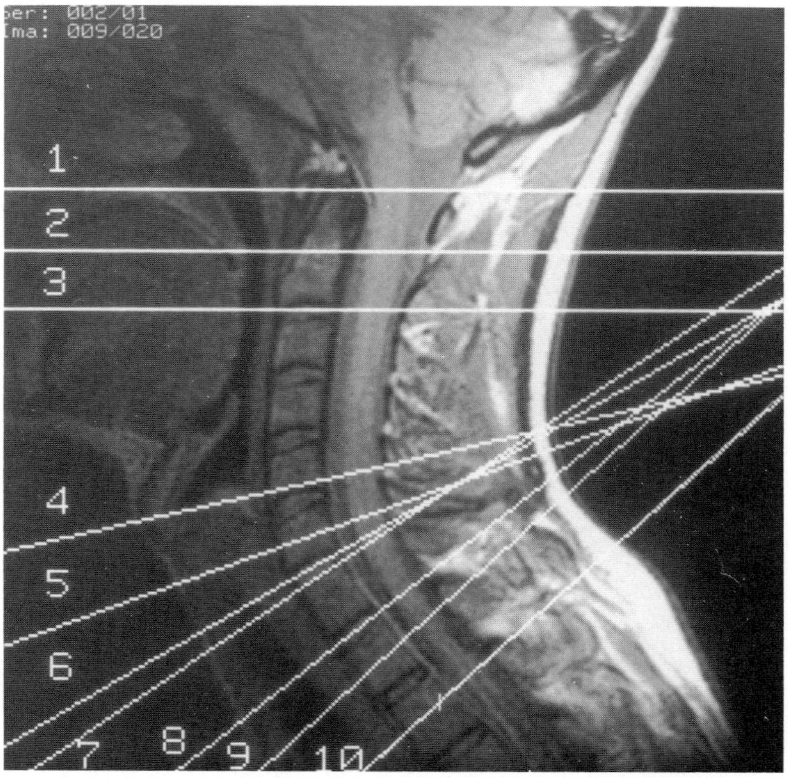

3-14 Sagittal scout MR scan of cervical spine for orientation of selected axial MR scans. Sections 3, 4, and 7 will be shown.

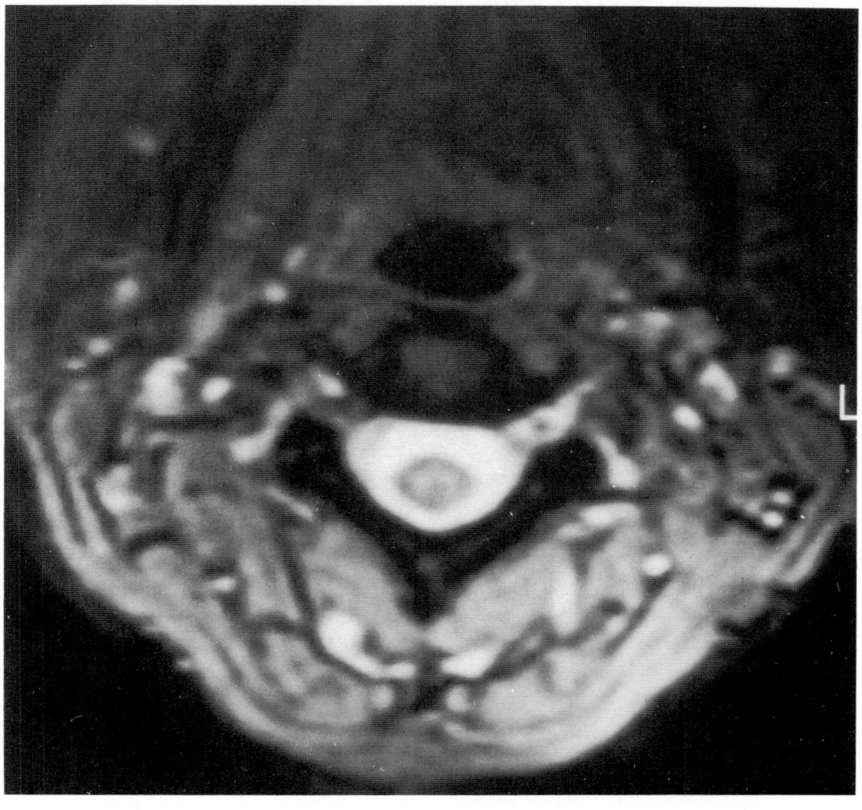

3-15 Axial MR scan through C-2–C-3 level (500/18, flip angle 15°) (section 3 in Fig. 3-14).

3/Cervical Spine, Axial MRI

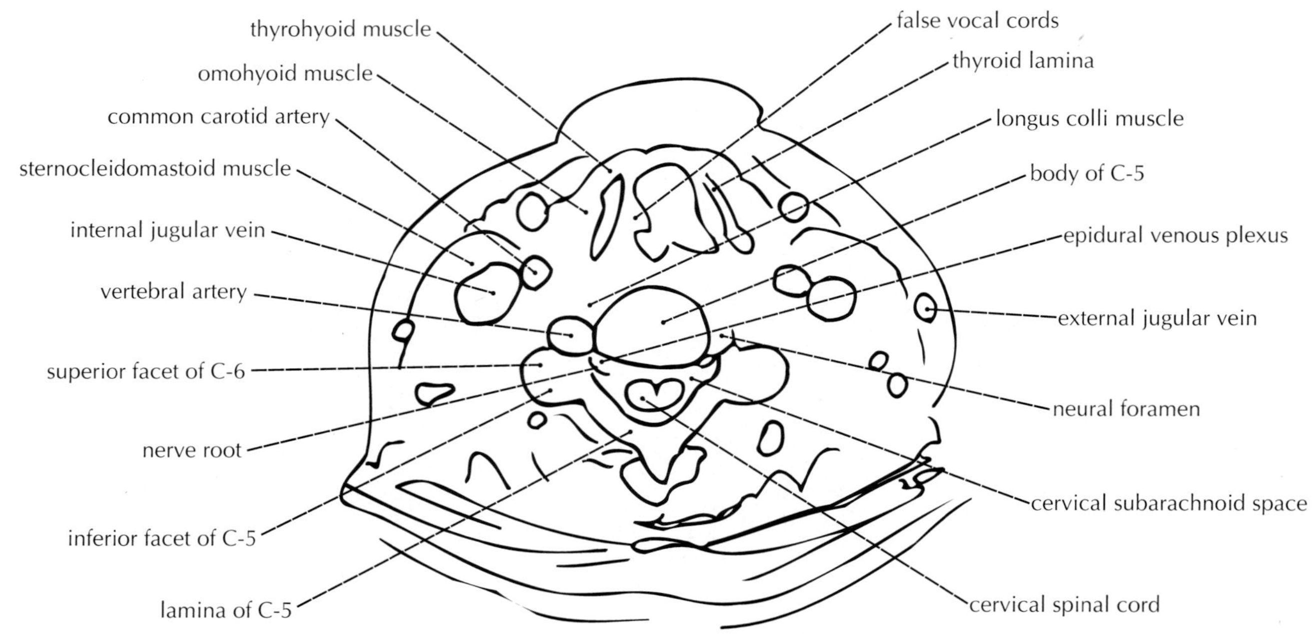

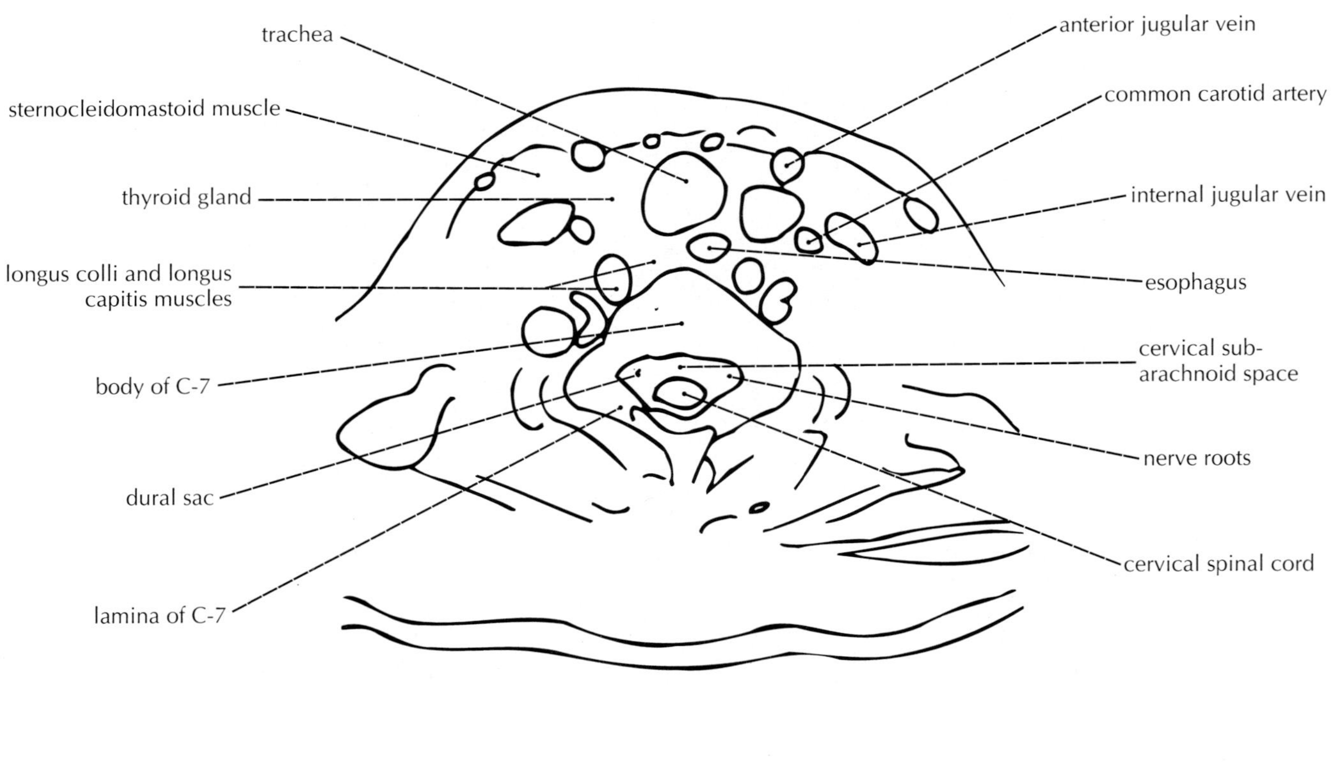

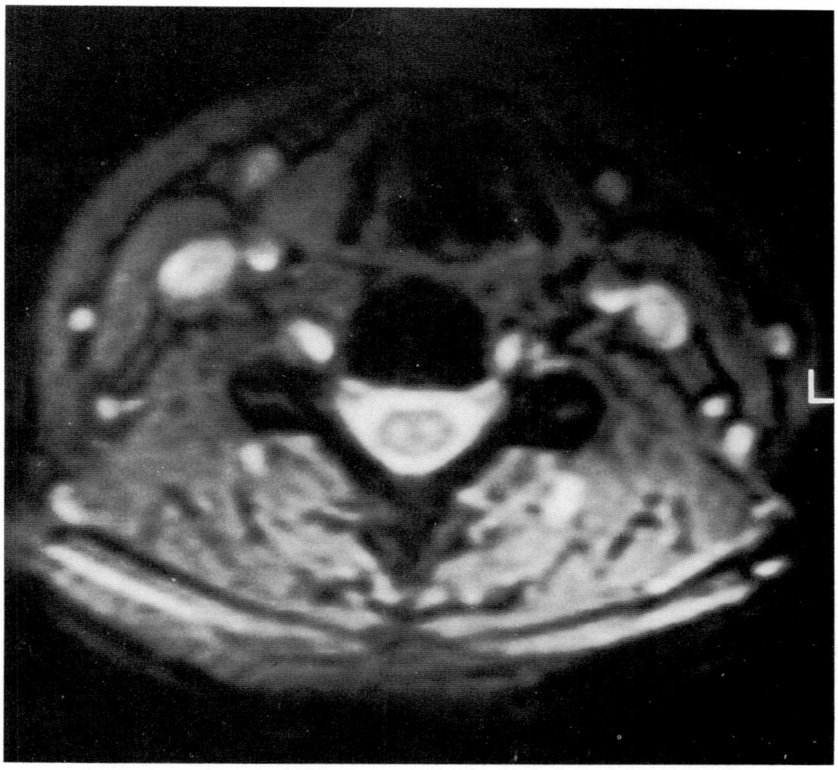

3-16 Axial MR scan through body of C-5 (500/18, flip angle 15°) (section 4 in Fig. 3-14).

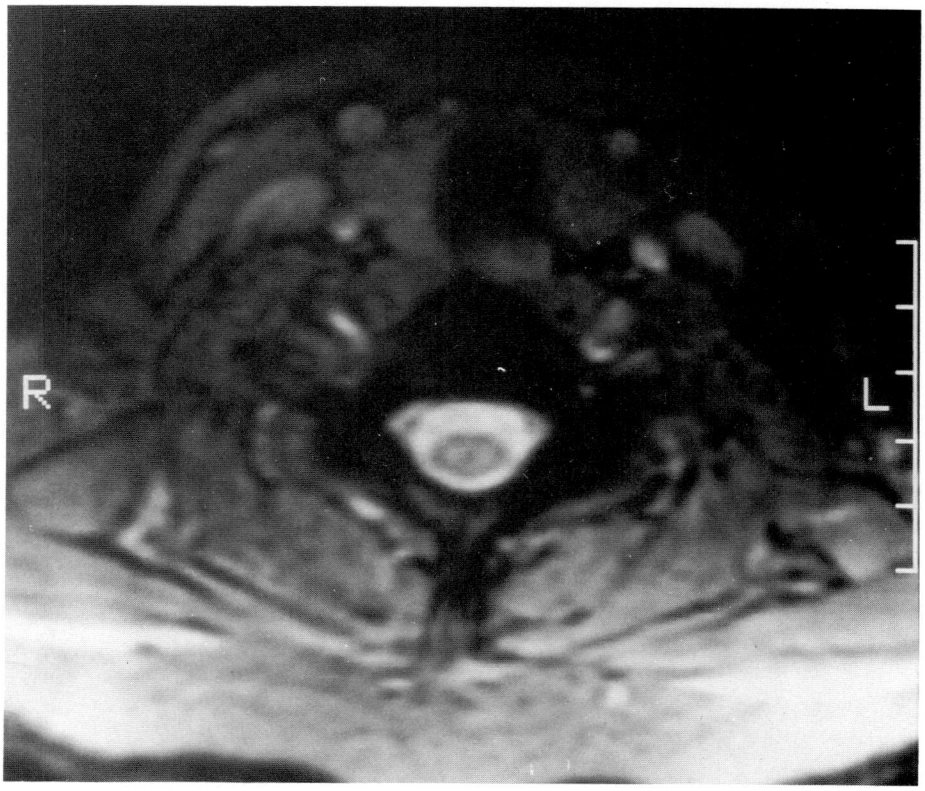

3-17 Axial MR scan through body of C-7 (500/18, flip angle 15°) (section 7 in Fig. 3-14).

3/Cervical Spine, Axial MRI

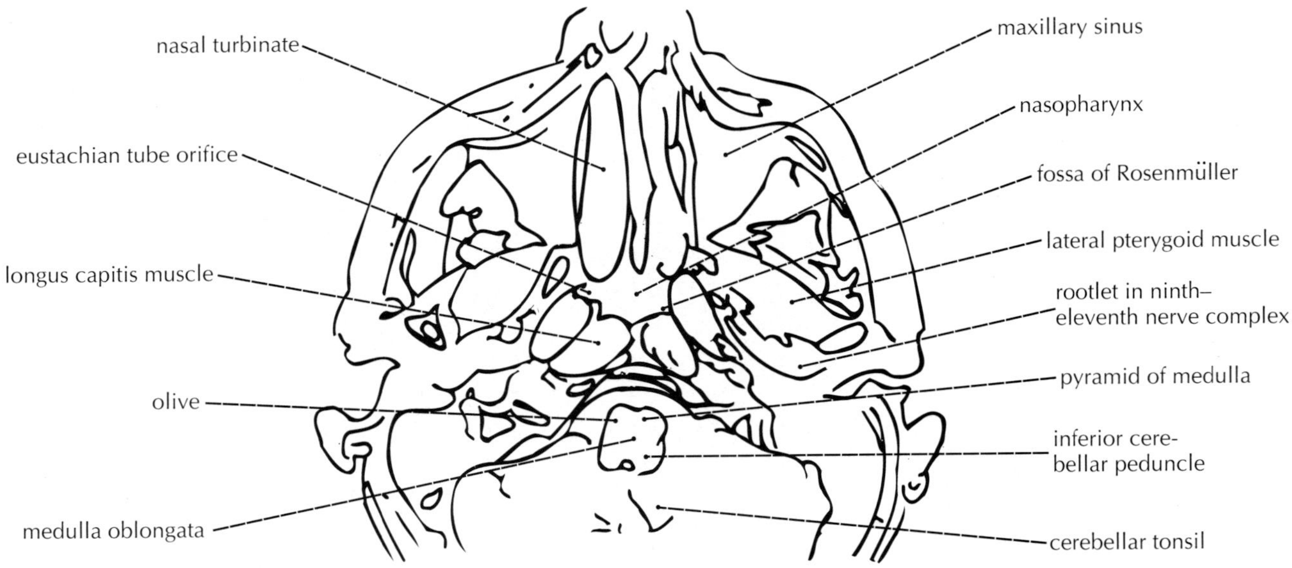

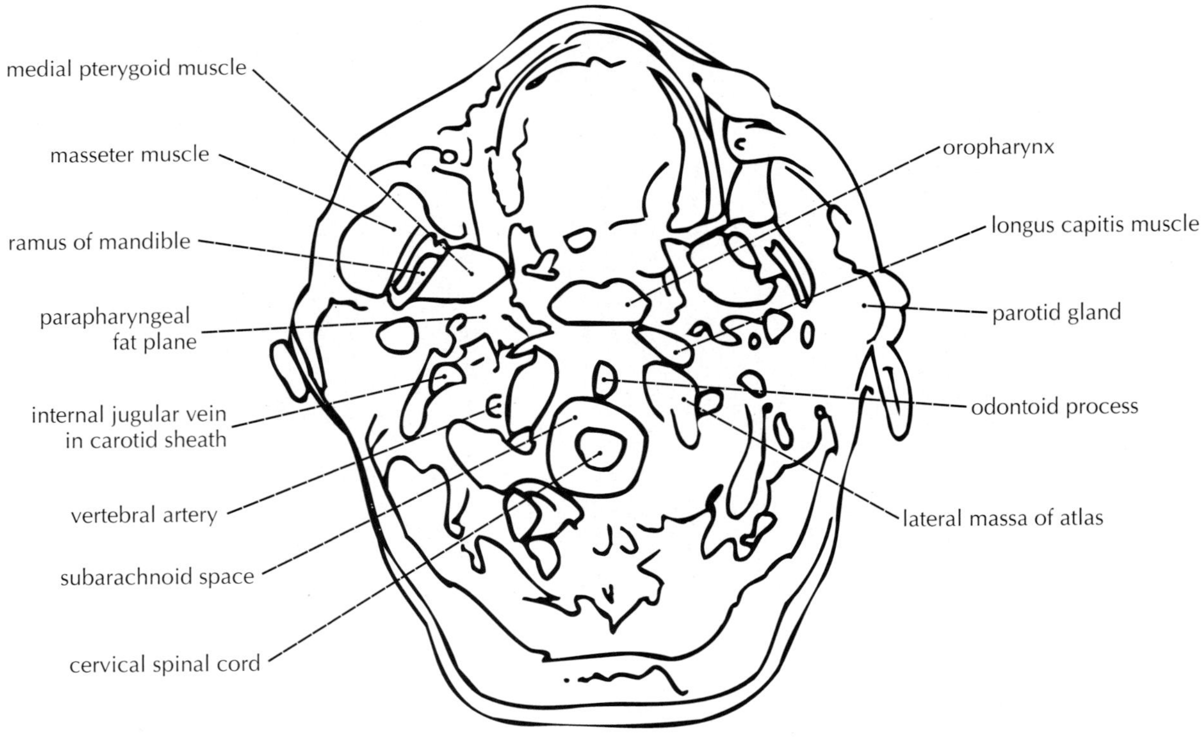

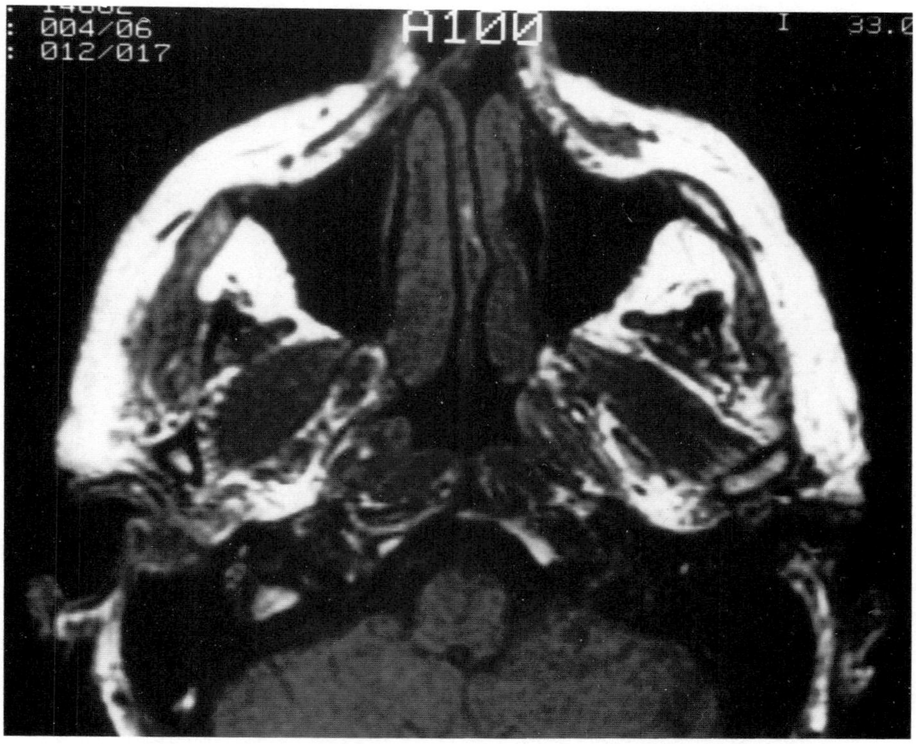

3-18 Axial MR scan through medulla and nasopharynx (600/20). Section 6 in Fig. 2-12.

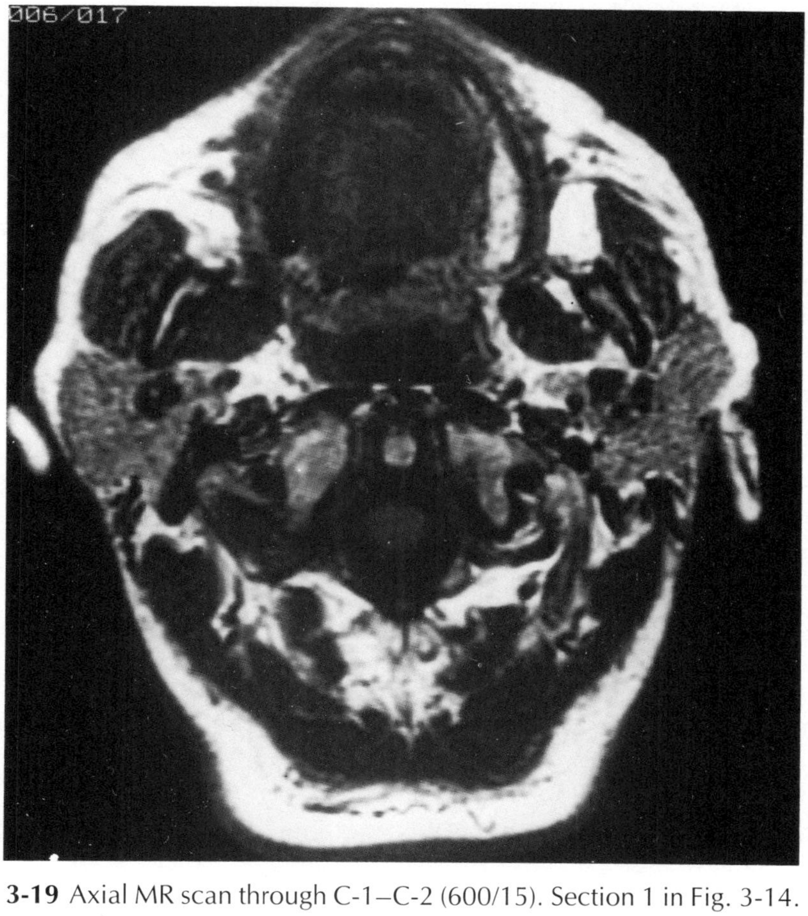

3-19 Axial MR scan through C-1–C-2 (600/15). Section 1 in Fig. 3-14.

3/Cervical Spine, Axial MRI

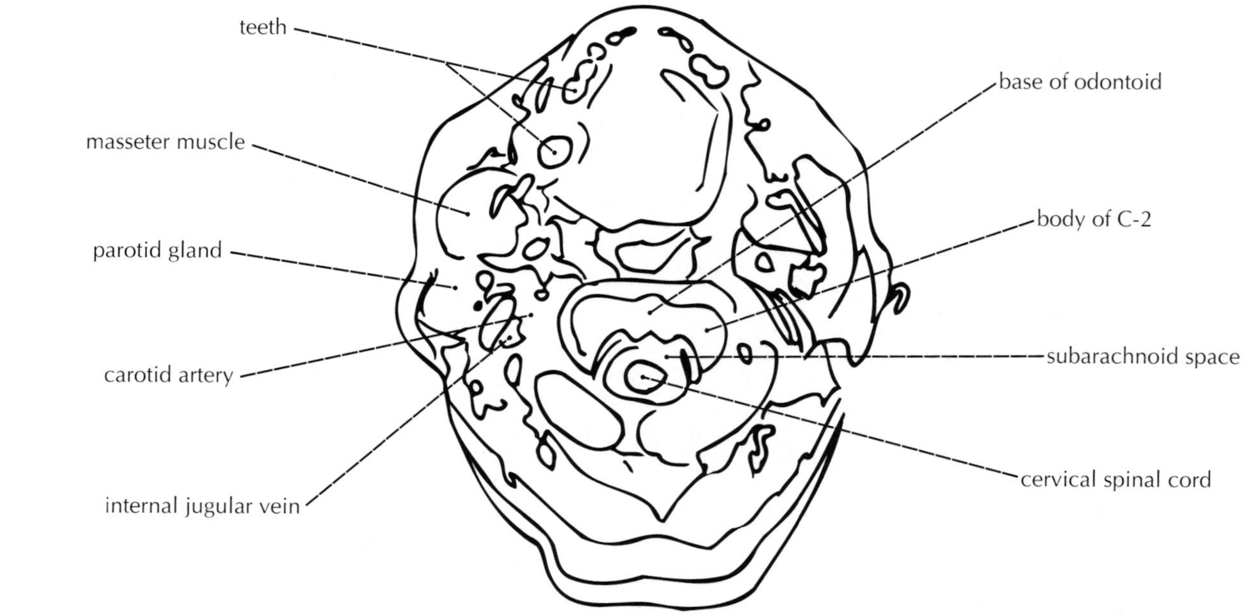

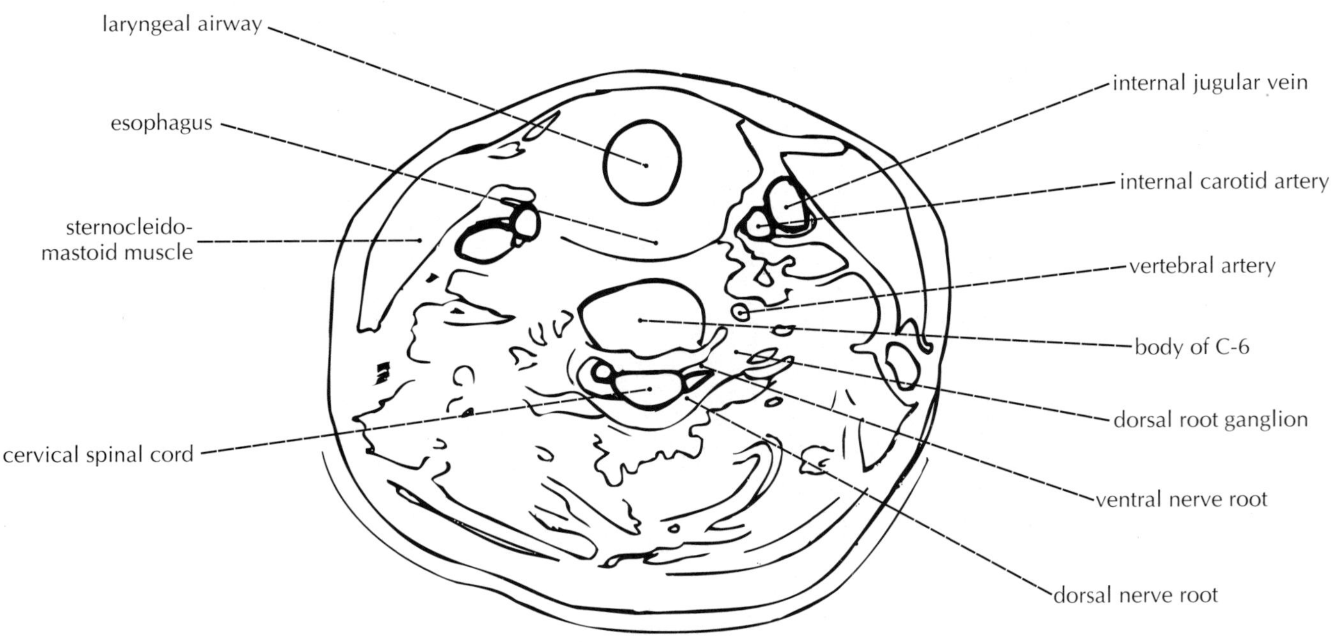

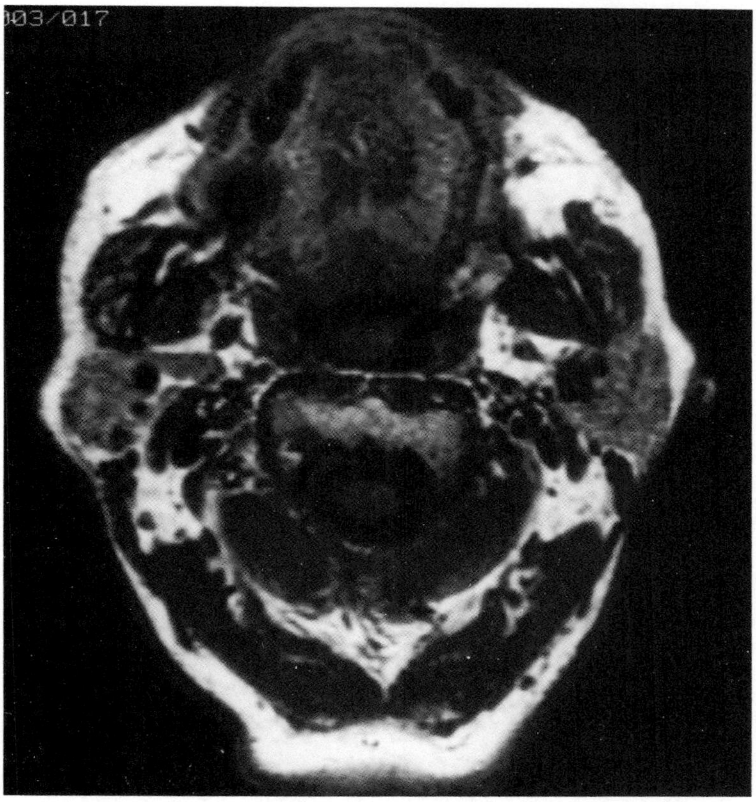

3-20 Axial MR scan through body of C-2 (600/15). Section 2 in Fig. 3-14.

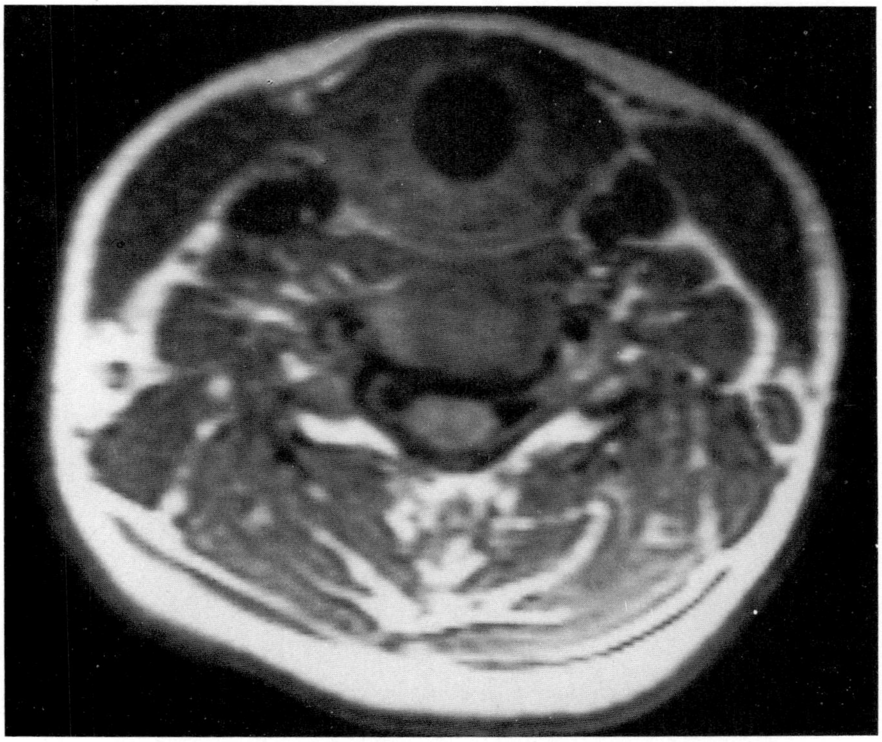

3-21 Axial MR scan through body of C-6 (800/20) (section 5 in Fig. 3-14).

3/Cervical Spine, Axial MRI

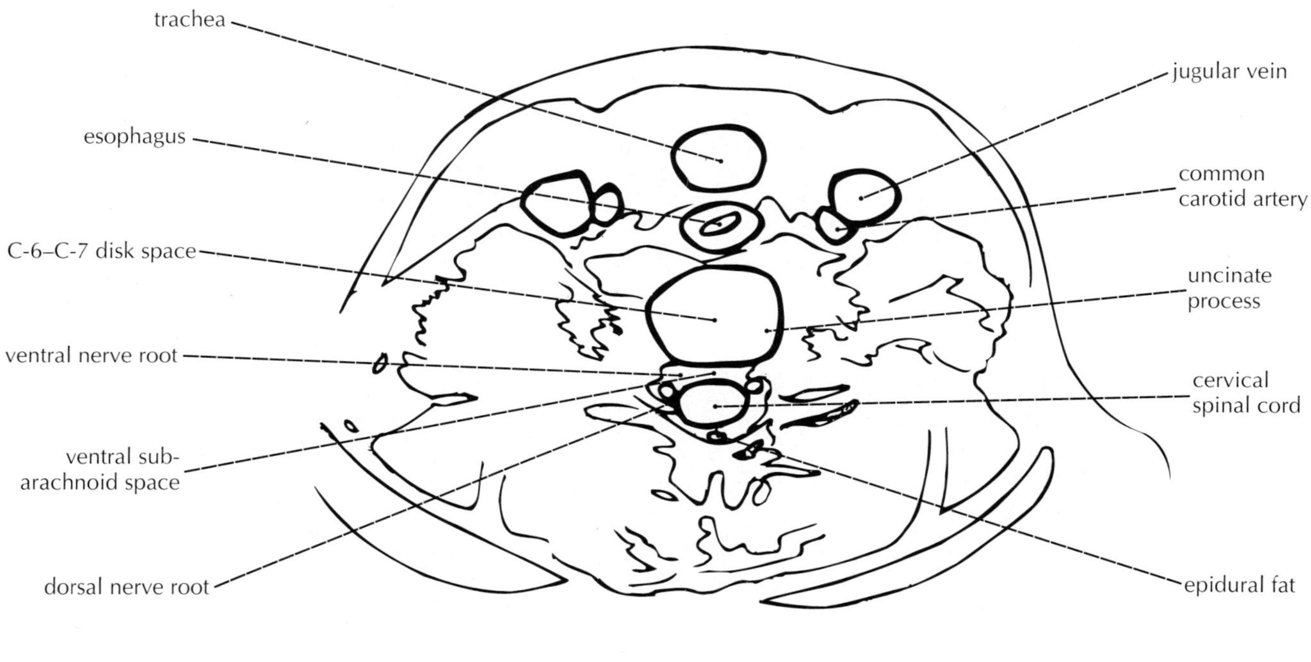

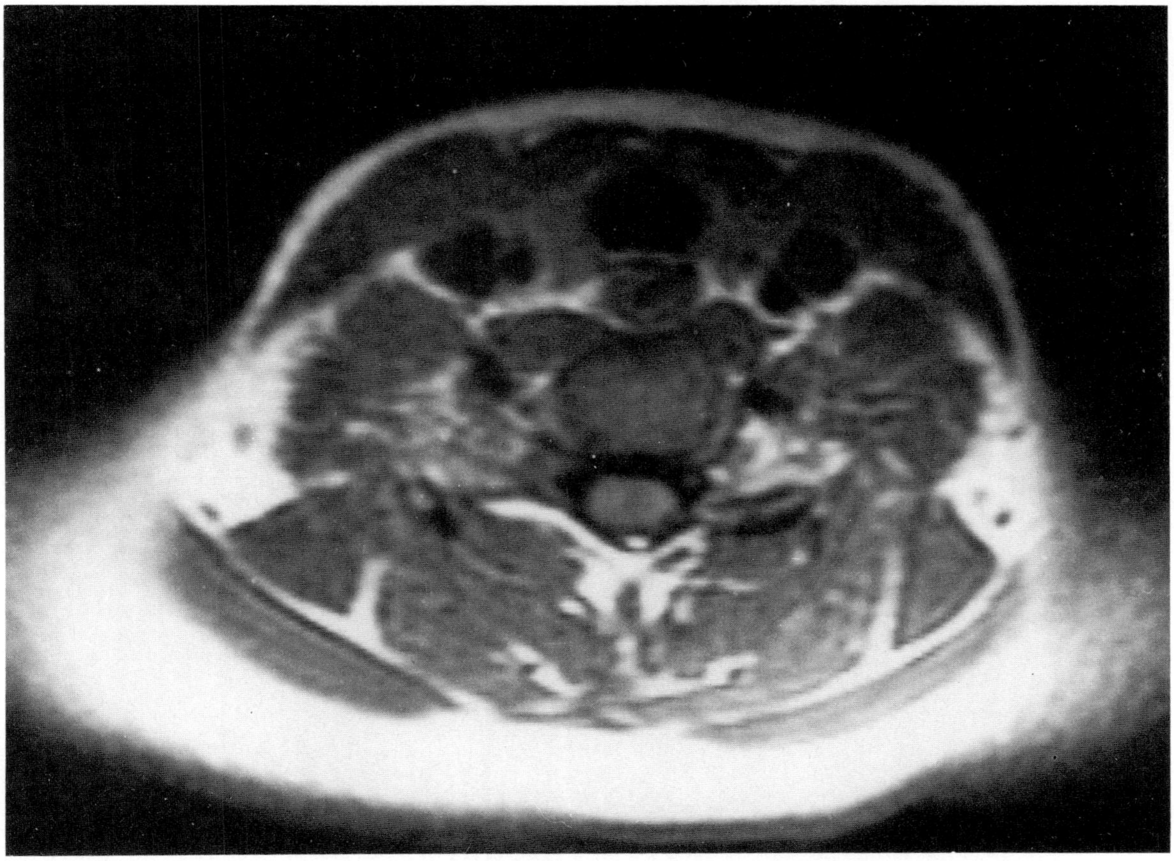

3-22 Axial MR scan through C-6–C-7 disk space (800/20) (section 6 in Fig. 3-14).

3/Neck, Arteriography

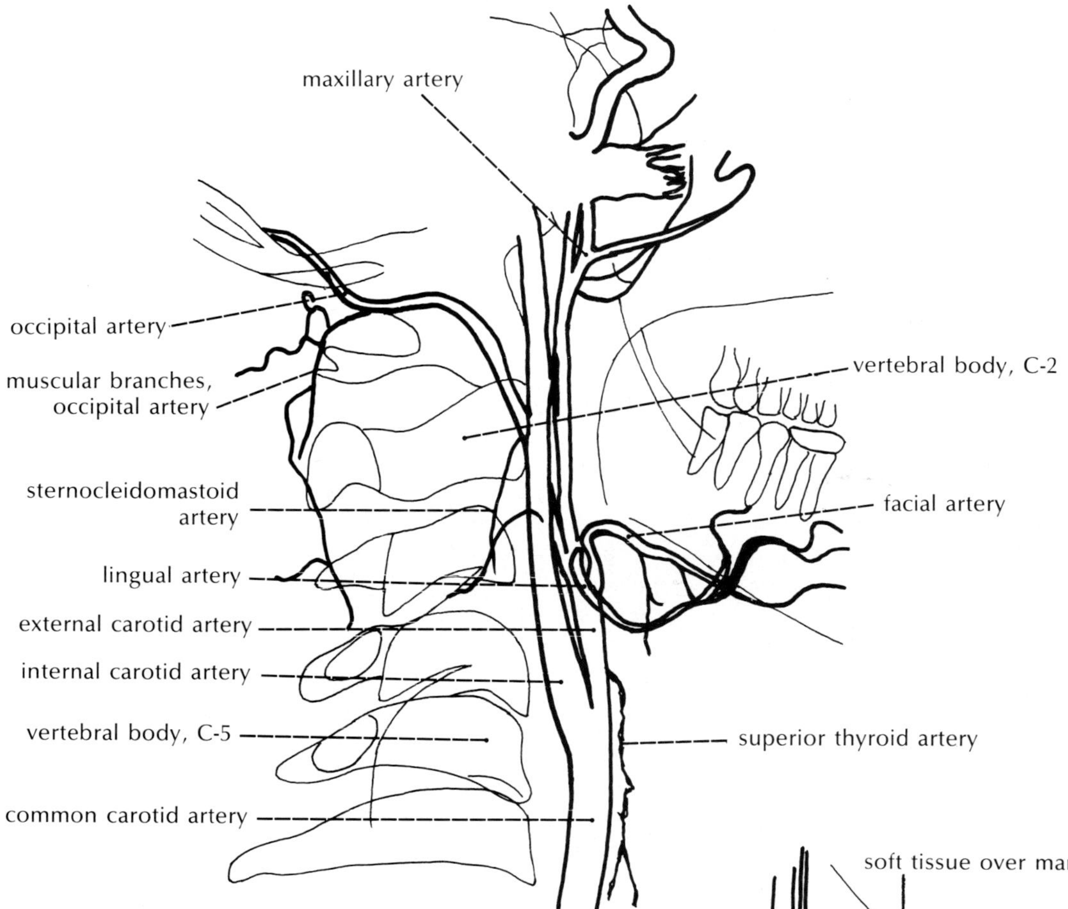

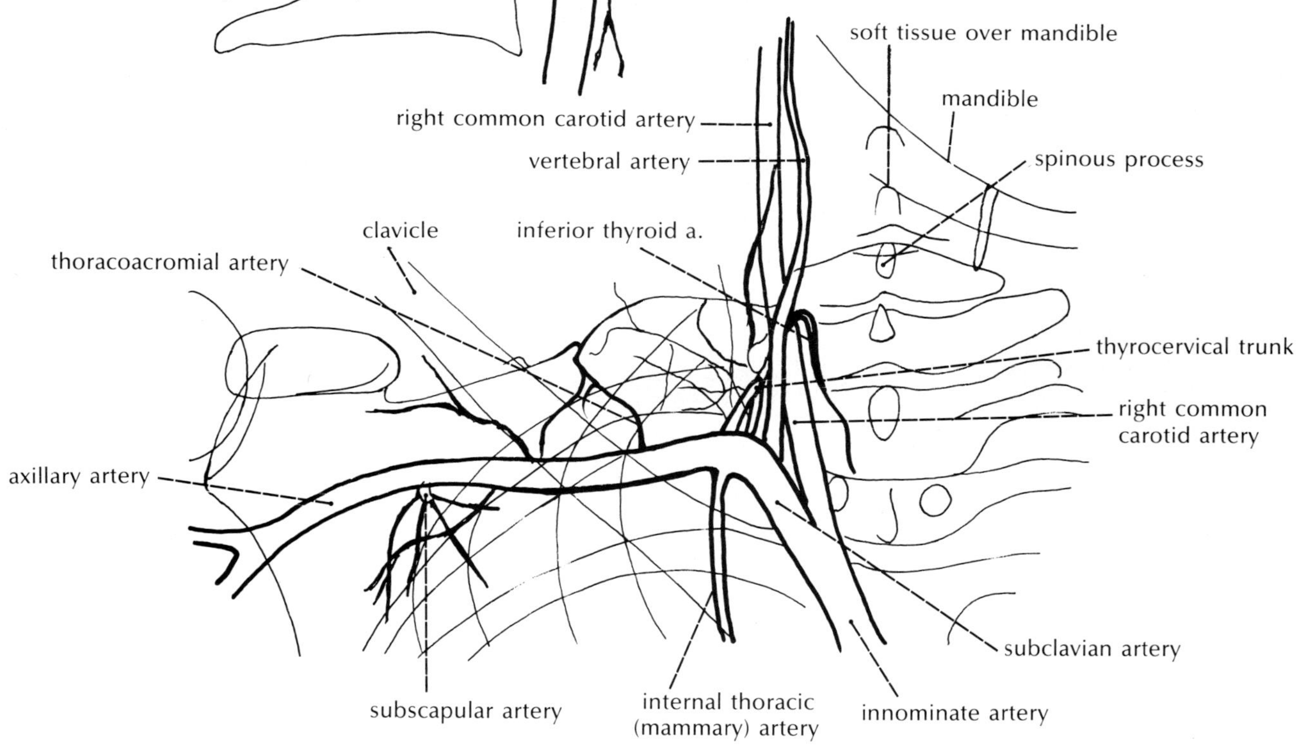

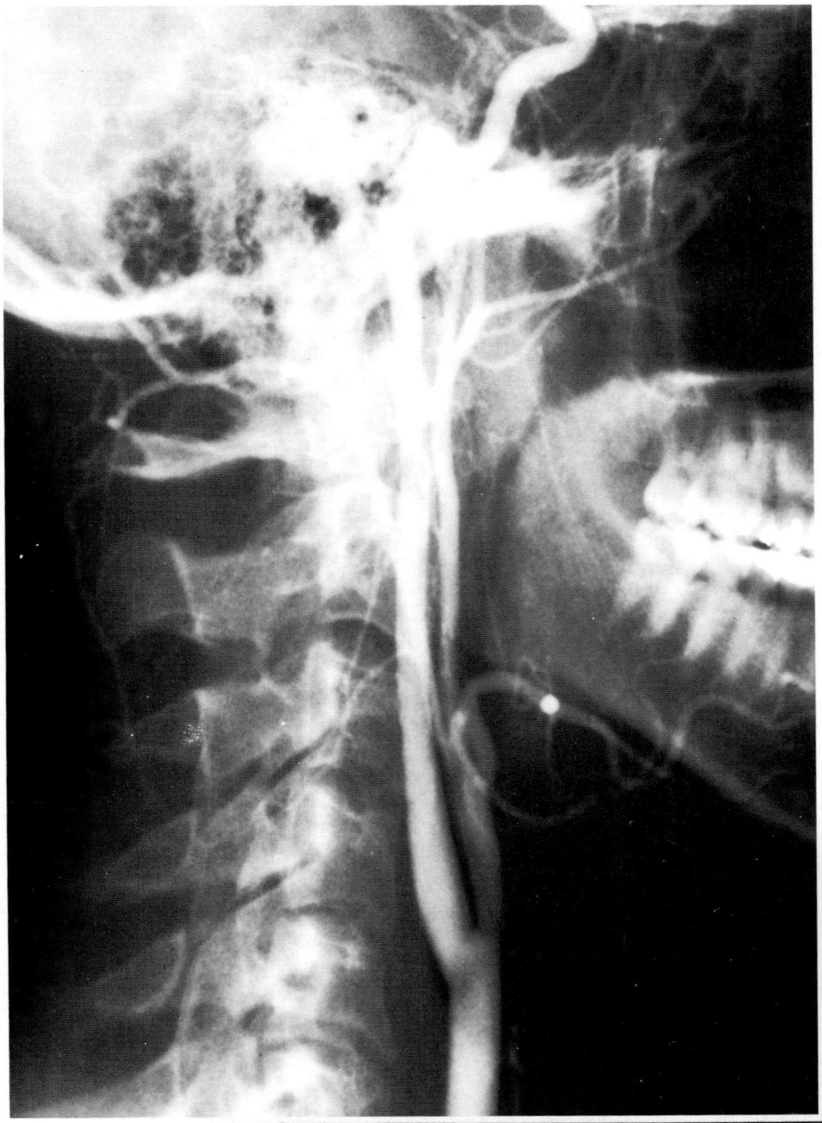

3-23 Arteries of the neck, lateral view.

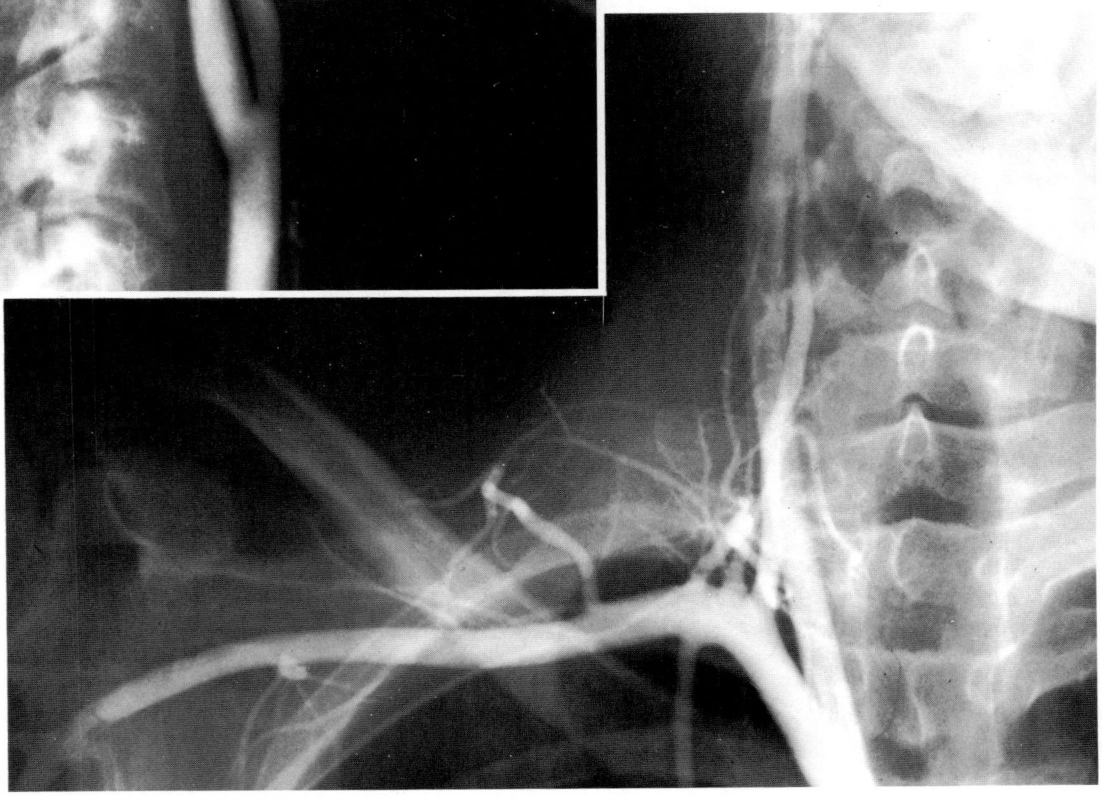

3-24 Arteries of the neck, AP view.

3/Neck, Angiography

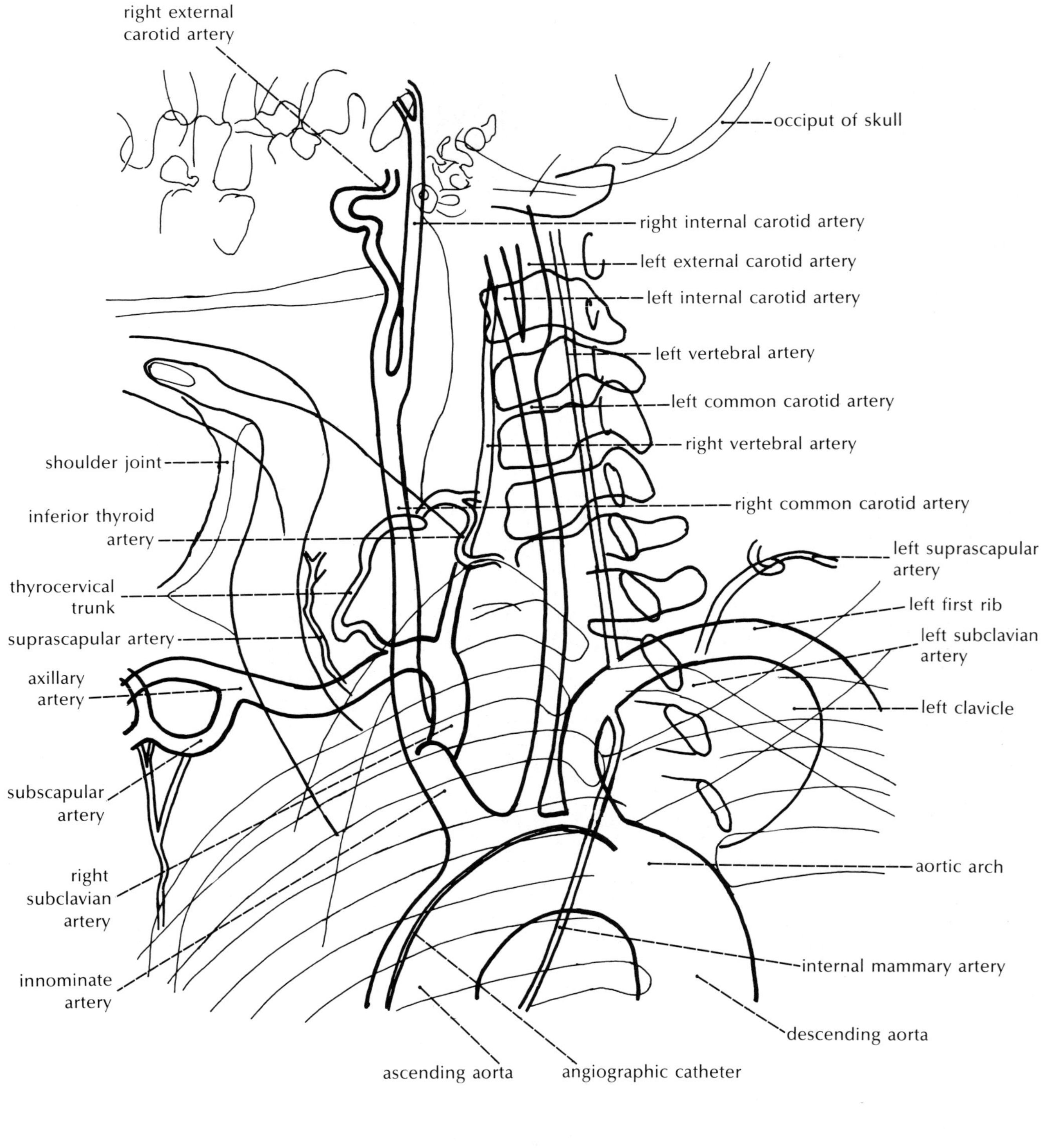

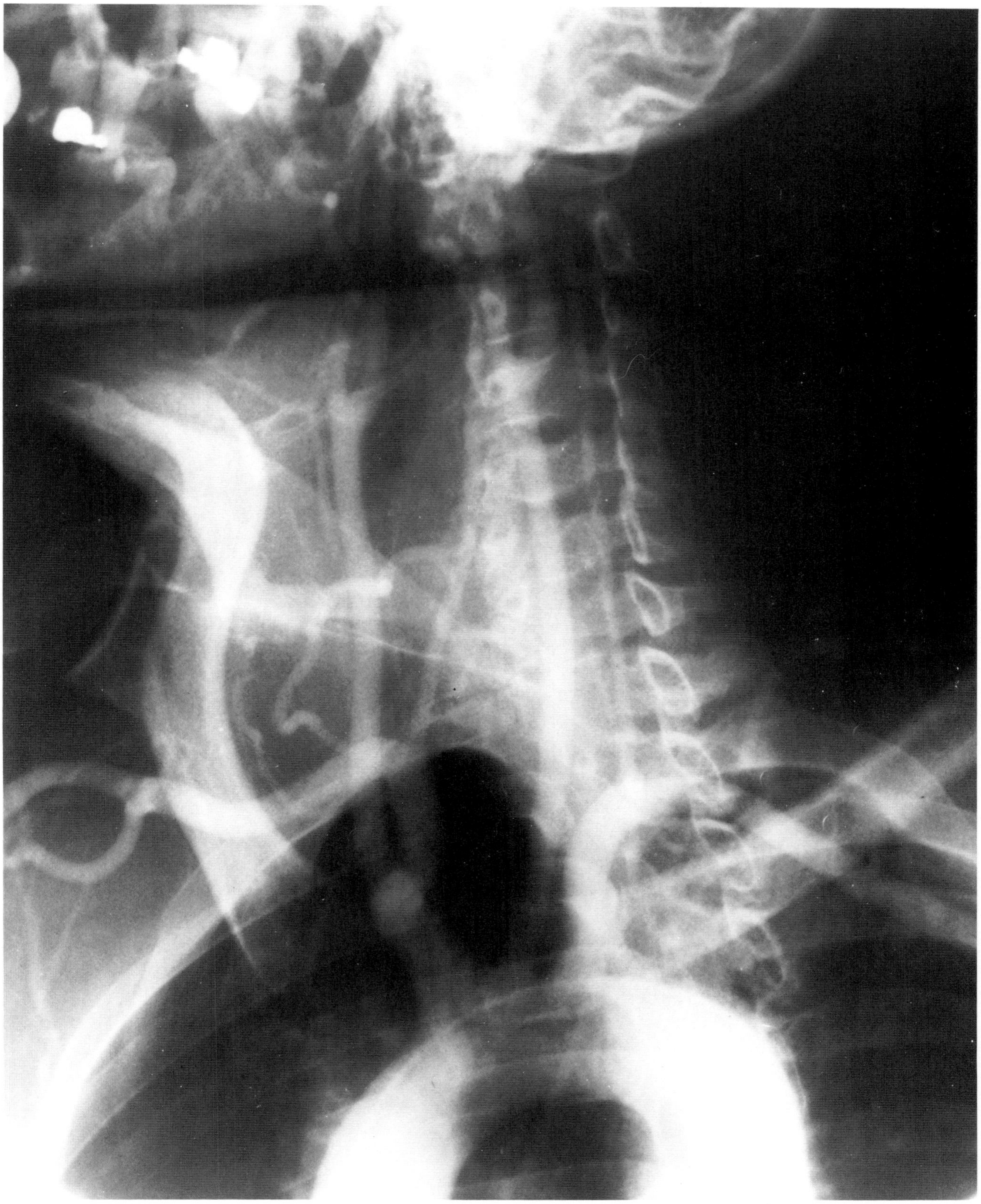

3-25 Angiogram of aortic arch and its branches. (Contrast medium injected from catheter in proximal aortic arch.)

3/Neck, MR Angiography

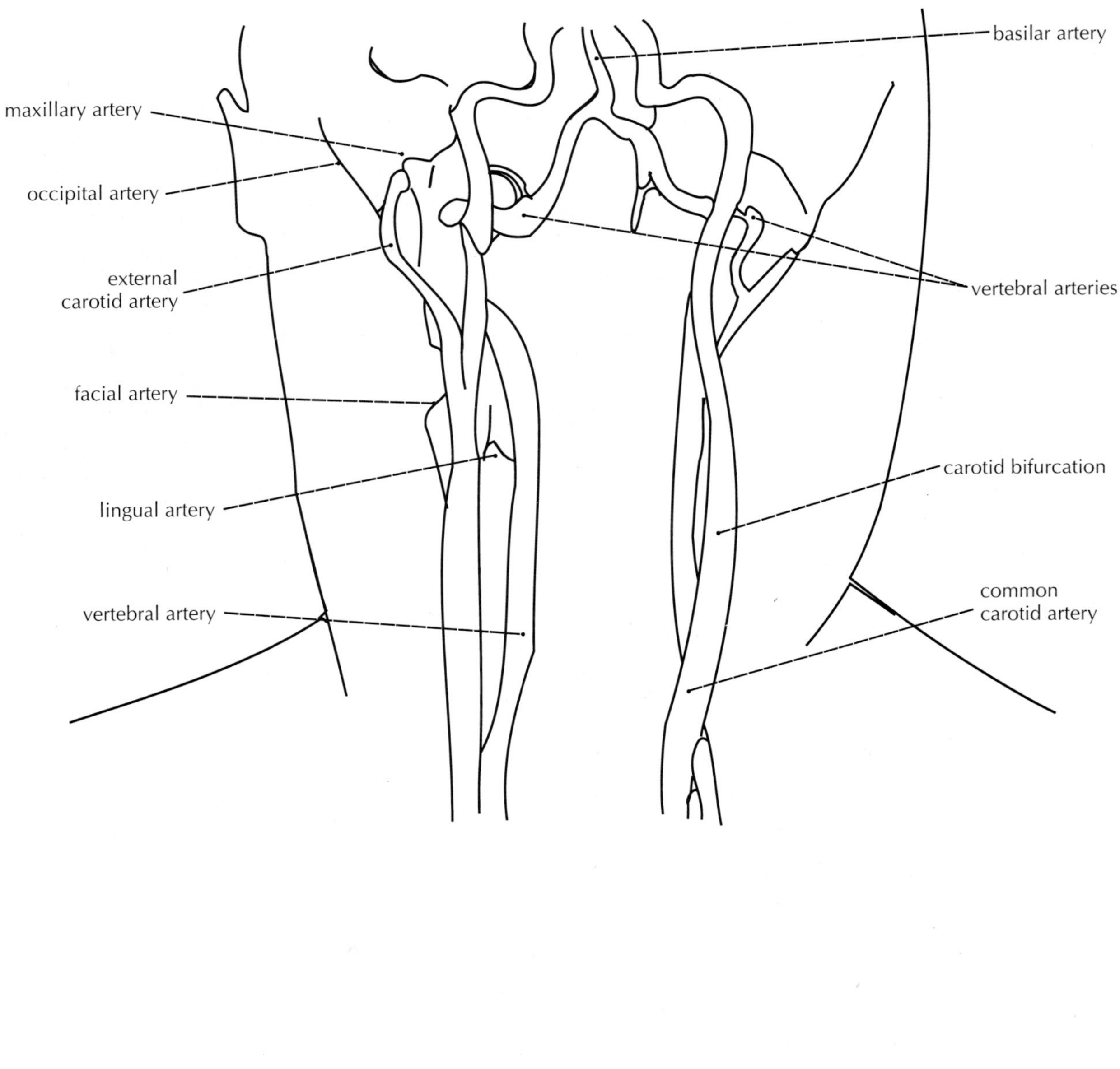

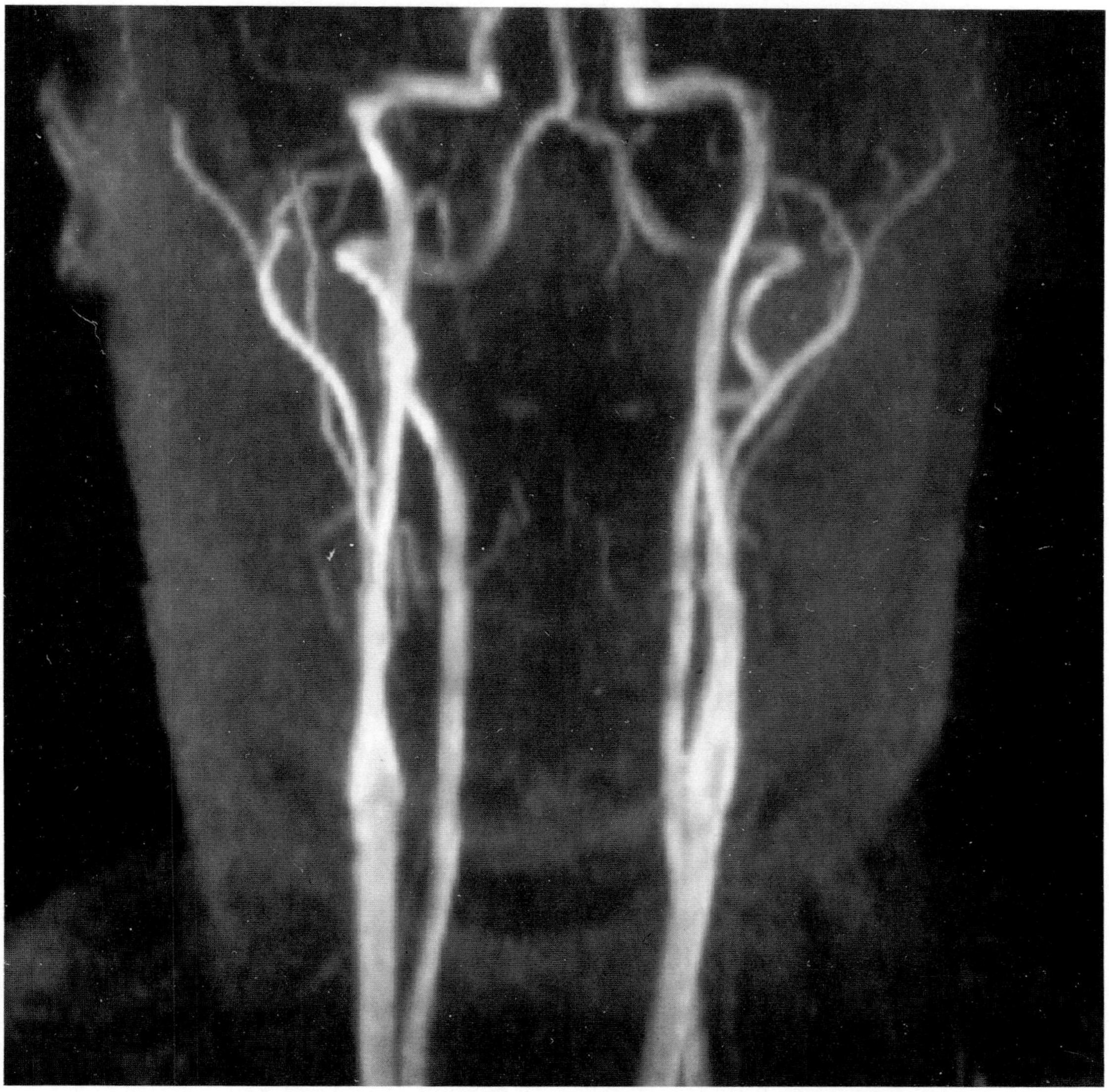

3-26 MR angiogram of neck vessels, frontal view (noncontrast study).

3/Neck, MR Angiography

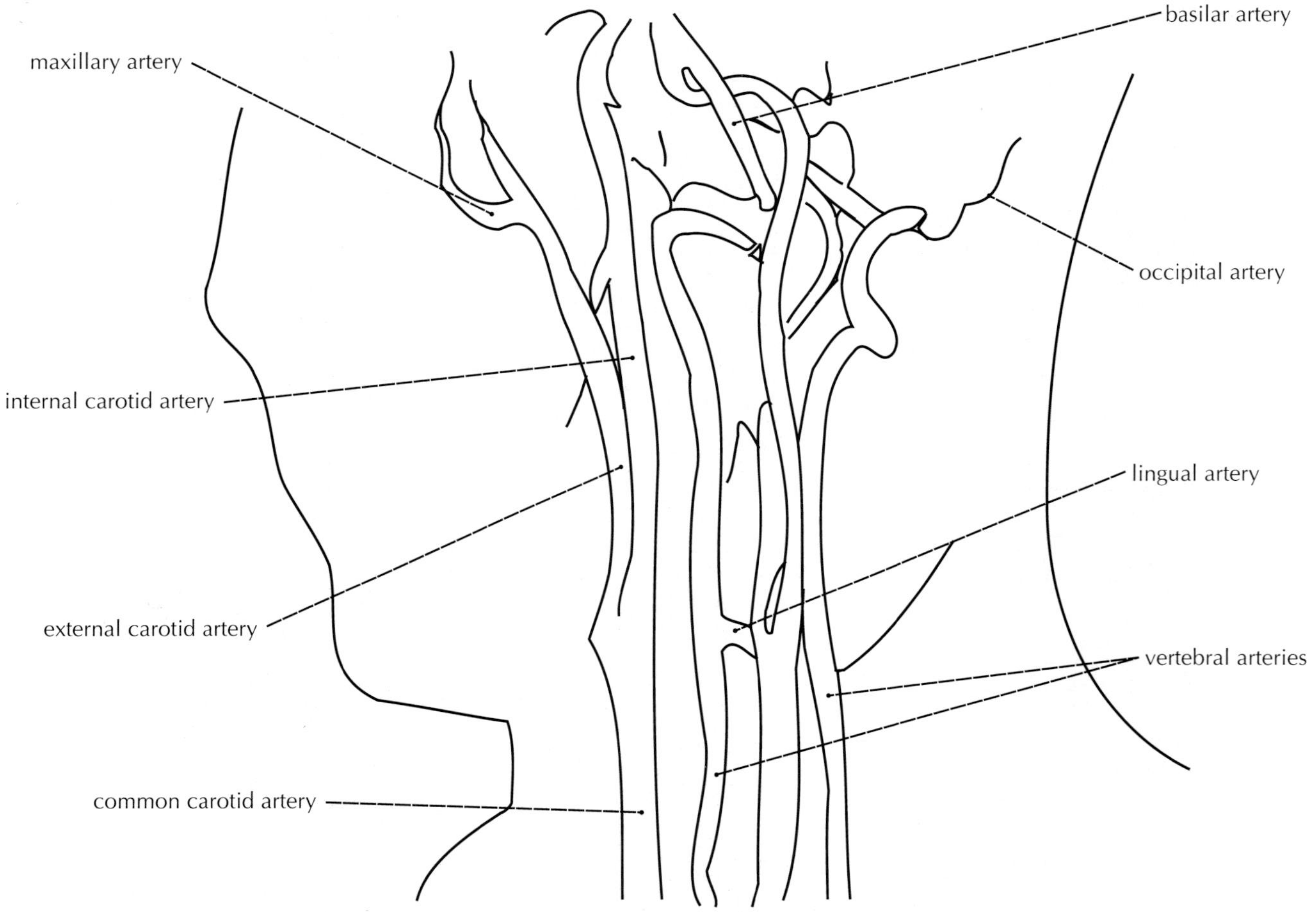

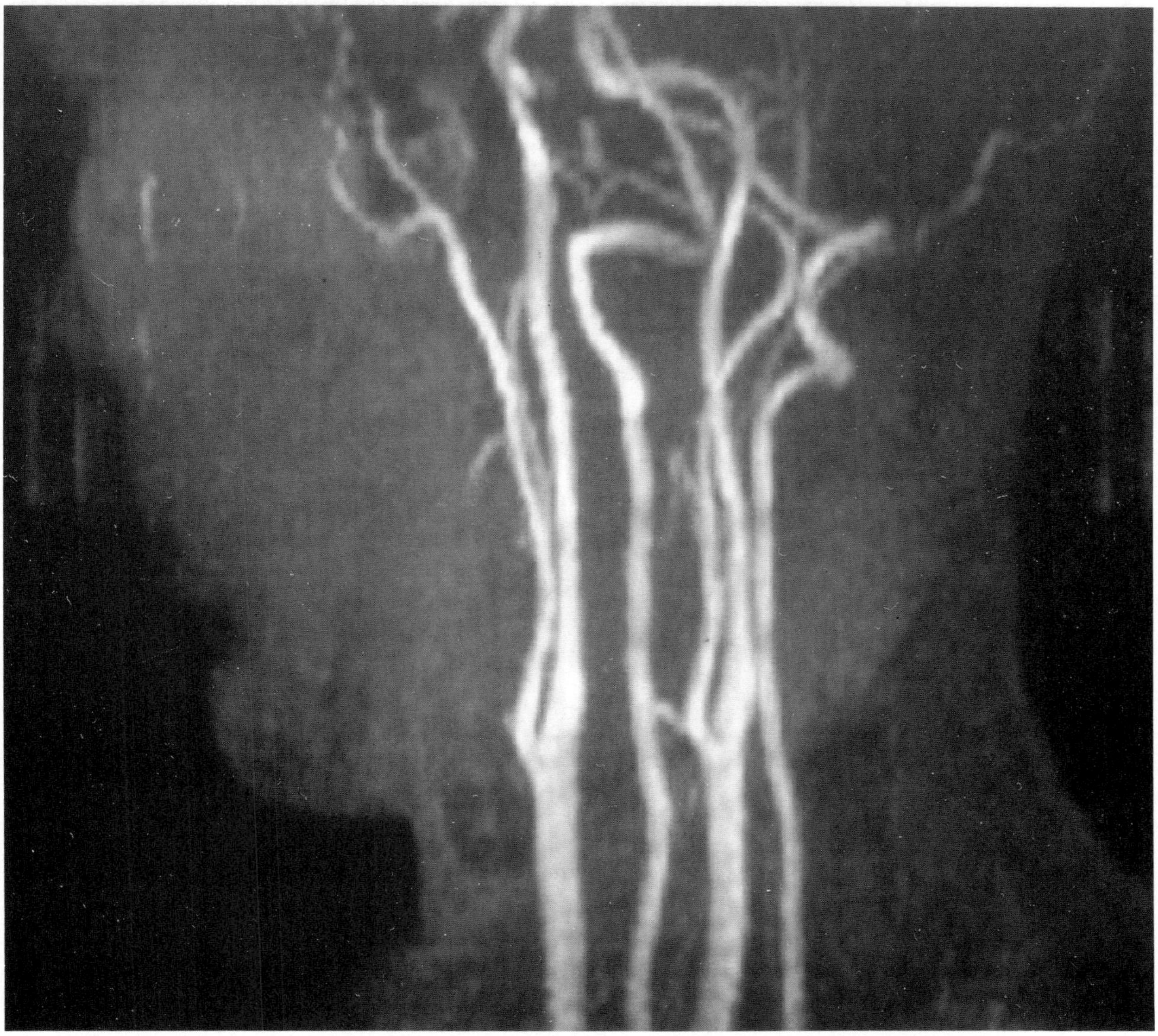

3-27 MR angiogram of neck vessels, oblique view (noncontrast study).

3/Cervical Spine, Myelography

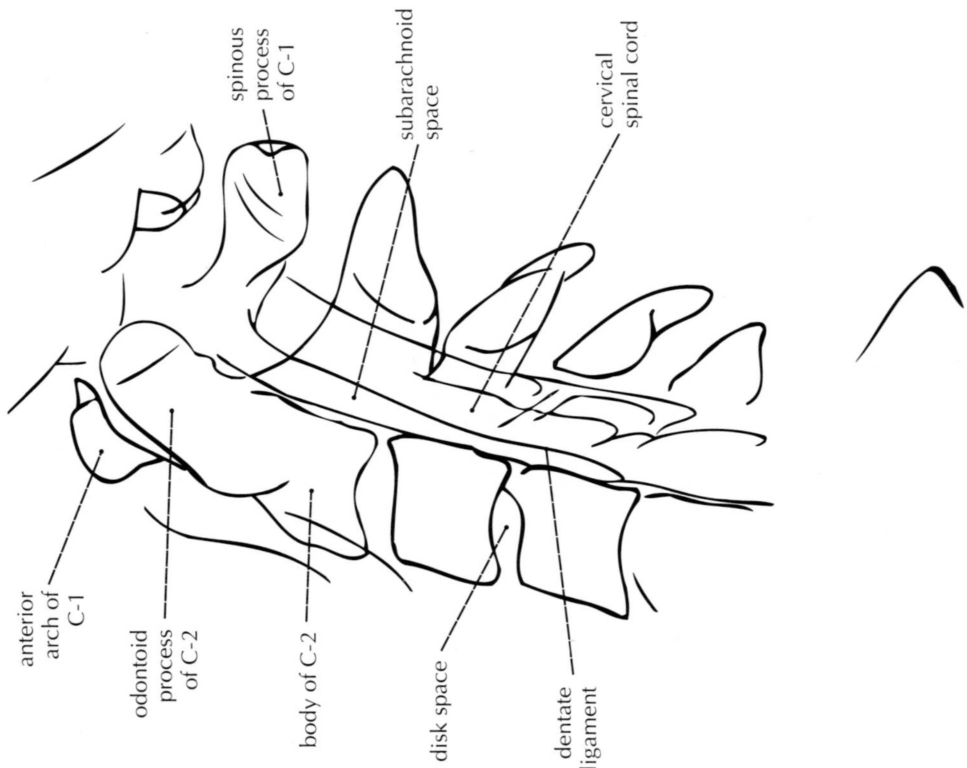

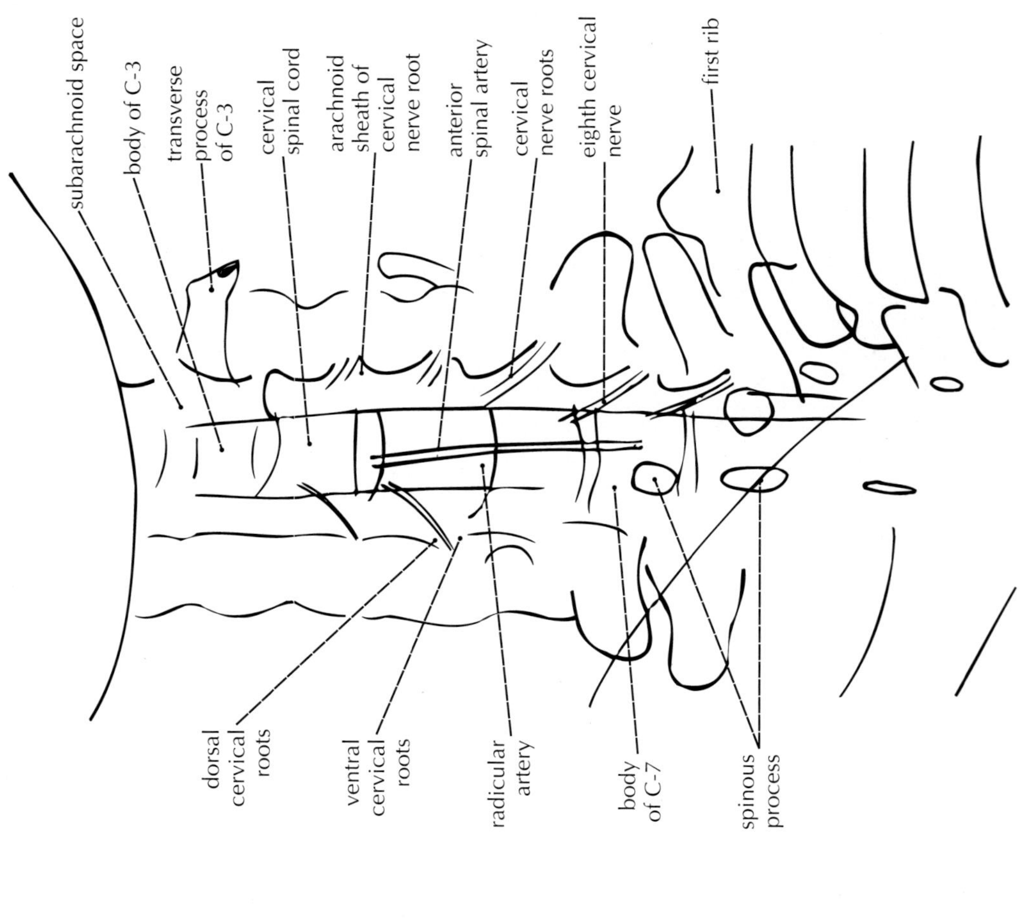

3/Cervical Spine, Myelography

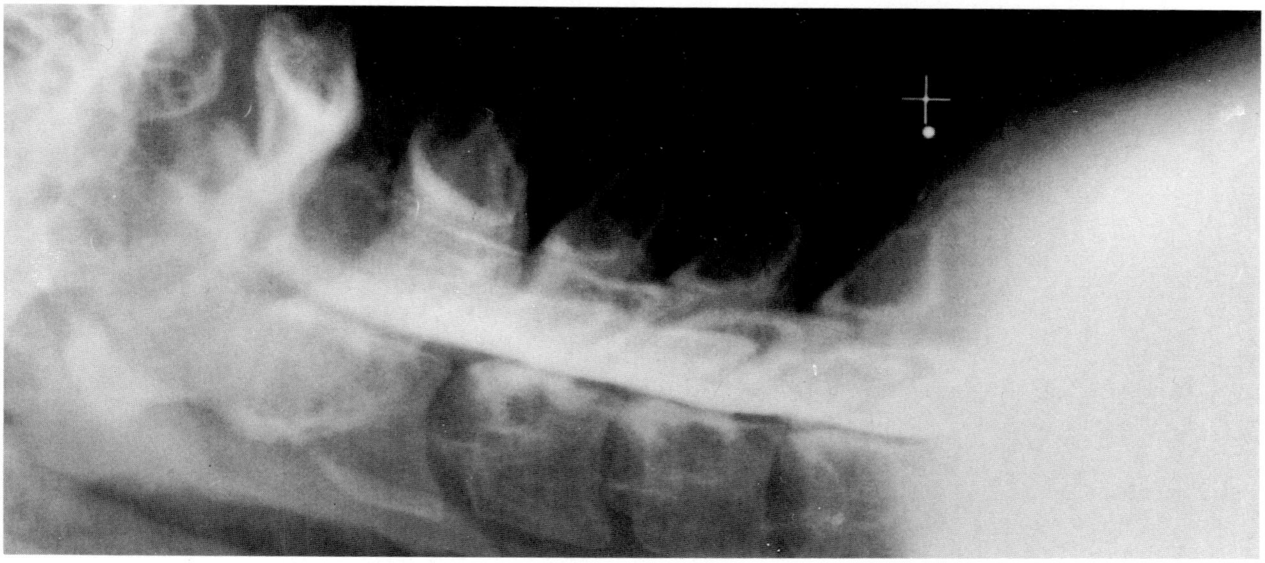

3-29 Cervical myelogram, lateral view.

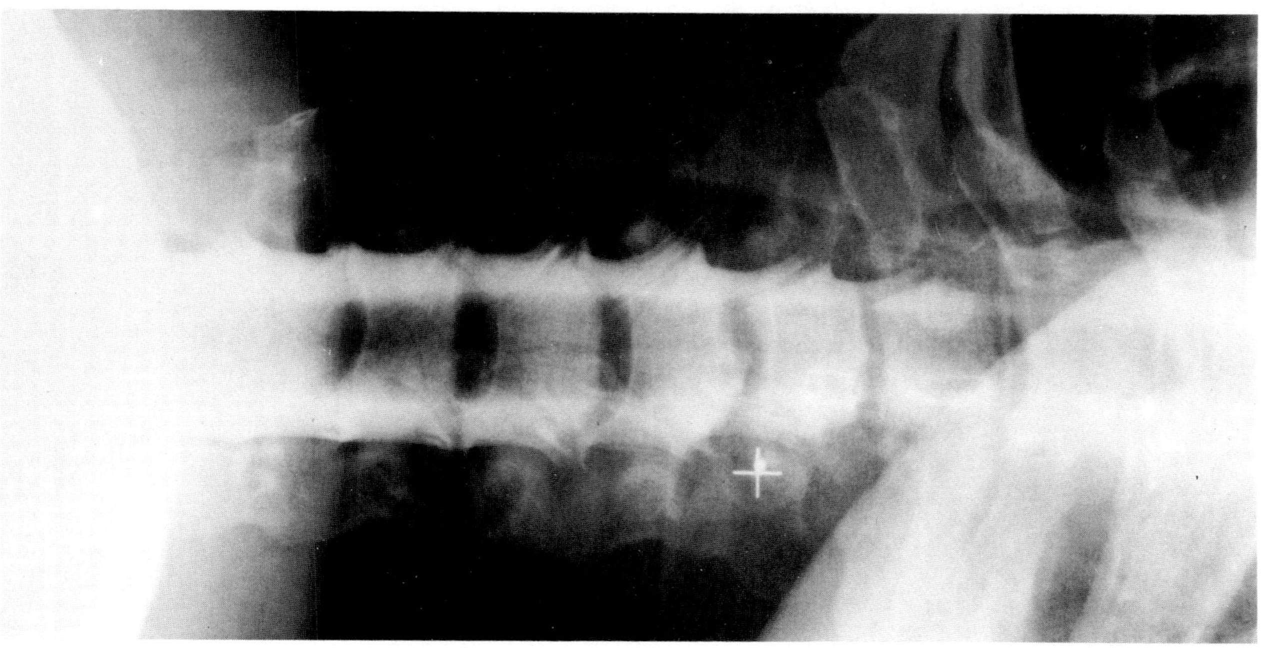

3-28 Cervical myelogram, AP view.

3/Cervical Spine, Myelography

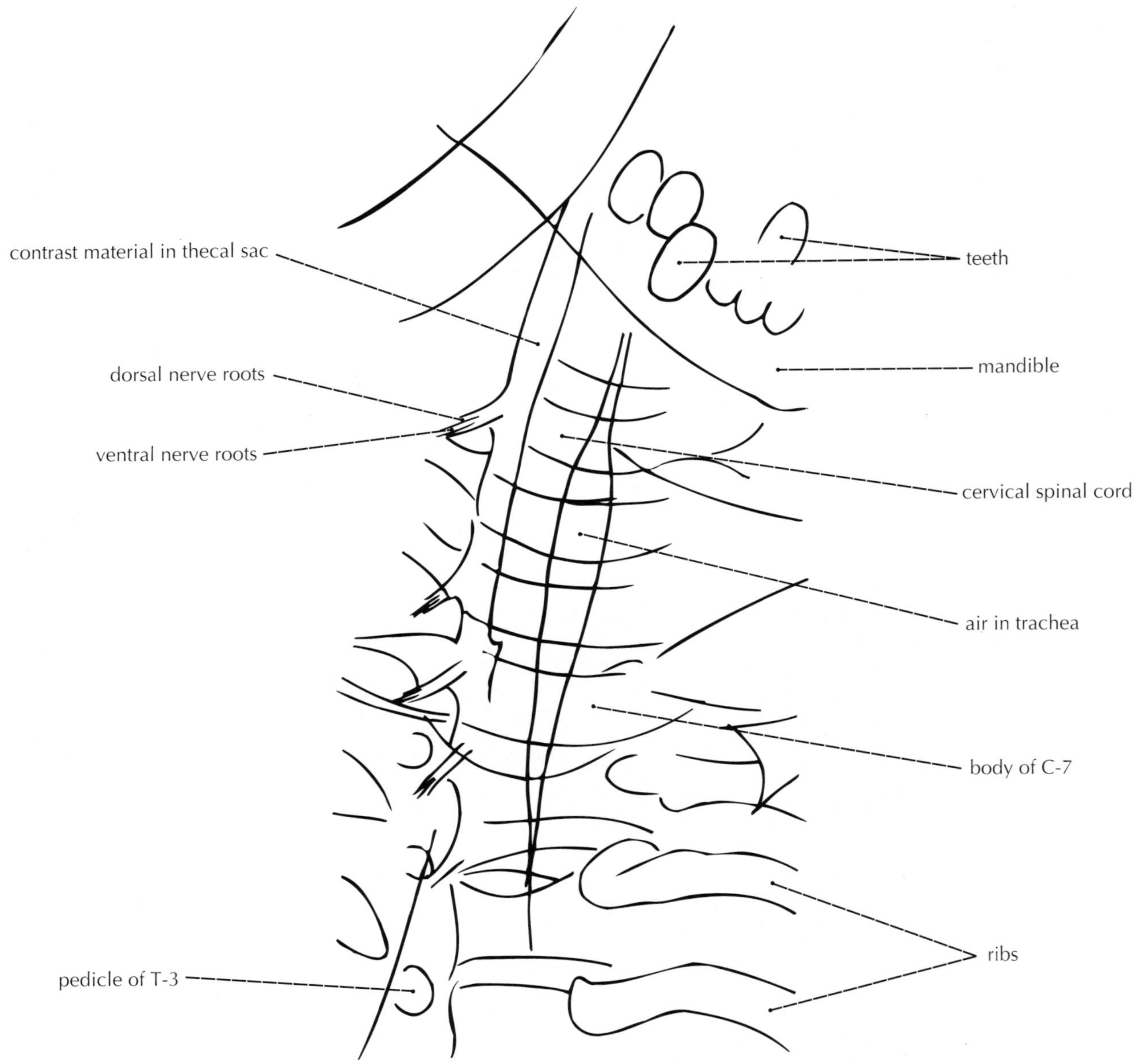

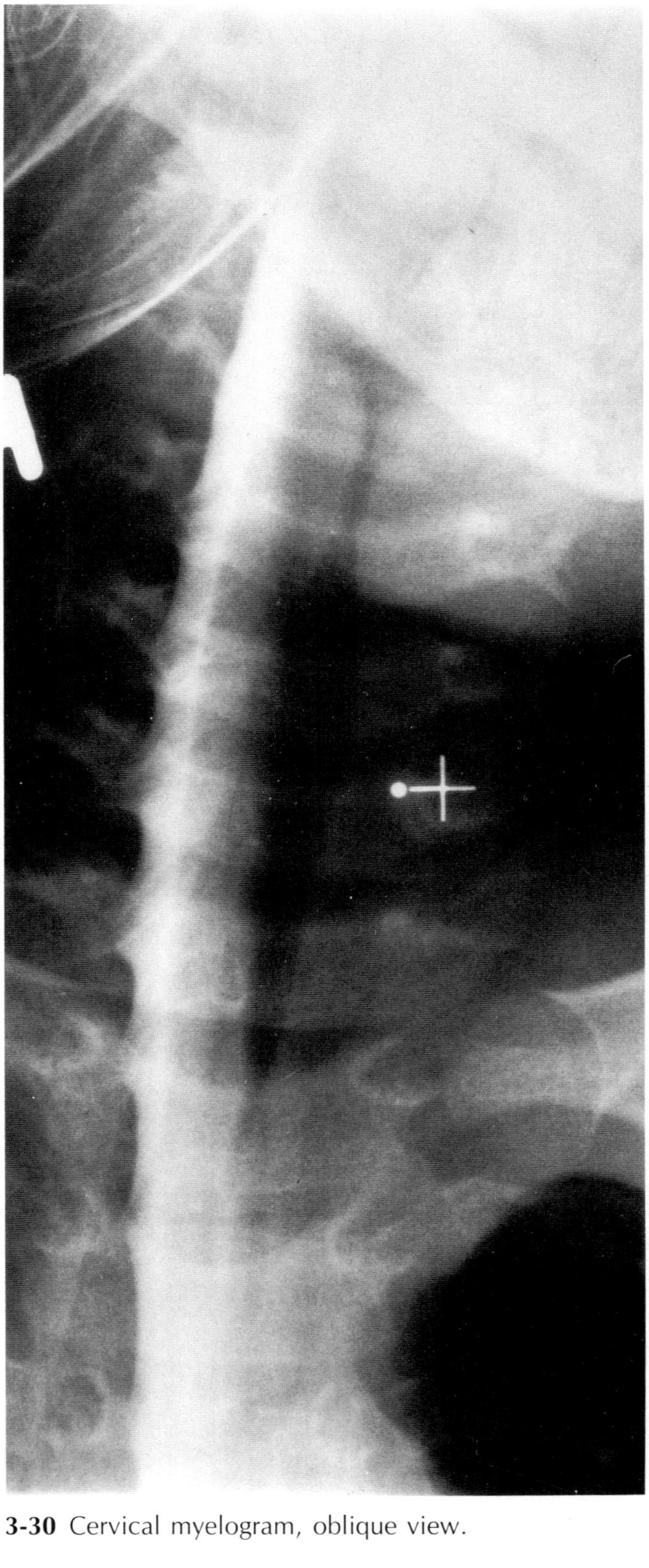

3-30 Cervical myelogram, oblique view.

4/Thoracic Spine □ Thoracic Spine, X-Ray

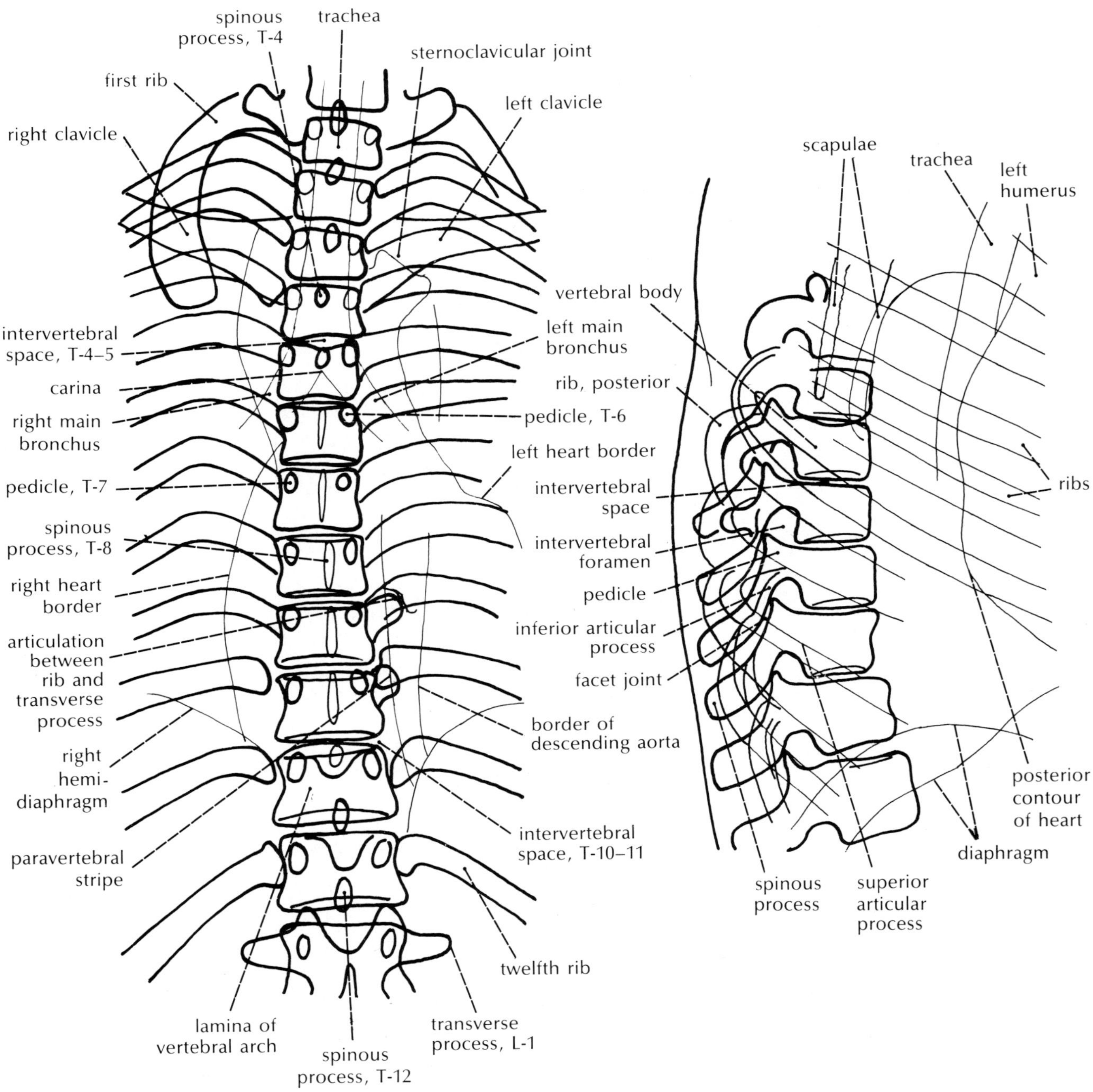

4/Thoracic Spine, X-Ray

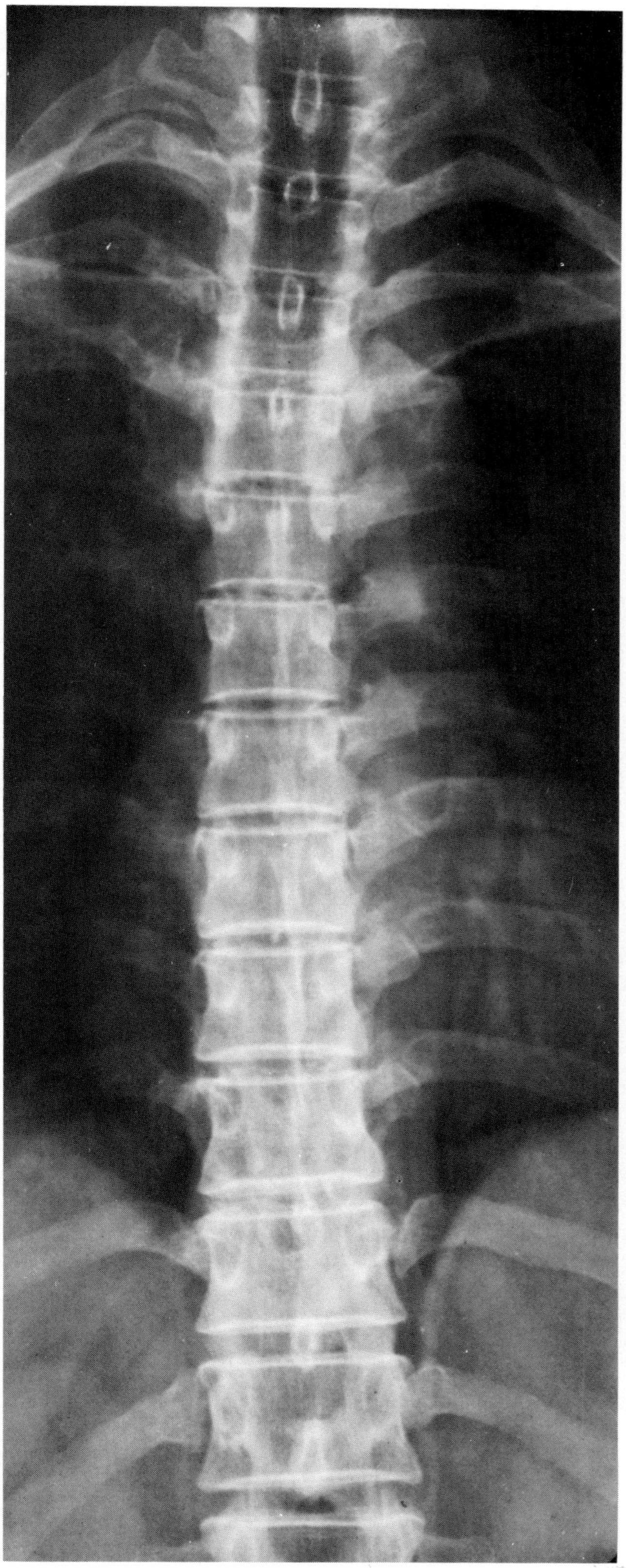

4-1 Thoracic spine, AP view.

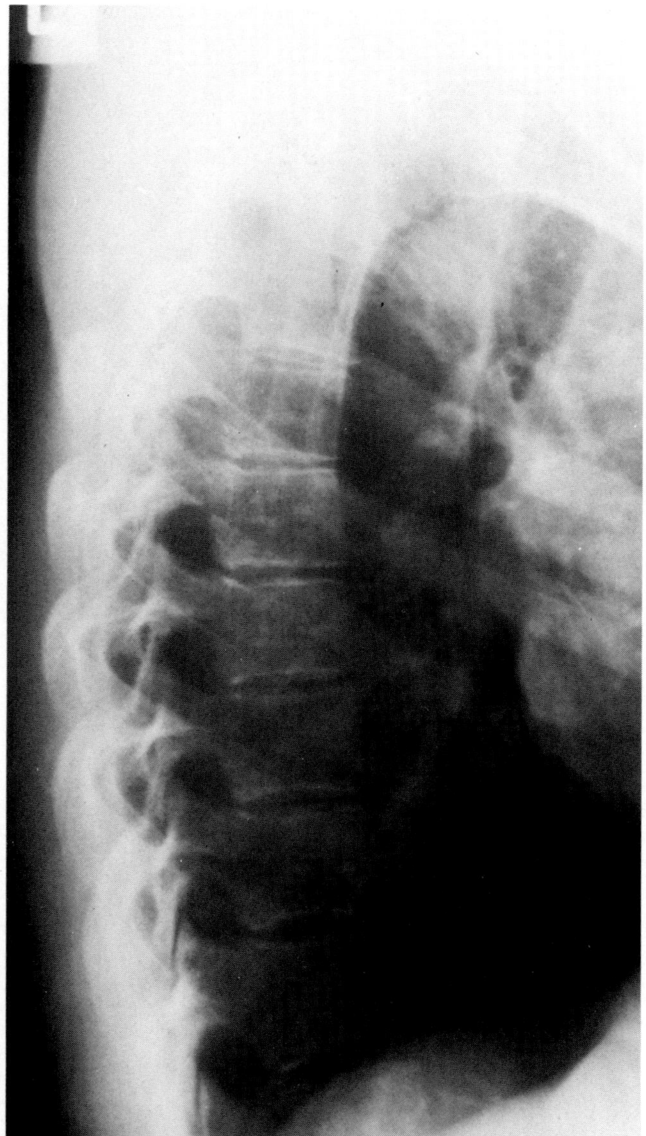

4-2 Thoracic spine, lateral view.

4/Thoracic Spine, Sagittal Scout CT and Axial CT

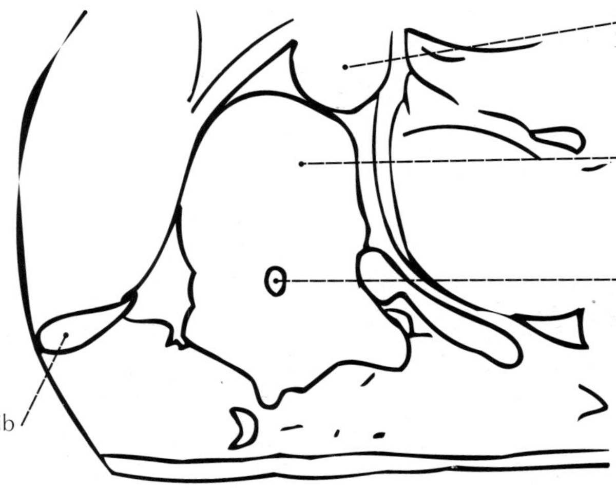

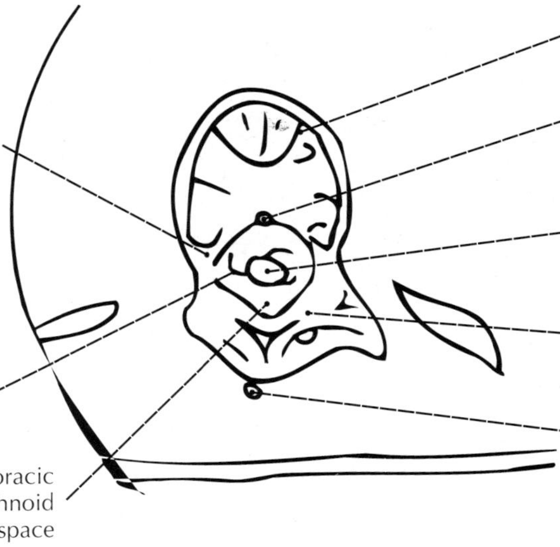

4/Thoracic Spine, Sagittal Scout CT and Axial CT

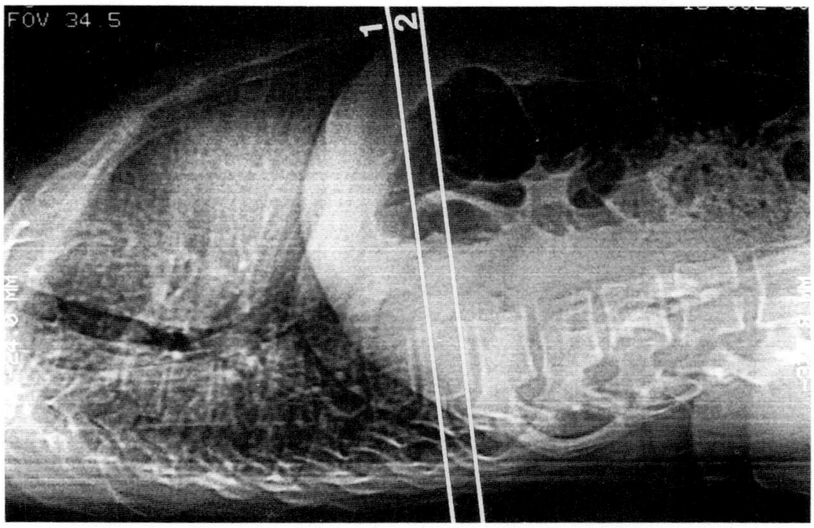

4-3 Sagittal scout CT for demonstration of the axial images.

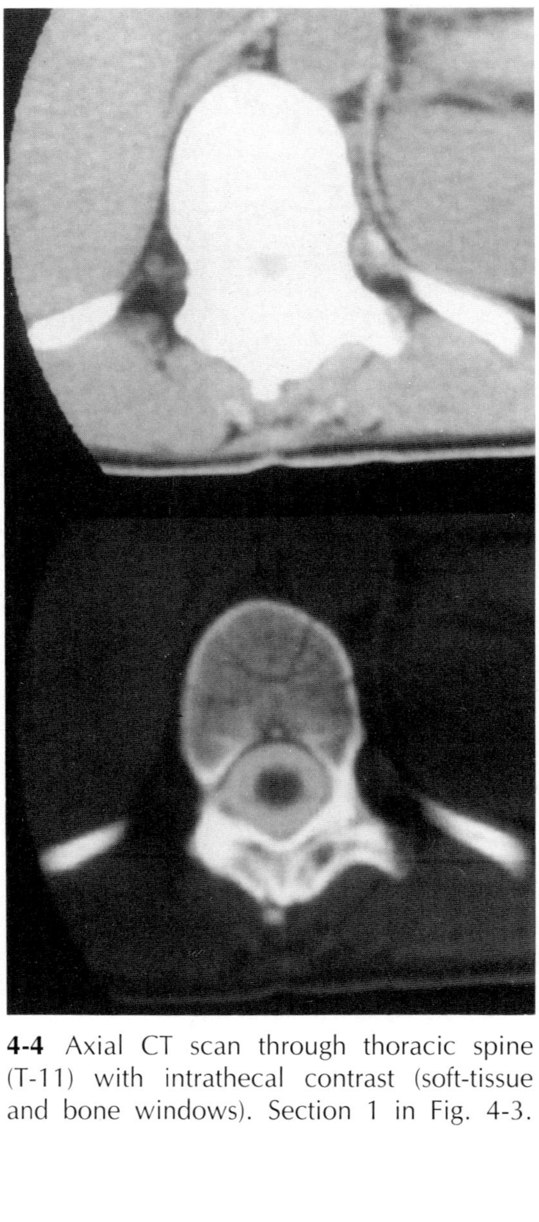

4-4 Axial CT scan through thoracic spine (T-11) with intrathecal contrast (soft-tissue and bone windows). Section 1 in Fig. 4-3.

4/Thoracic Spine, Axial CT

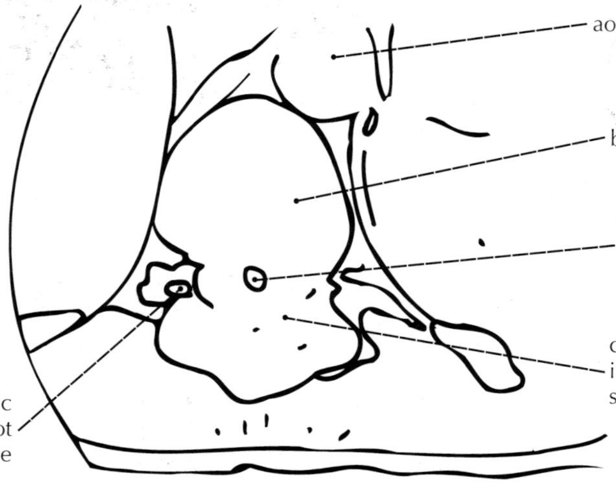

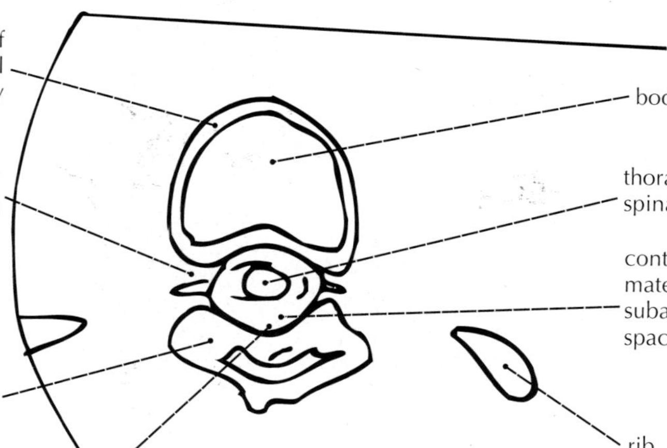

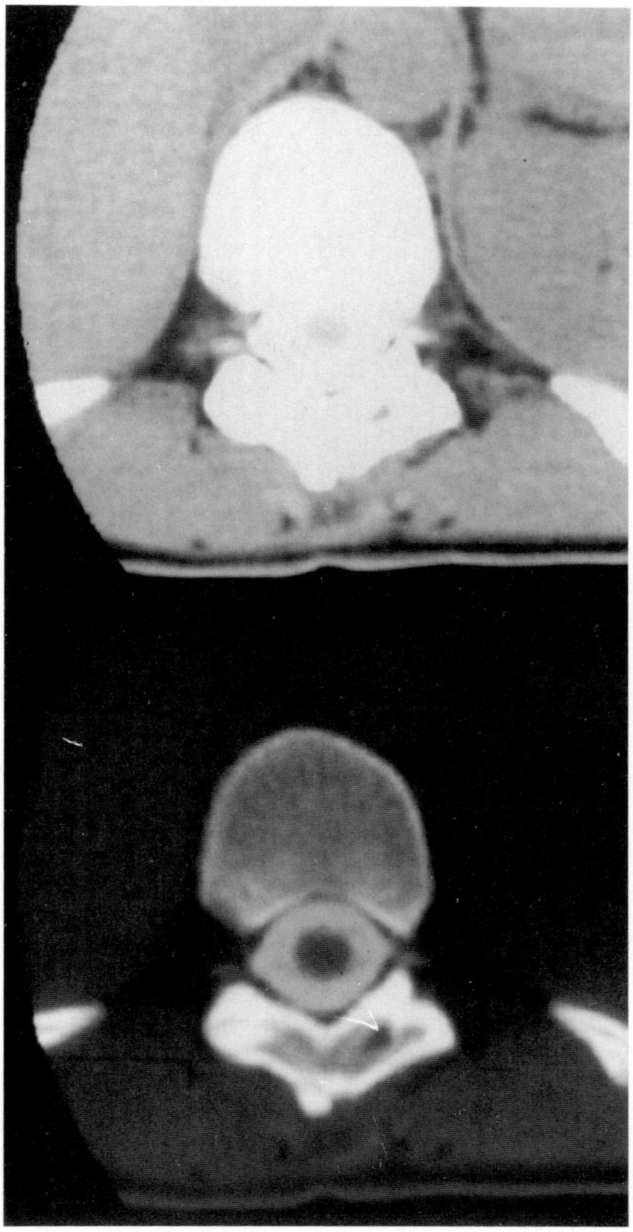

4-5 Axial CT scan through thoracic spine (T-11) at neural foramen, with intrathecal contrast (soft-tissue and bone windows). Section 2 in Fig. 4-3.

4/Thoracic Spine, Sagittal MRI

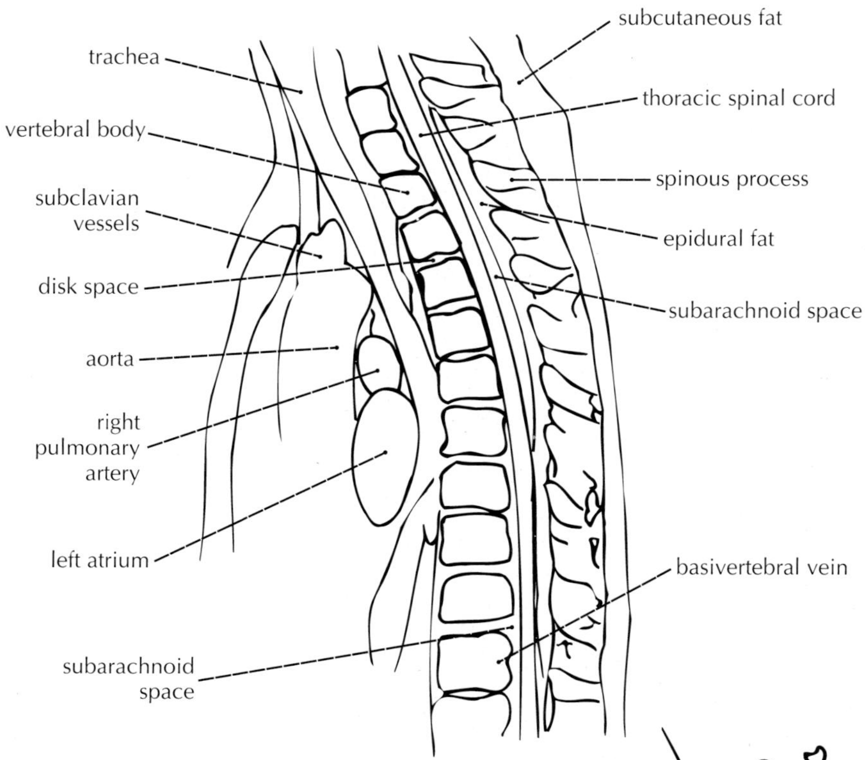

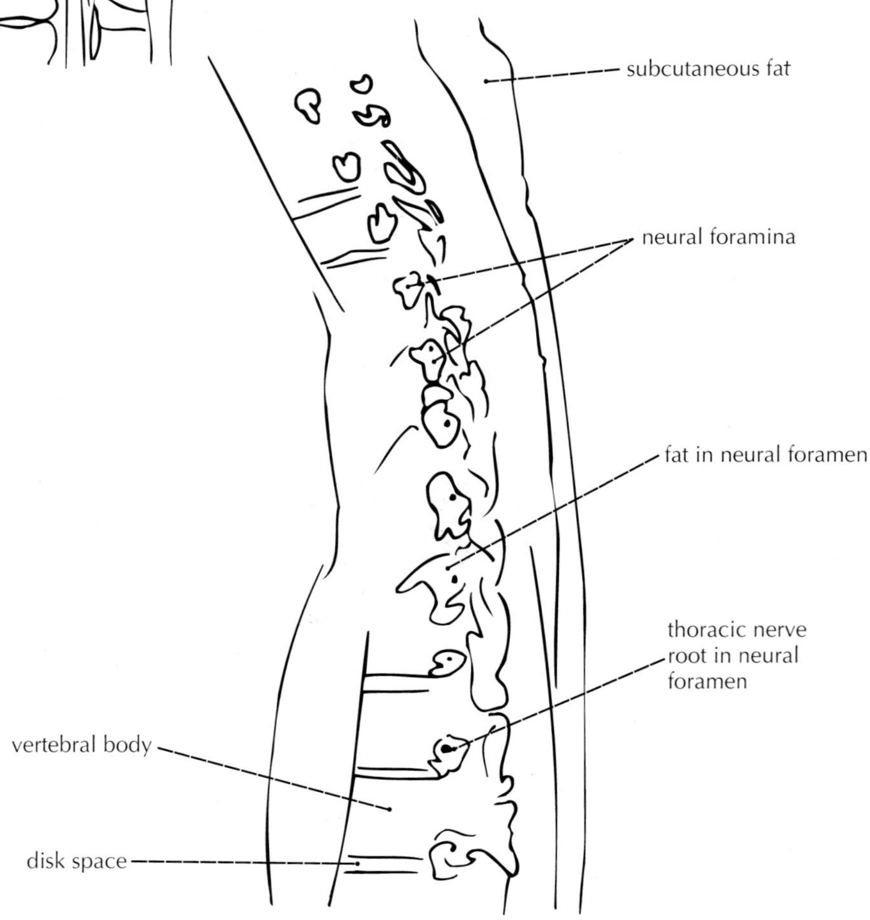

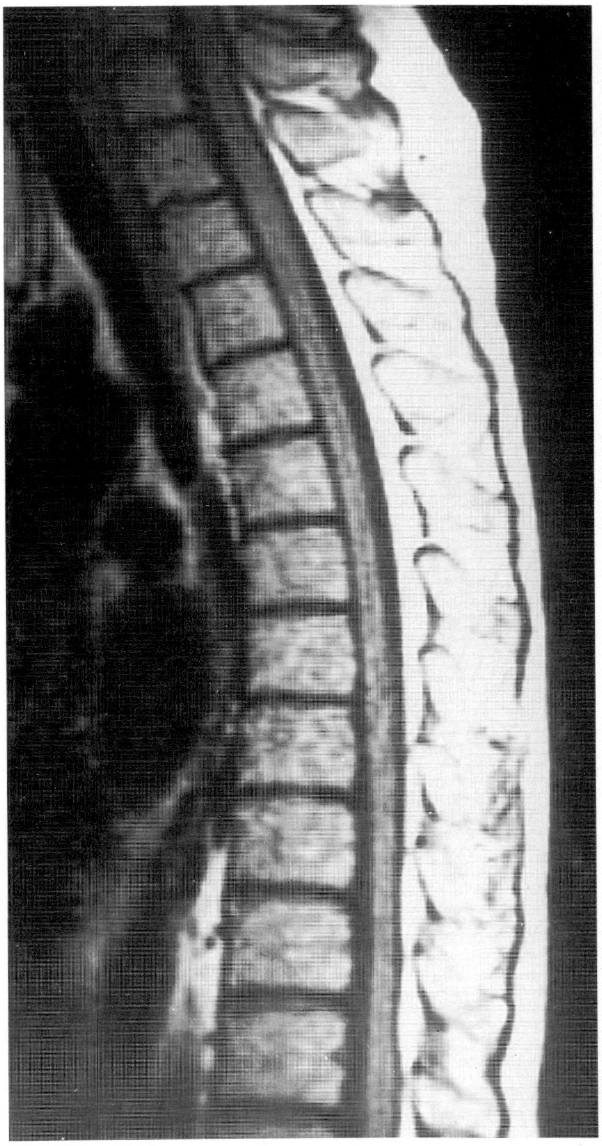

4-6 Midline sagittal MR scan through thoracic spine (600/20).

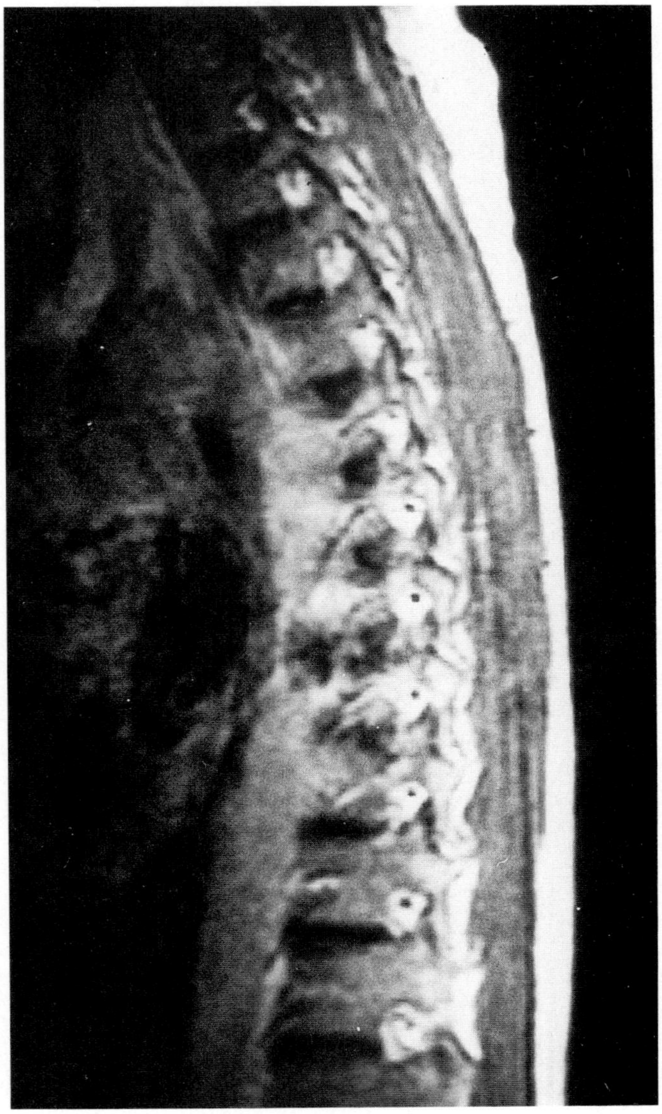

4-7 Paramidline sagittal MR scan through thoracic spine (2000/30).

4/Thoracic Spine, Sagittal MRI

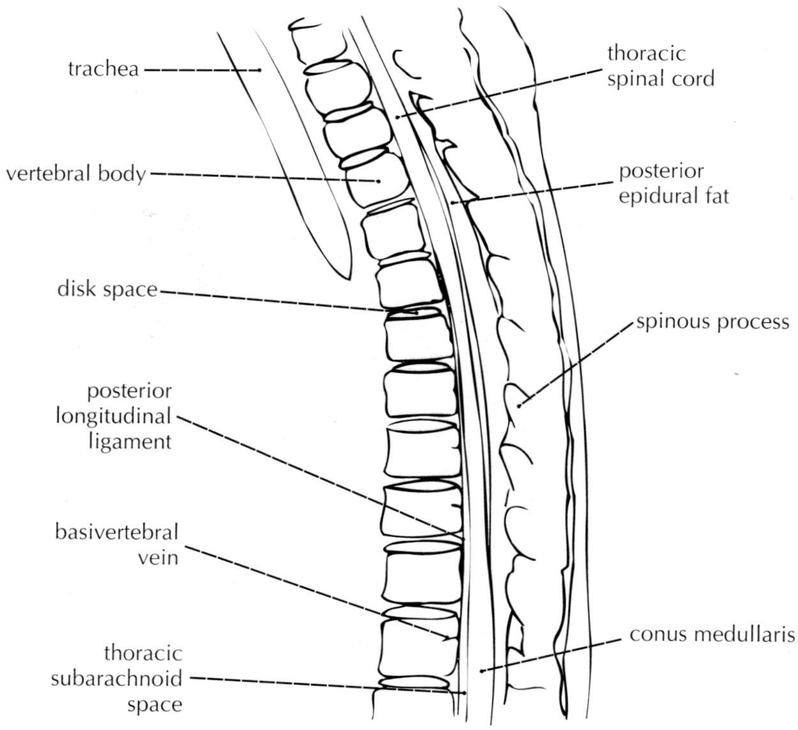

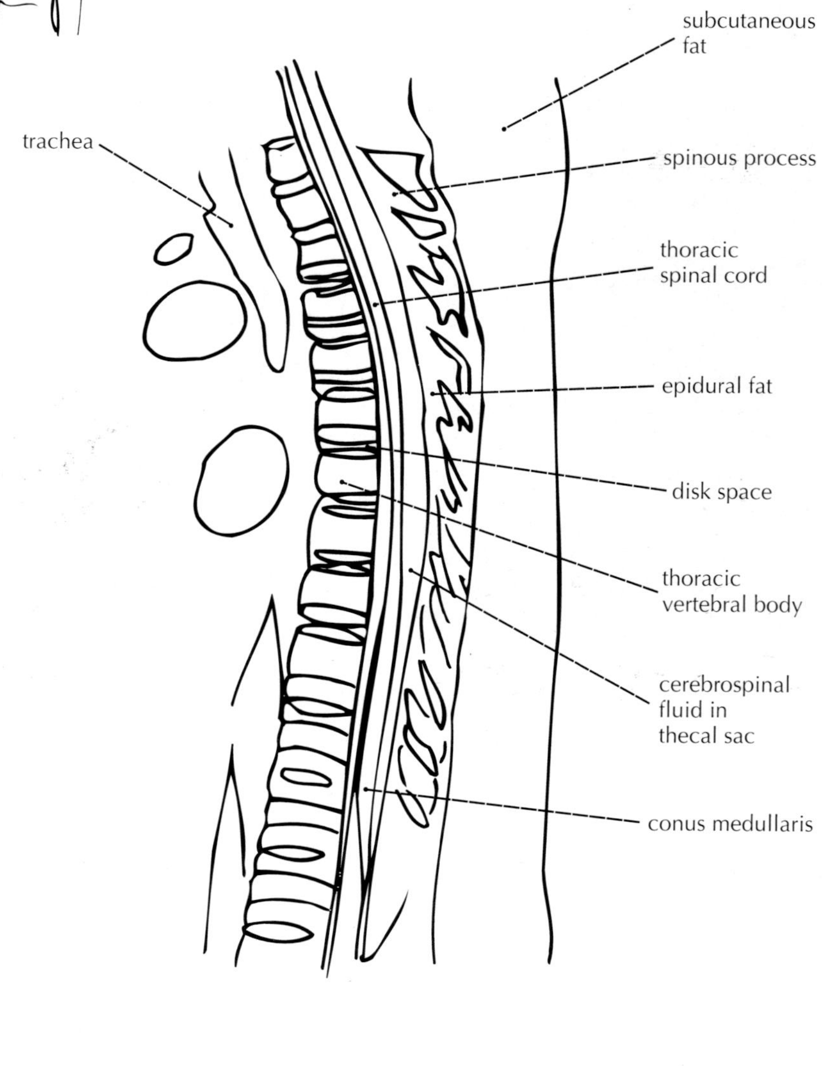

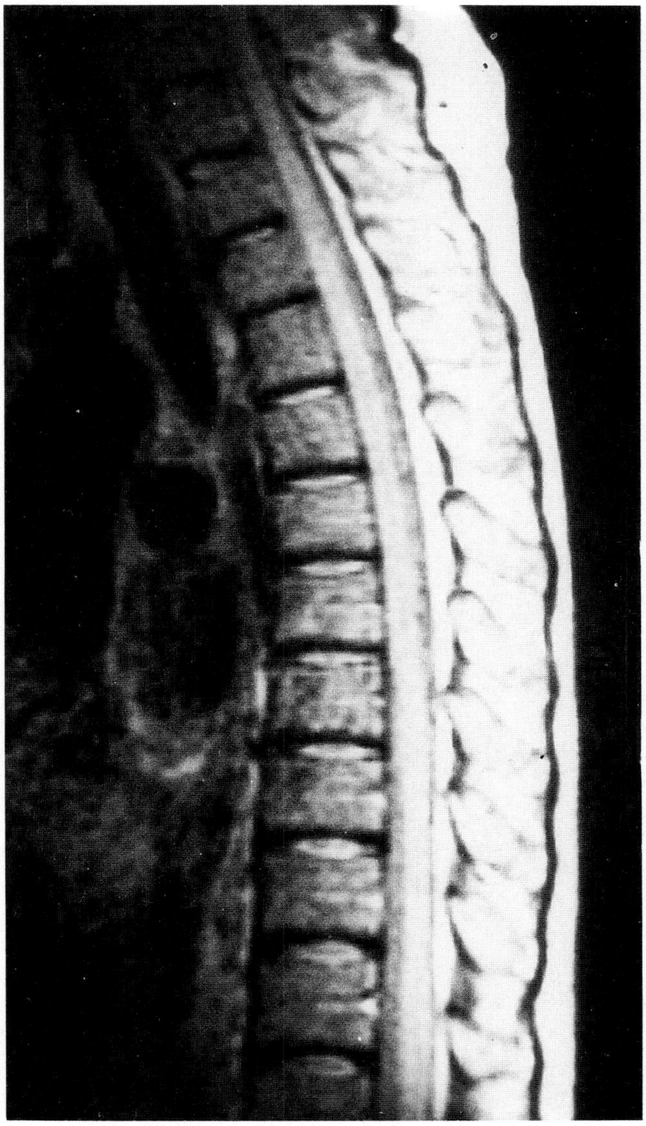

4-8 Midline sagittal MR scan through thoracic spine (2000/30).

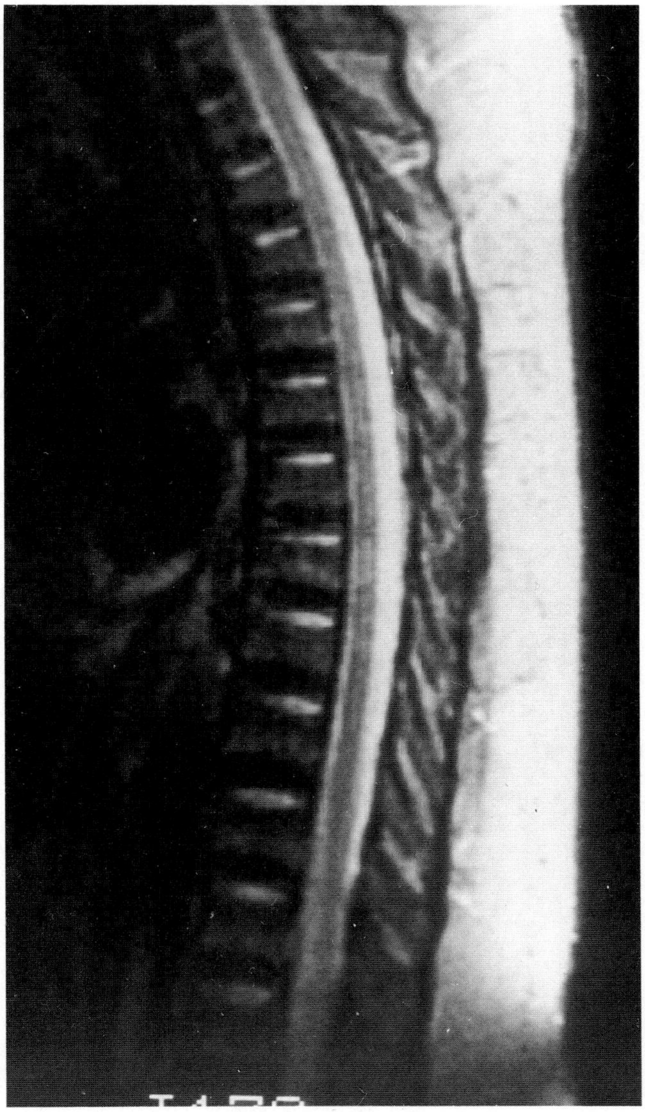

4-9 Midline sagittal MR scan through thoracic spine (2000/90).

4/Thoracic Spine, Sagittal Scout MRI and Coronal MRI

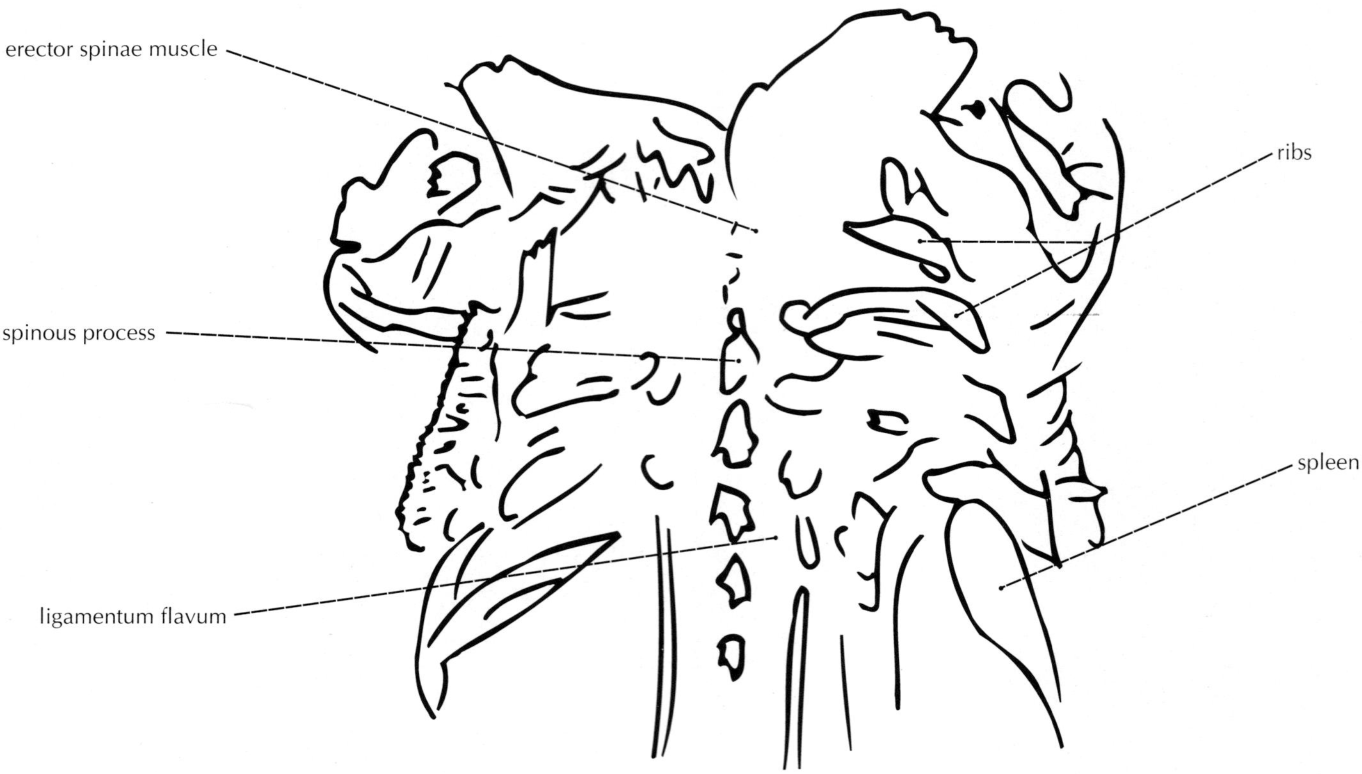

4/Thoracic Spine, Sagittal Scout MRI and Coronal MRI

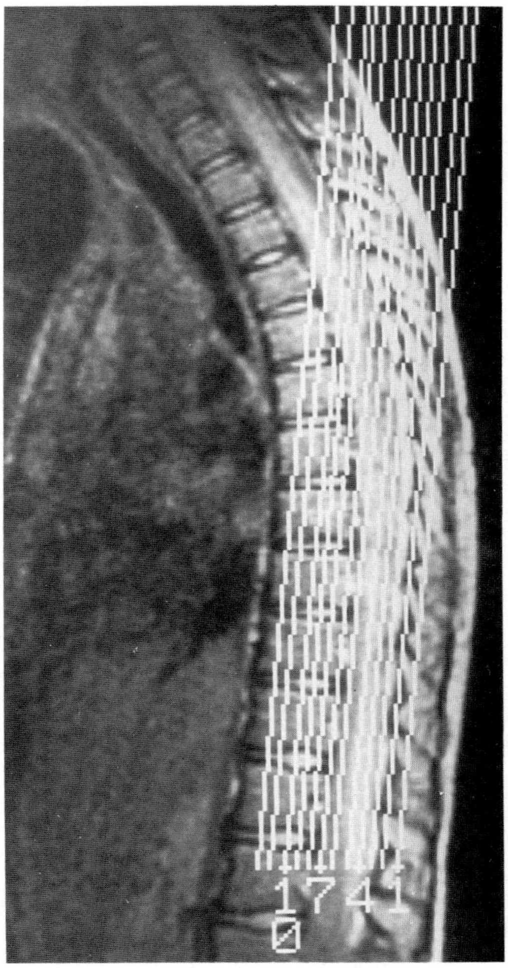

4-10 Sagittal scout MR scan for orientation of coronal MR scans of thoracic spine. Sections 1, 5, and 9 will be demonstrated (Figs. 4-11–4-13).

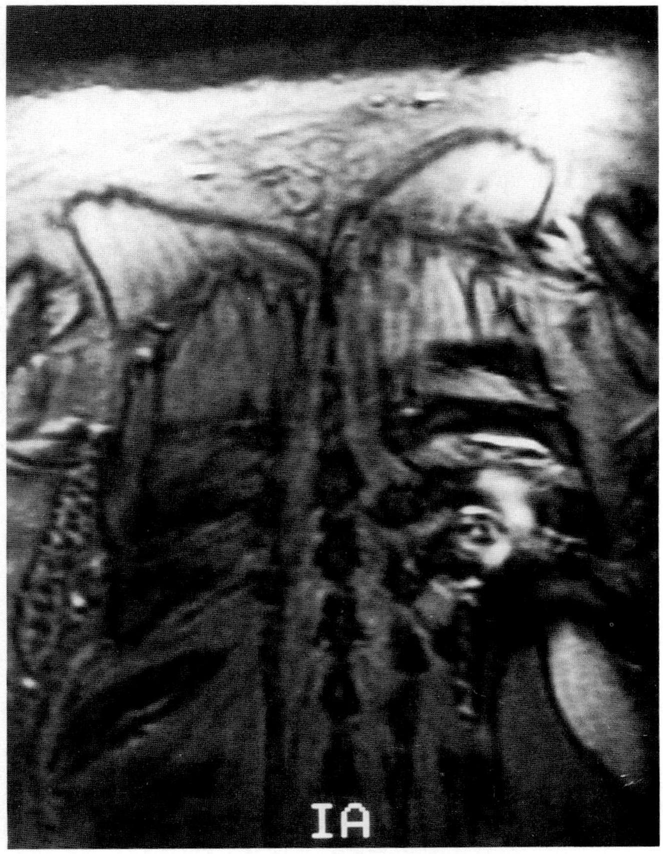

4-11 Coronal MR scan through posterior thoracic spine (500/18, flip angle 15°) (section 1 in Fig. 4-10).

4/Thoracic Spine, Coronal MRI

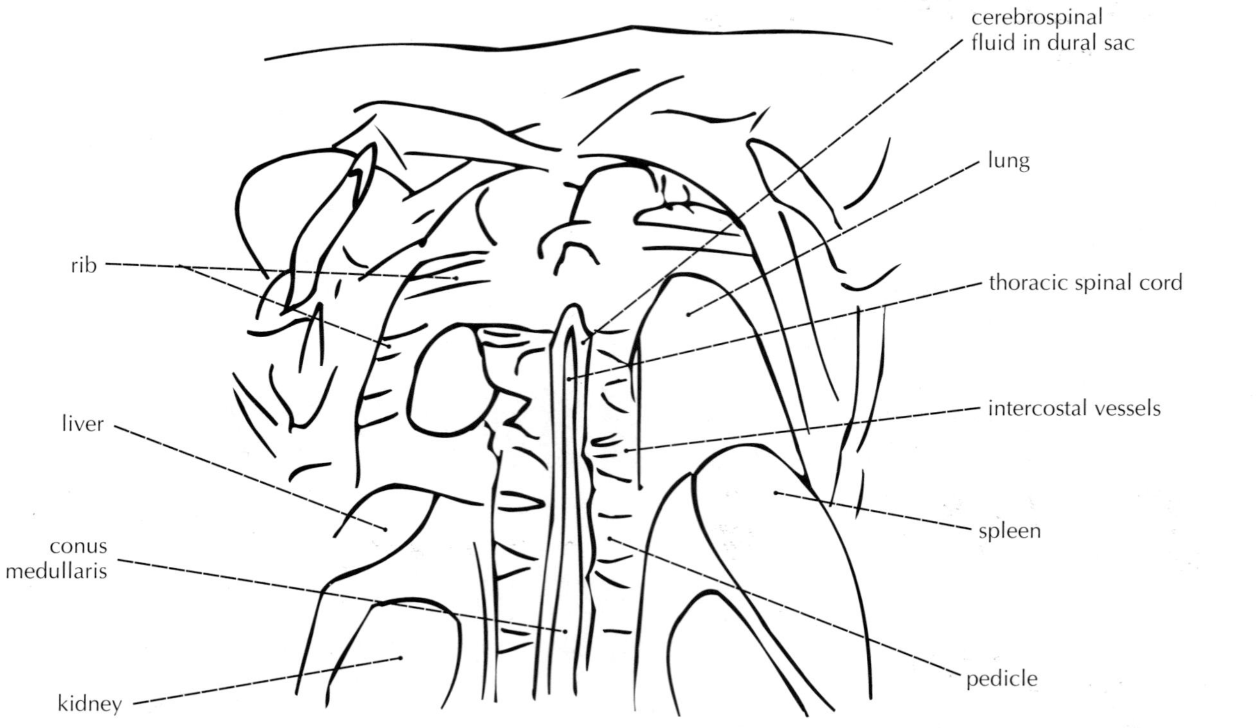

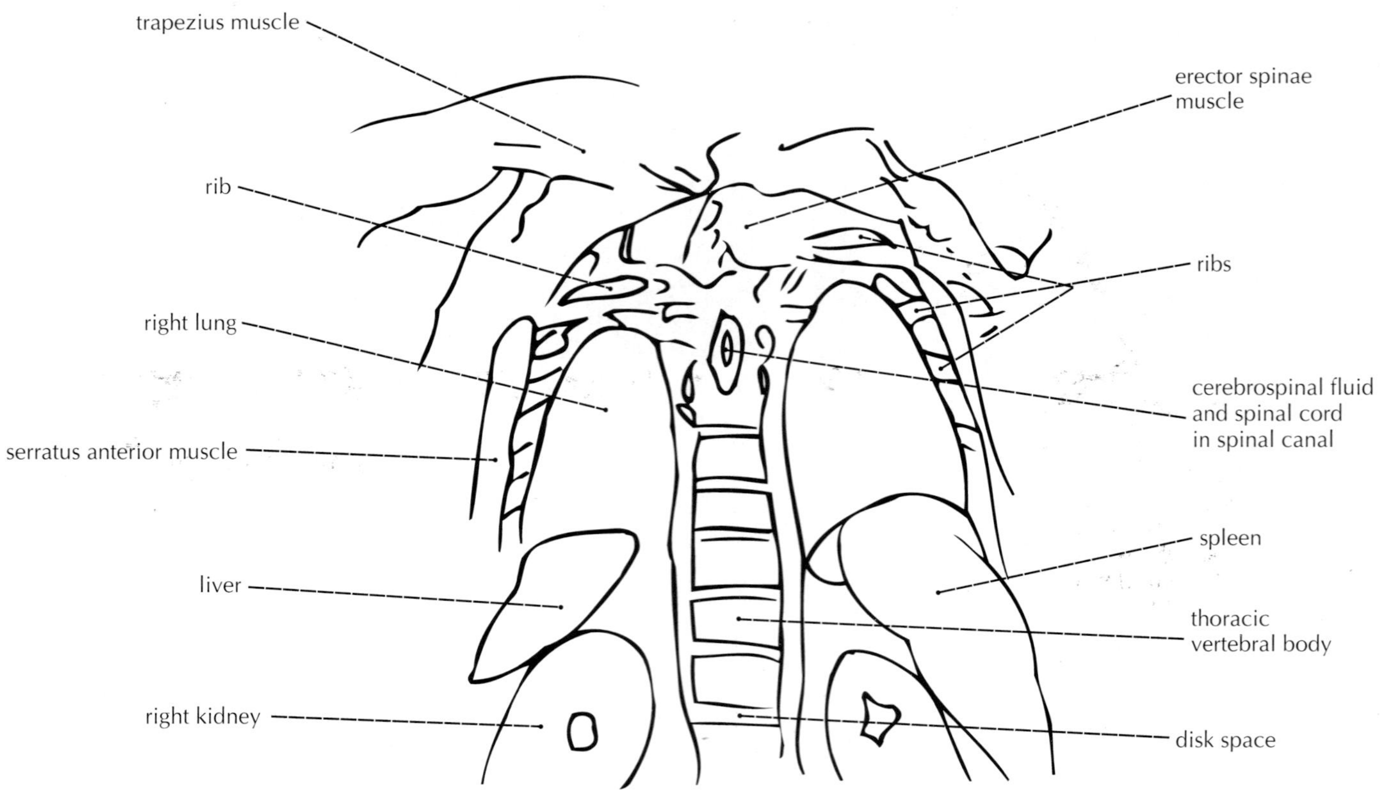

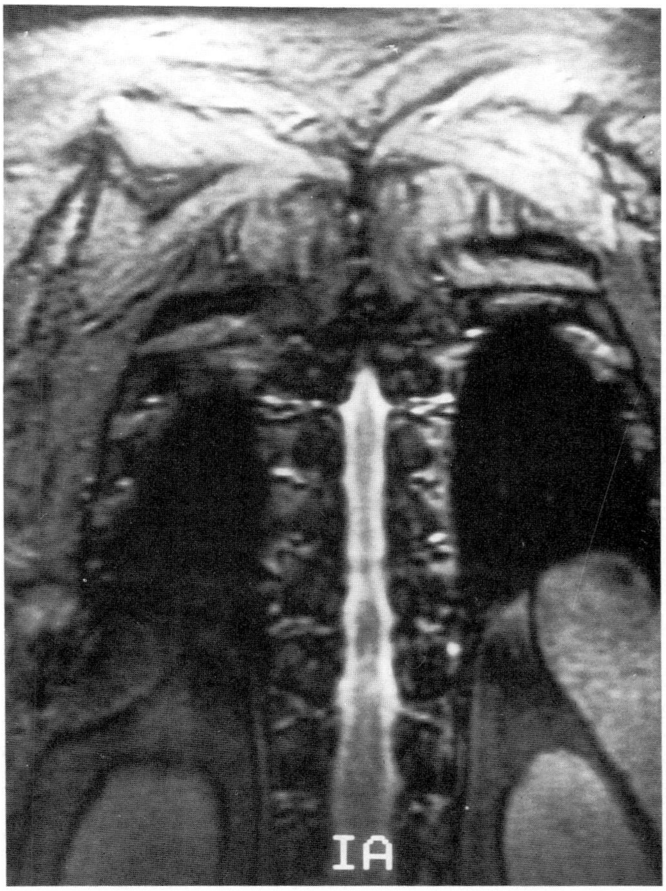

4-12 Coronal MR scan through thoracic spine (500/18, flip angle 15°) (section 5 in Fig. 4-10).

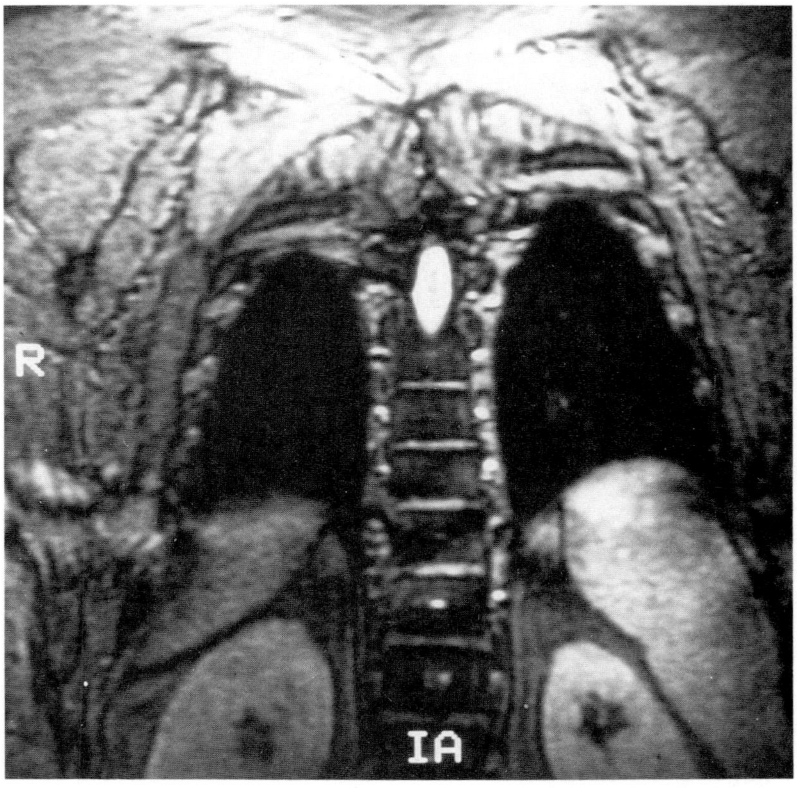

4-13 Coronal MR scan through thoracic spine (500/18, flip angle 15°) (section 9 in Fig. 4-10).

4/Thoracic Spine, Sagittal Scout MRI and Axial MRI

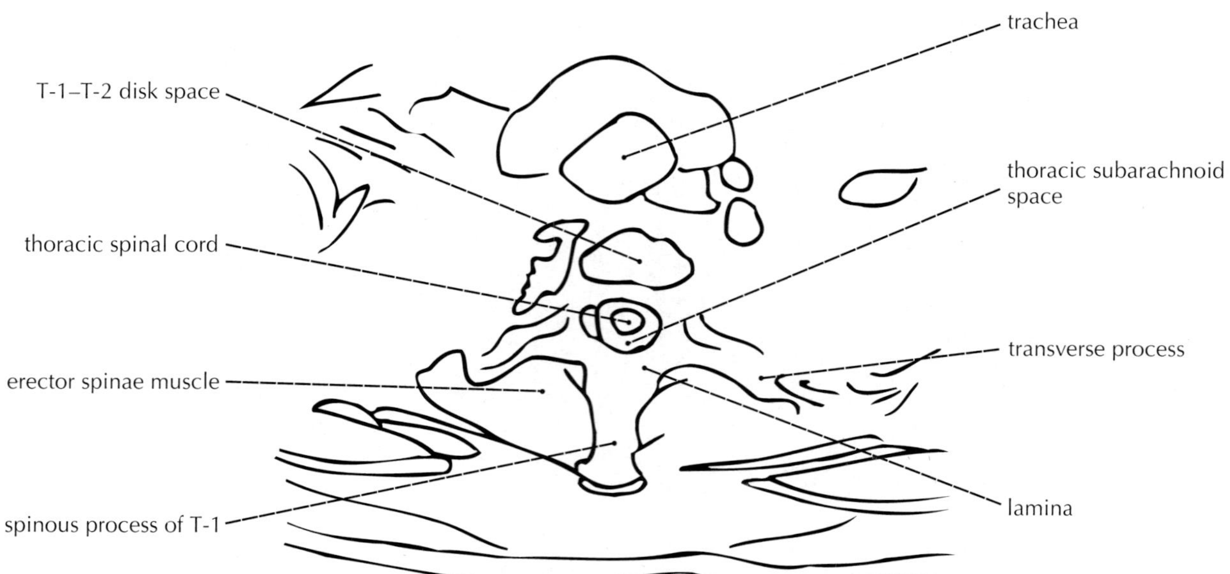

4/Thoracic Spine, Sagittal Scout MRI and Axial MRI

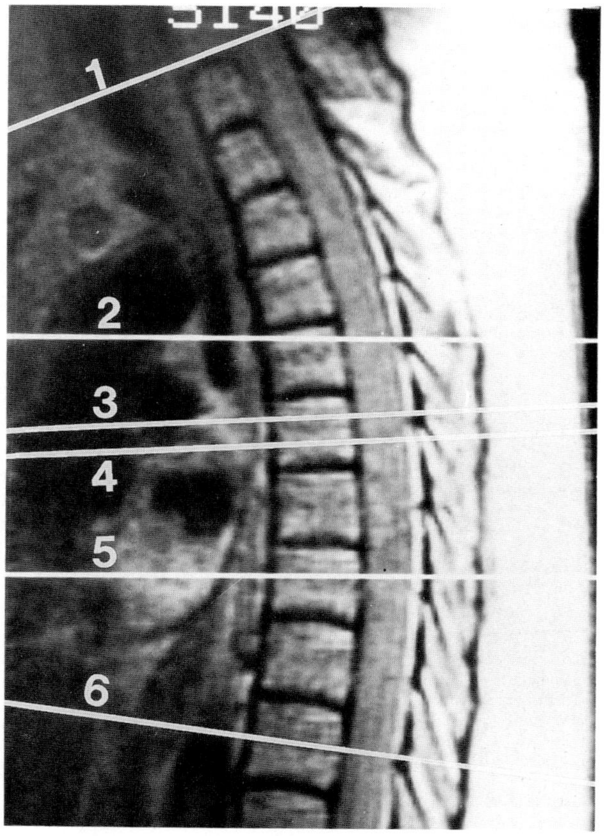

4-14 Sagittal scout MR for demonstration of the axial images.

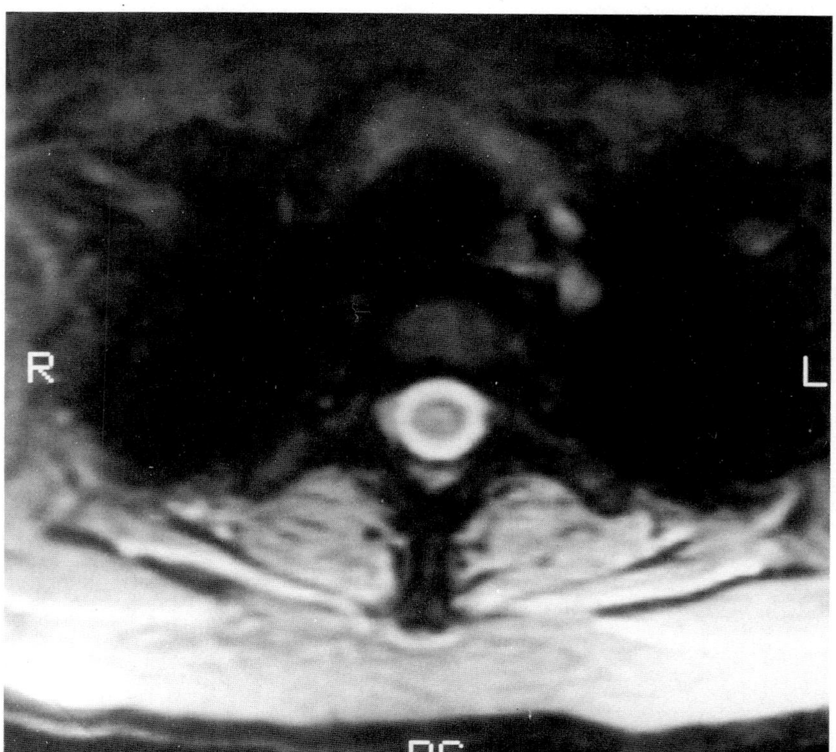

4-15 Axial MR scan through T-1–T-2 disk space (500/18, flip angle 15°). Section 1 in Fig. 4-14.

4/Thoracic Spine, Axial MRI

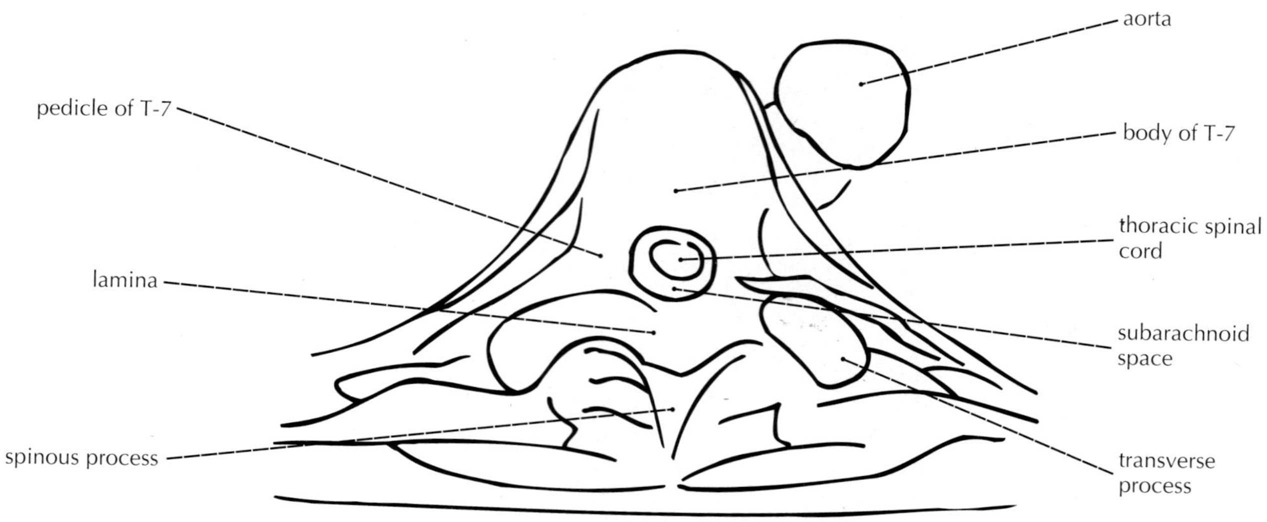

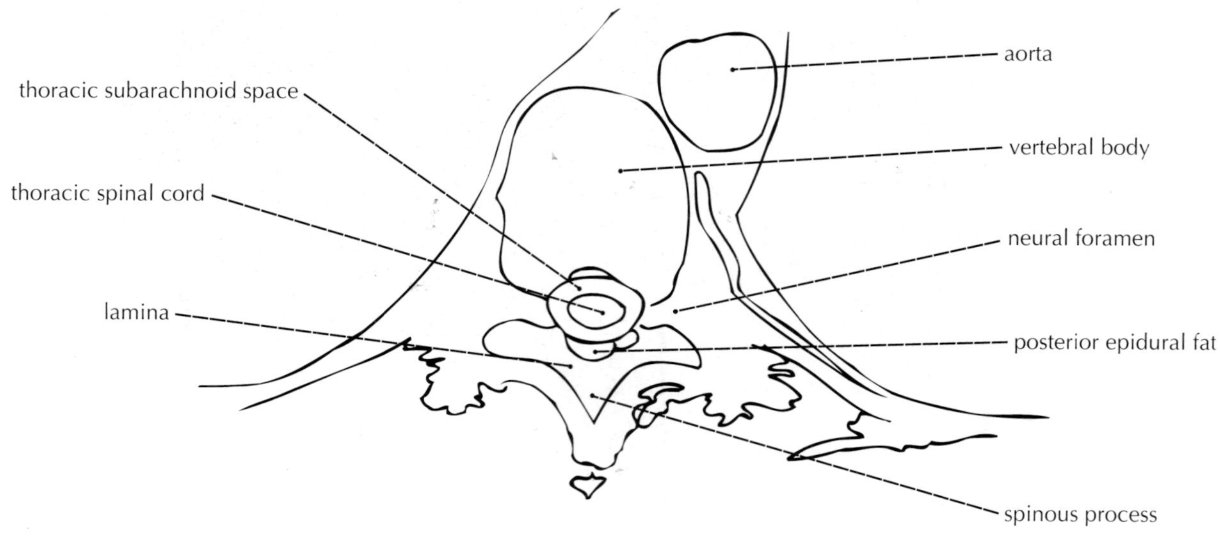

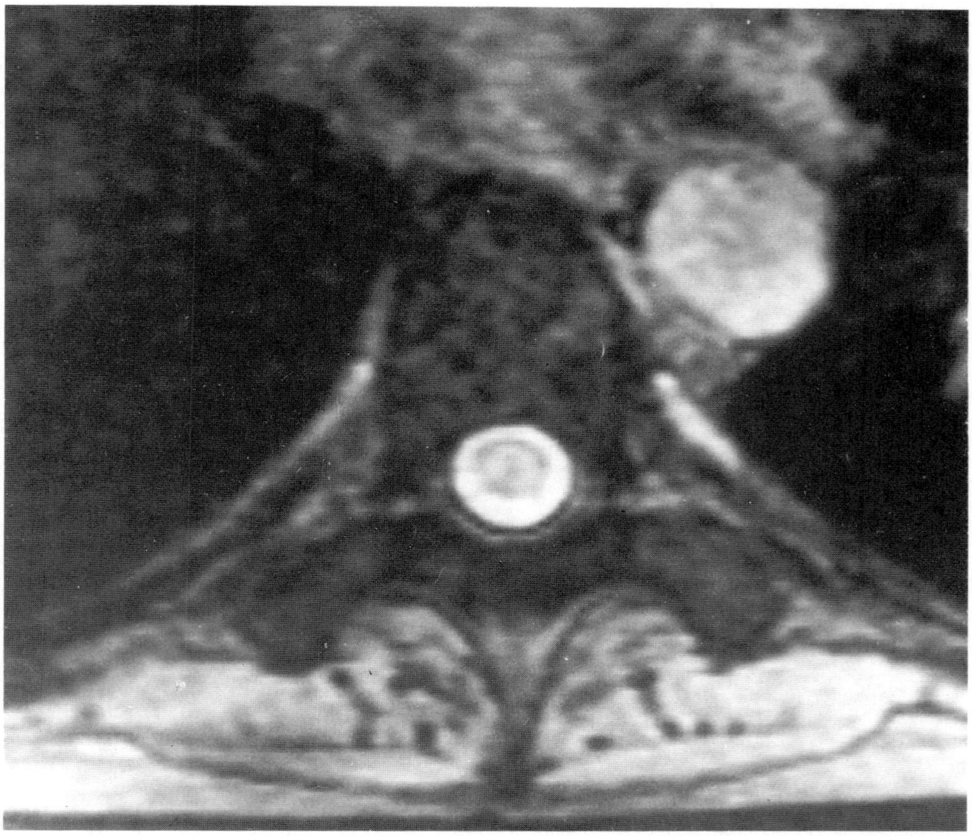

4-16 Axial MR scan through body of T-7 (500/18, flip angle 15°). Section 3 in Fig. 4-14.

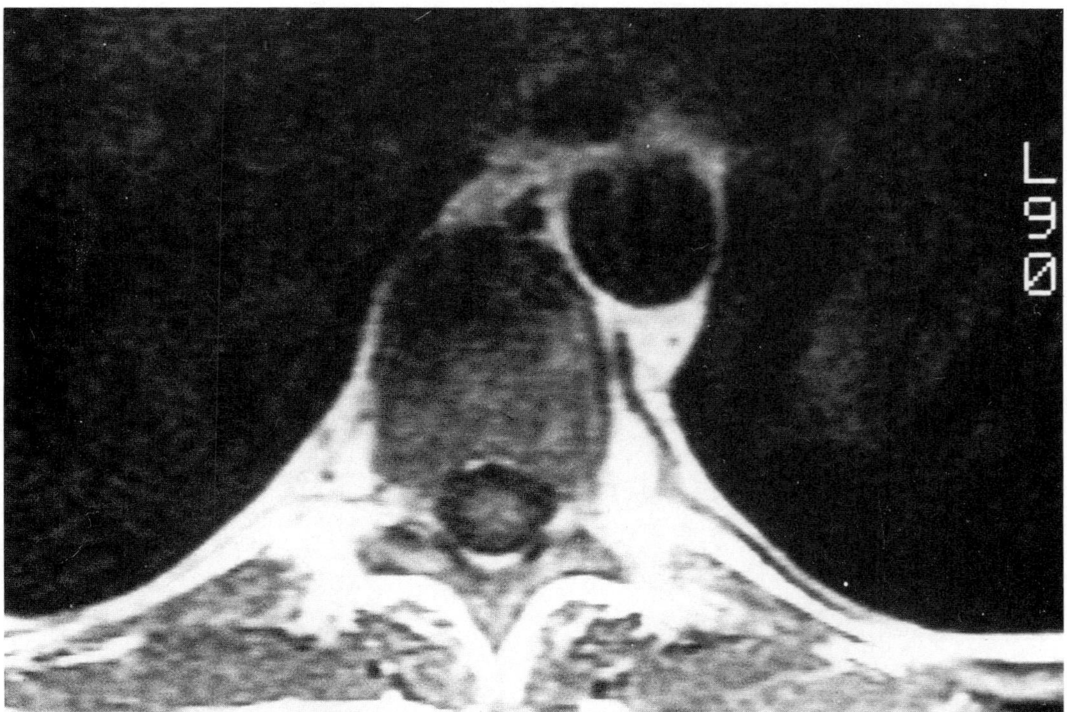

4-17 Axial MR scan through T-7 (500/20). Section 4 in Fig. 4-14.

4/Thoracic Spine, Axial MRI

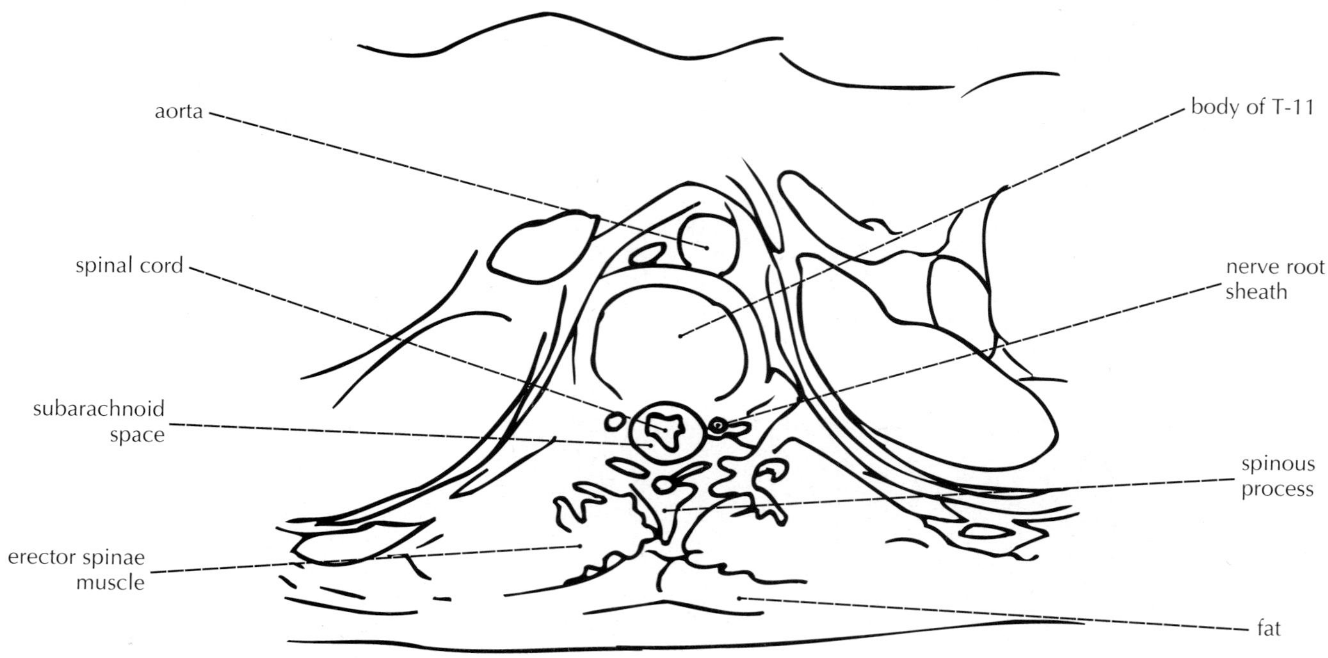

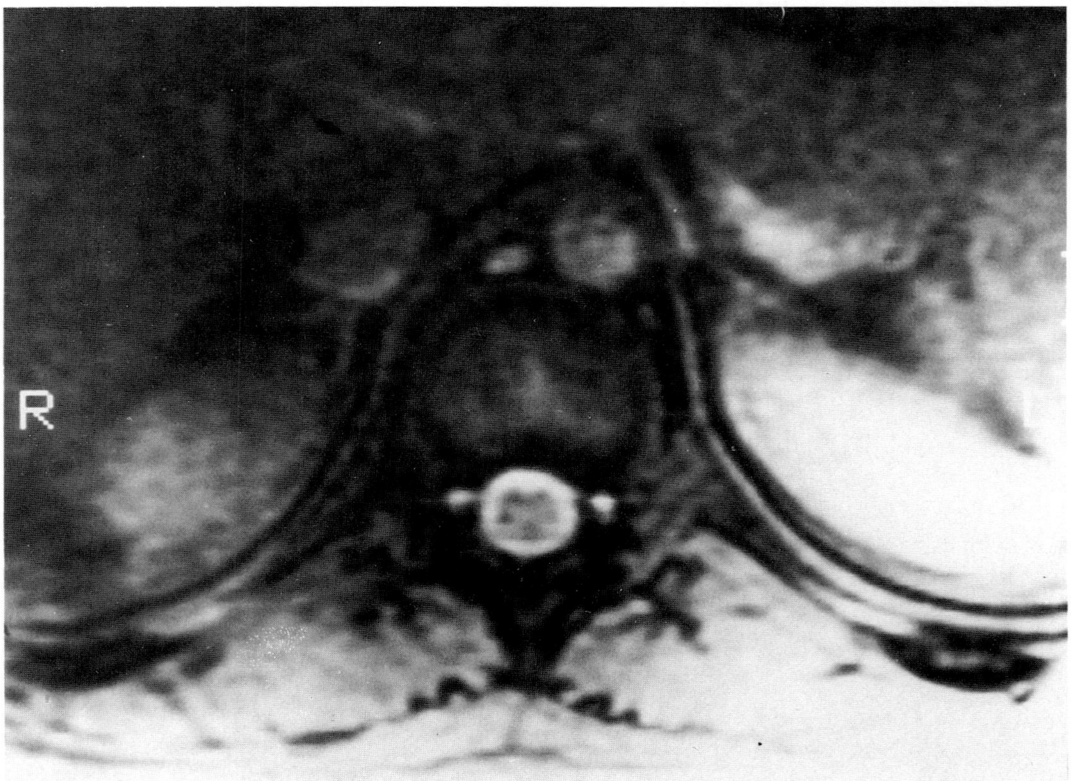

4-18 Axial MR scan through body of T-11 (500/18, flip angle 15°). Section 6 in Fig. 4-14.

4/Thoracic Spine, Myelography

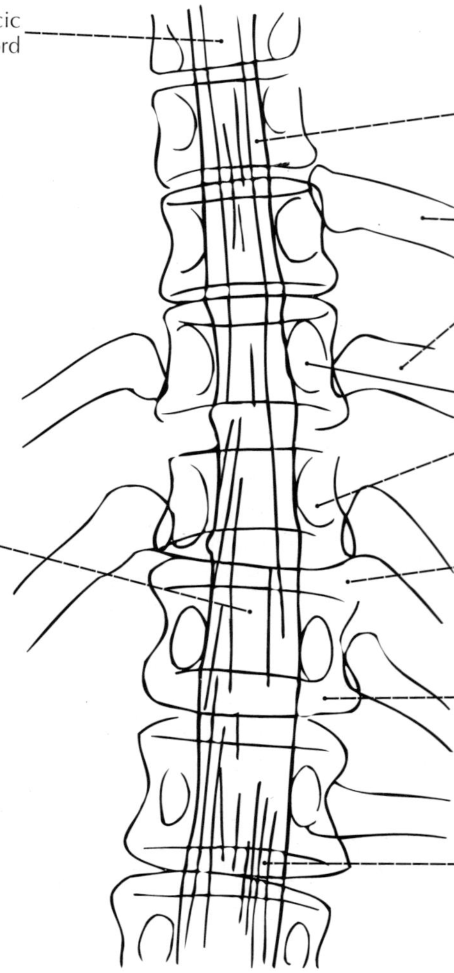

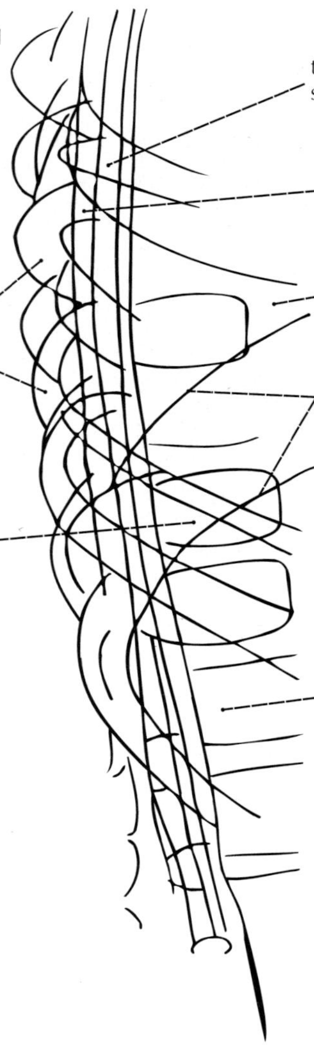

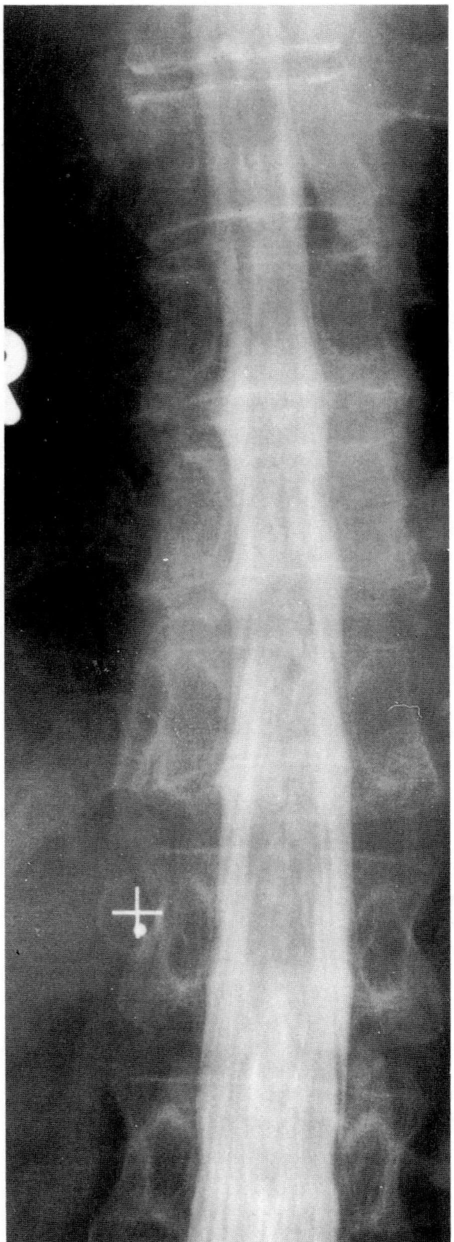

4-19 Myelogram of thoracic region with conus medullaris, AP view.

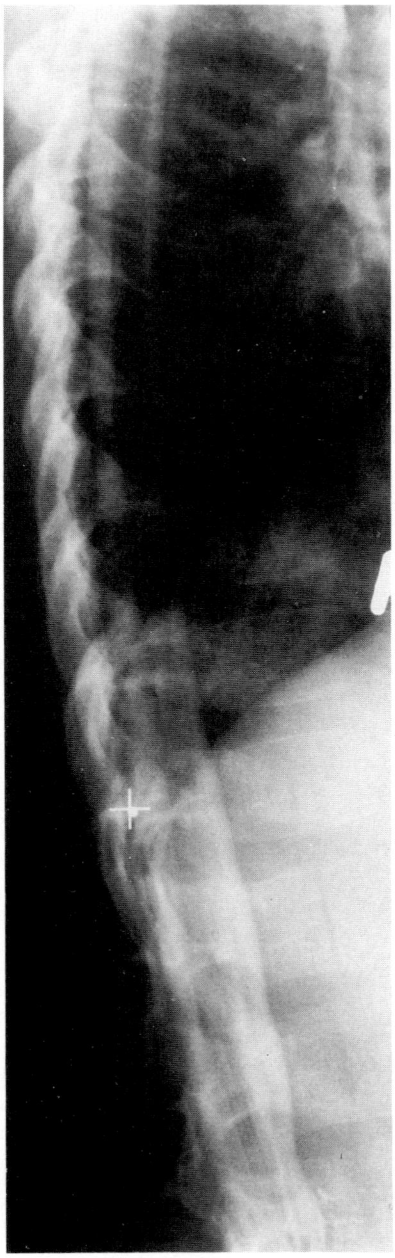

4-20 Myelogram of lumbothoracic junction, lateral view.

5/Lumbosacral Spine □ Lumbar Spine, X-Ray

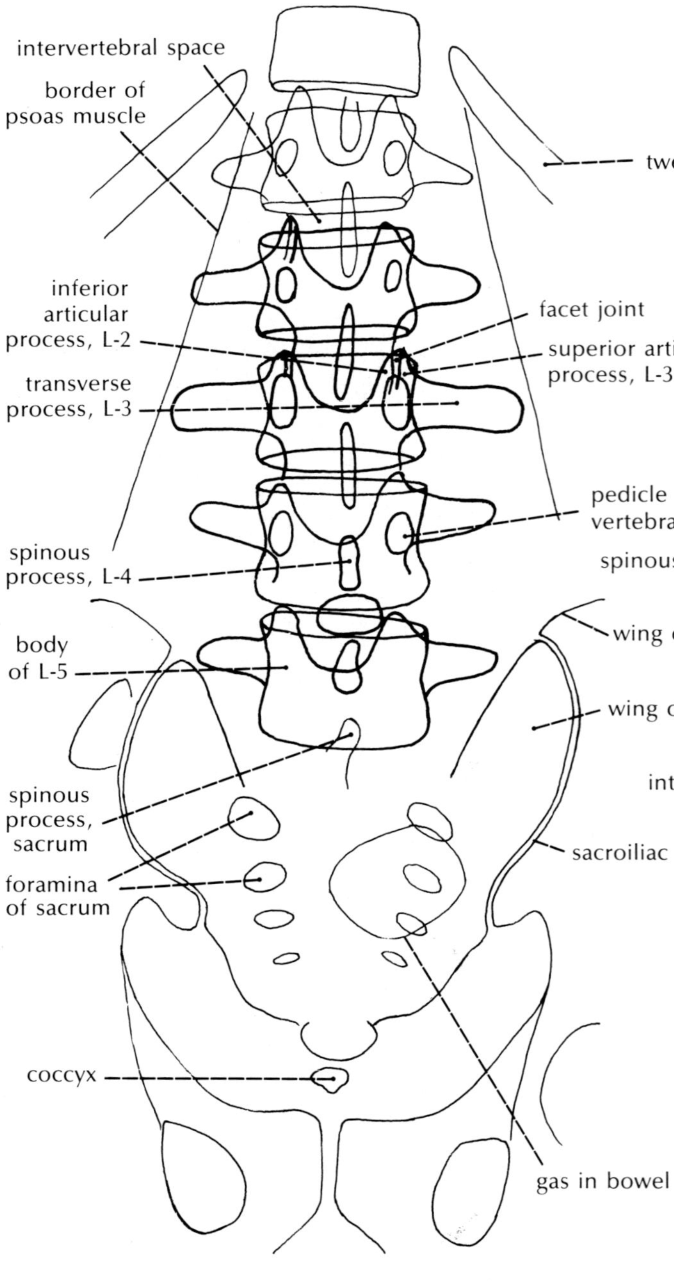

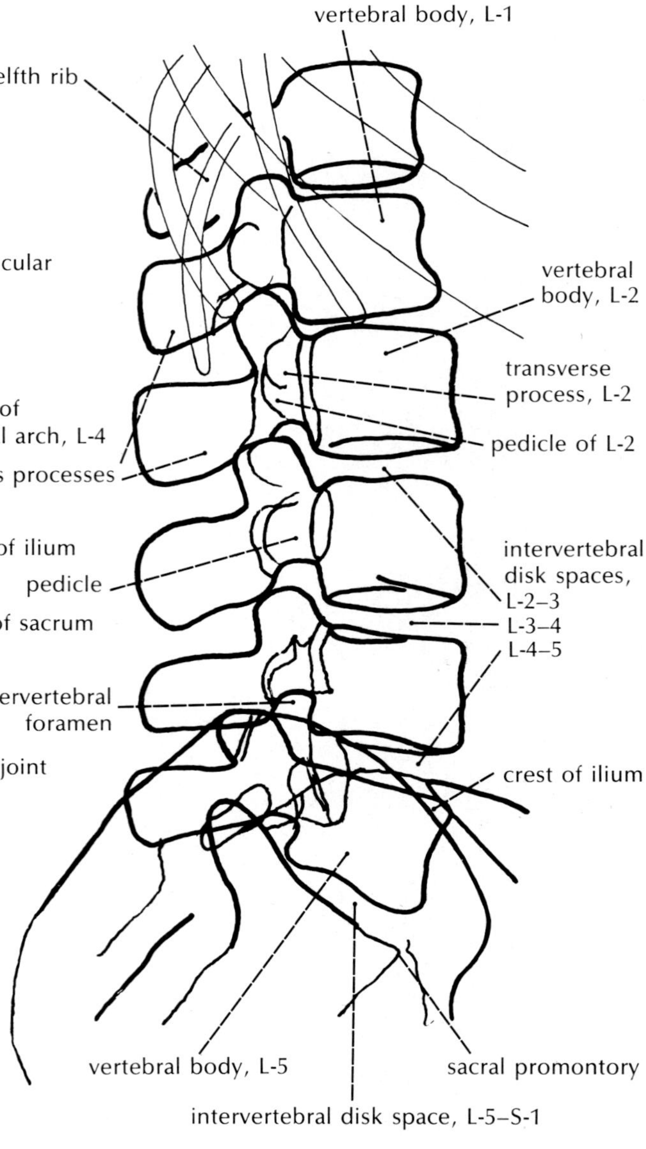

5/Lumbar Spine, X-Ray

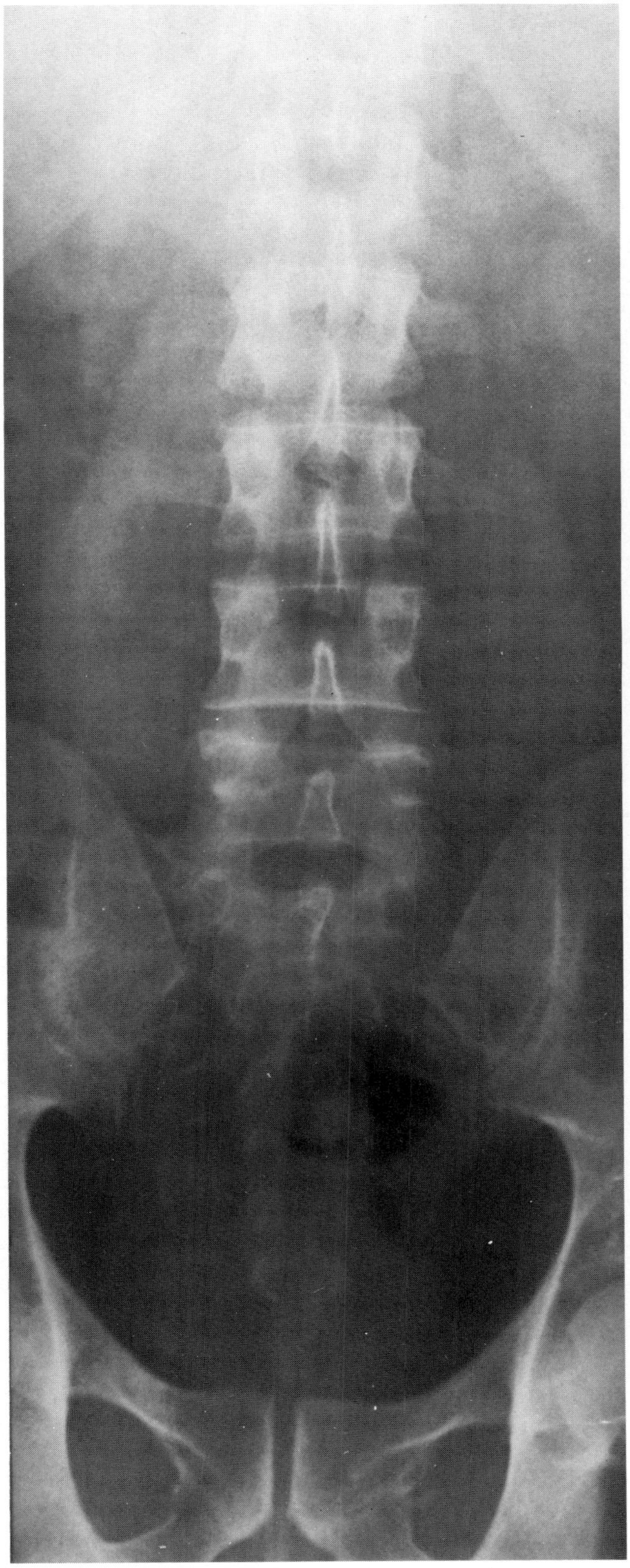

5-1 Lumbar spine, AP view.

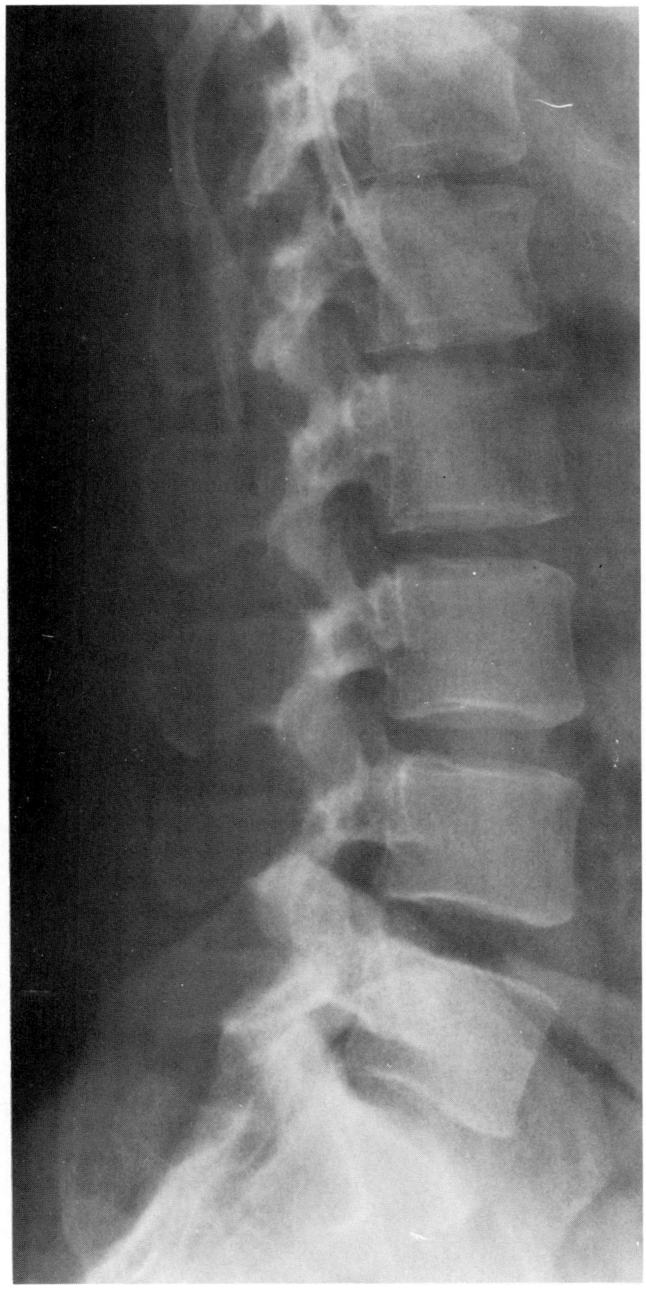

5-2 Lumbar spine, lateral view.

5/Lumbar Spine and Sacroiliac Joint, X-Ray

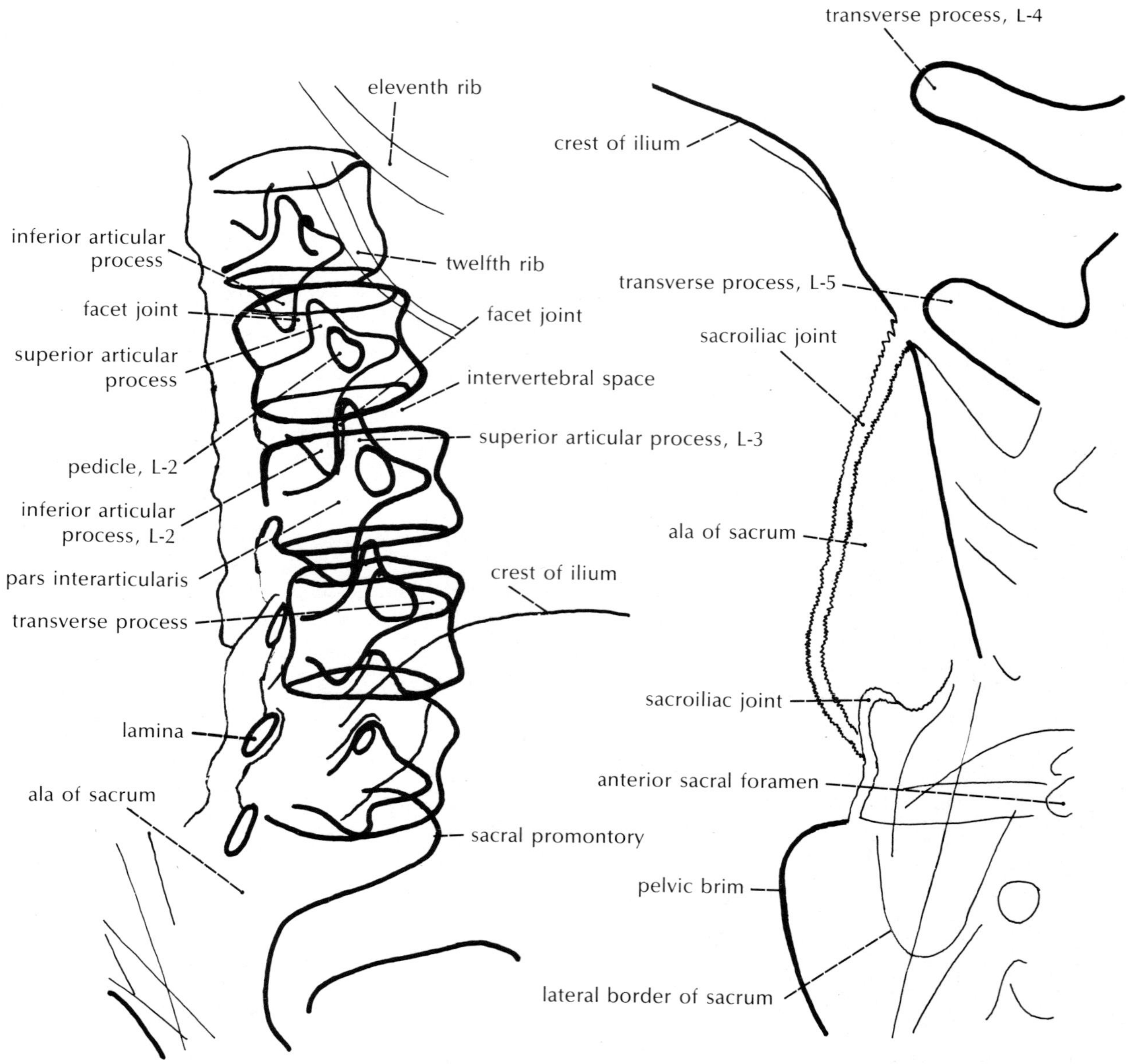

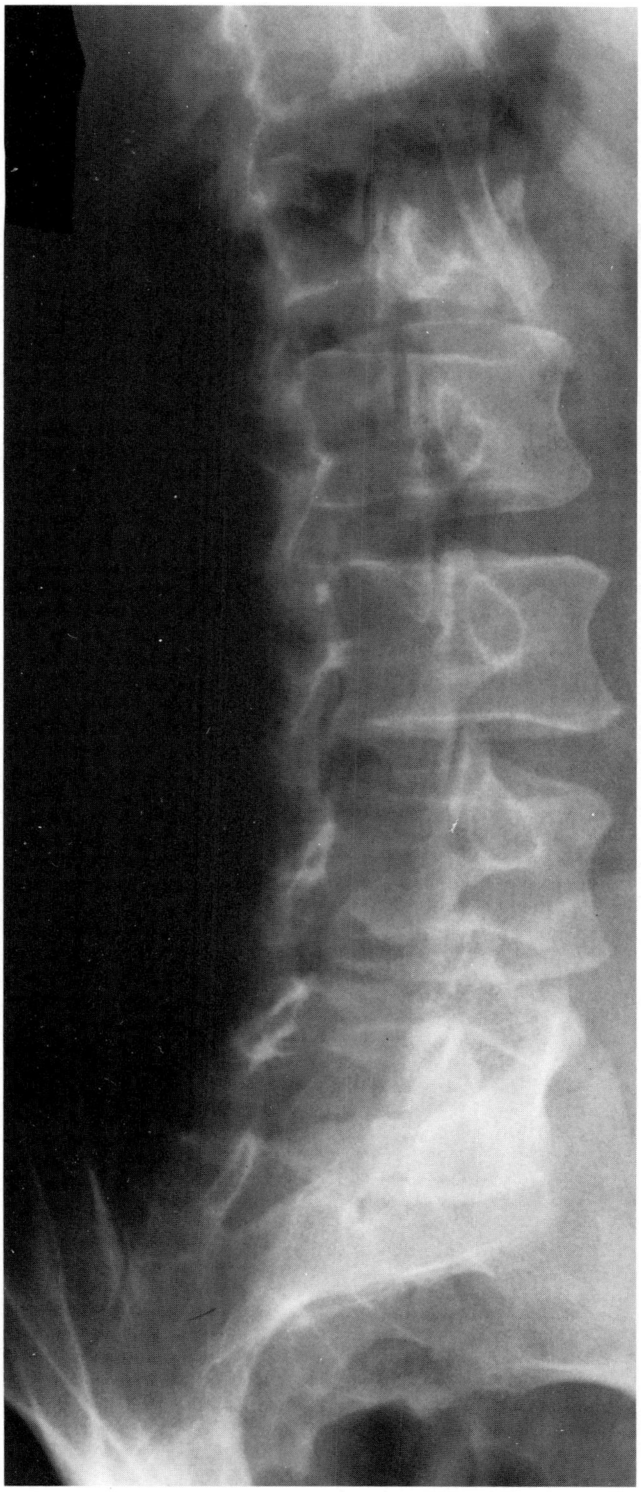

5-3 Lumbar spine, oblique view (reduced in size compared with Fig. 5-4).

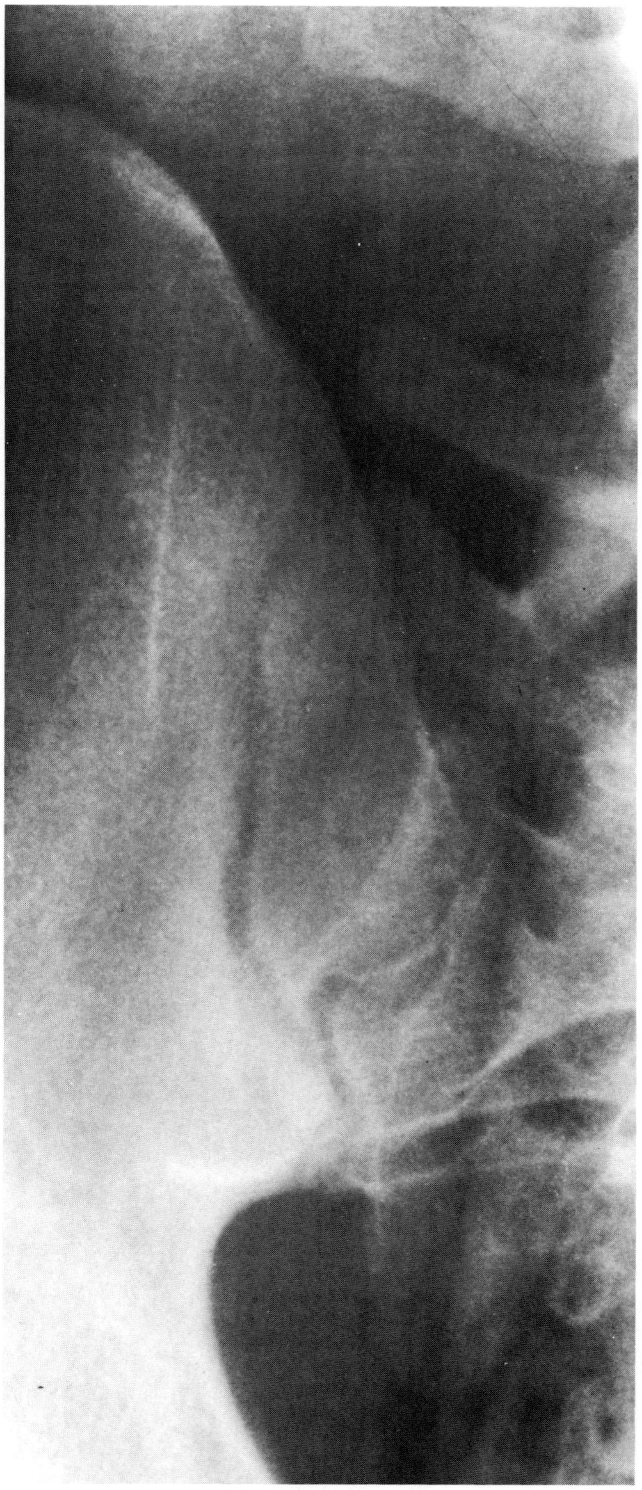

5-4 Sacroiliac joint, oblique view.

5/Sacrum and Coccyx, X-Ray

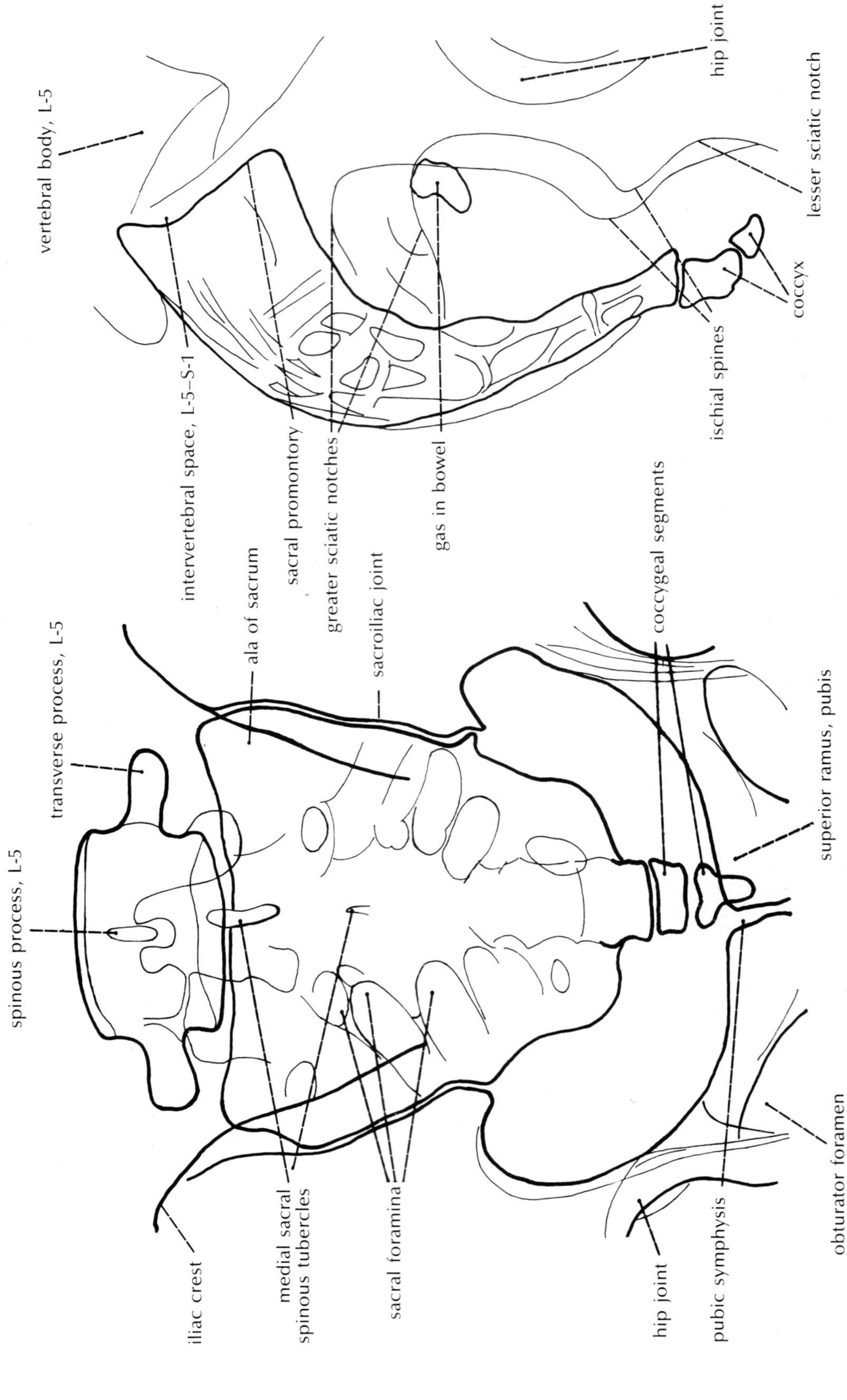

5/Sacrum and Coccyx, X-Ray

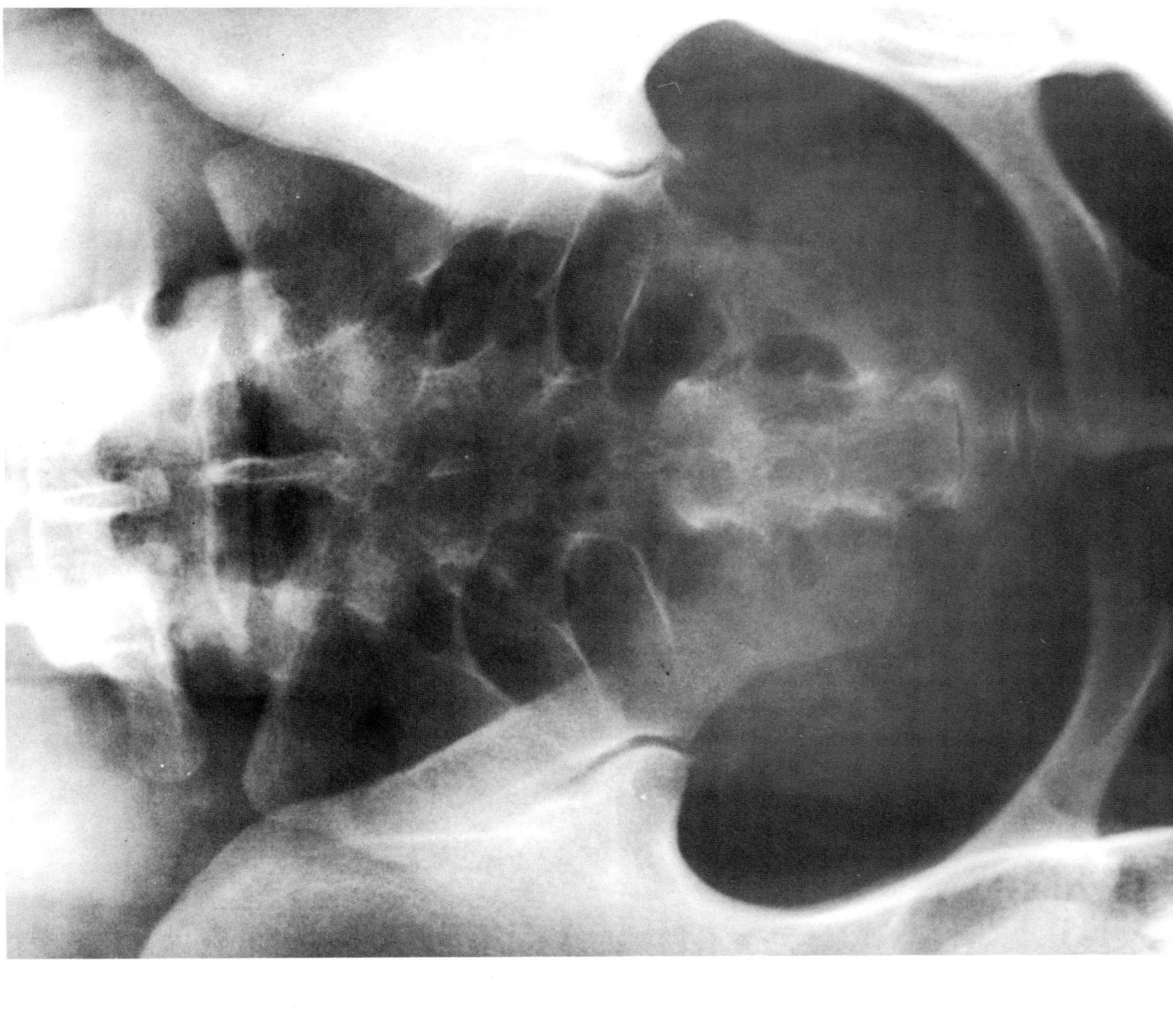

5-5 Sacrum and coccyx, AP view.

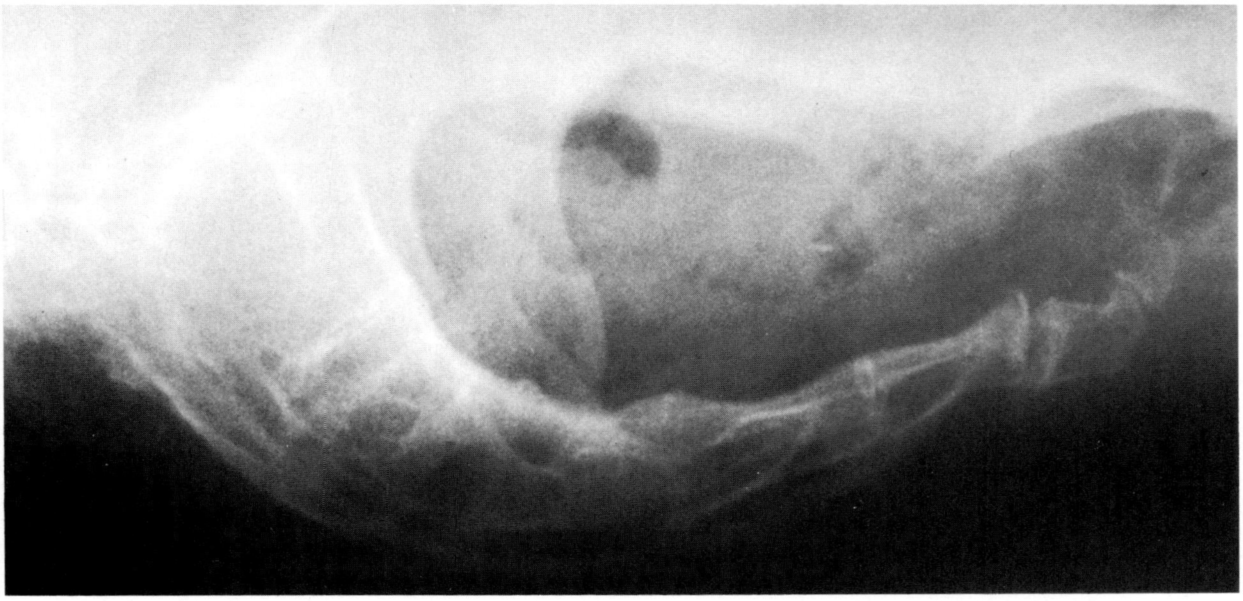

5-6 Sacrum and coccyx, lateral view.

5/Lumbosacral Spine, Sagittal Scout CT and Axial CT

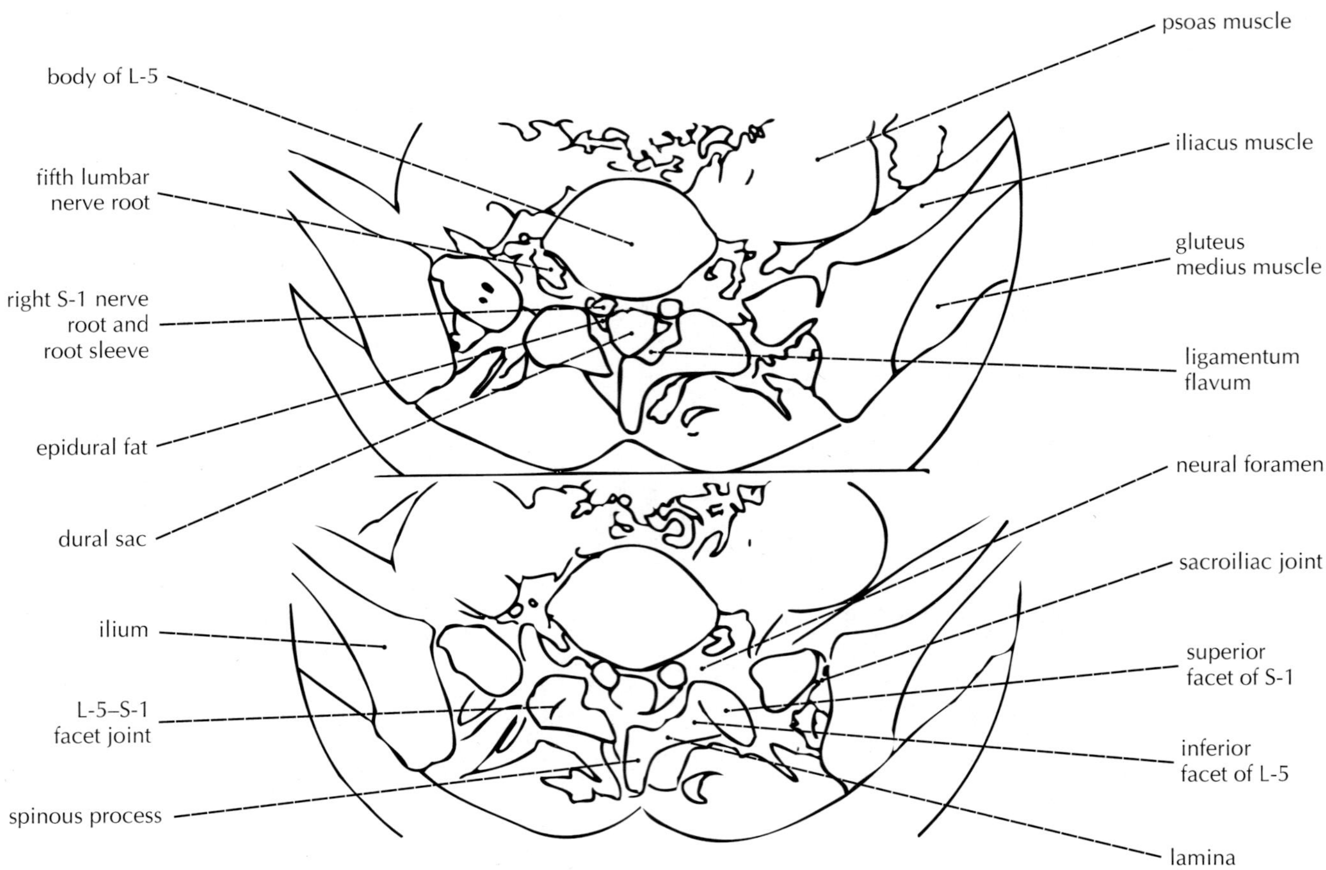

5/Lumbosacral Spine, Sagittal Scout CT and Axial CT

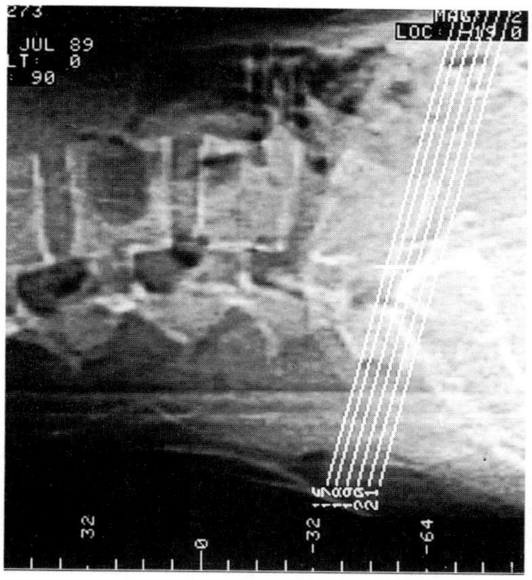

5-7 Sagittal scout CT scan for orientation of axial CT scans at L-5–S-1 disk space. Section 16 (the uppermost section) will be demonstrated in Fig. 5-8.

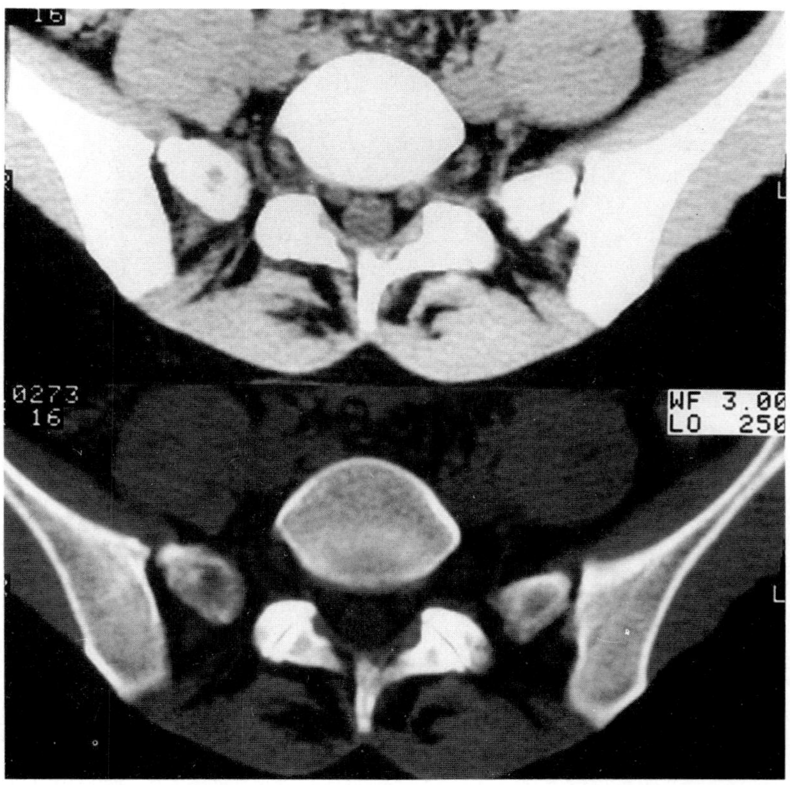

5-8 Axial CT scan through L-5–S-1 level (soft-tissue and bone windows) (section 16 in Fig. 5-7).

5/Lumbosacral Spine, Sagittal Scout CT and Axial CT

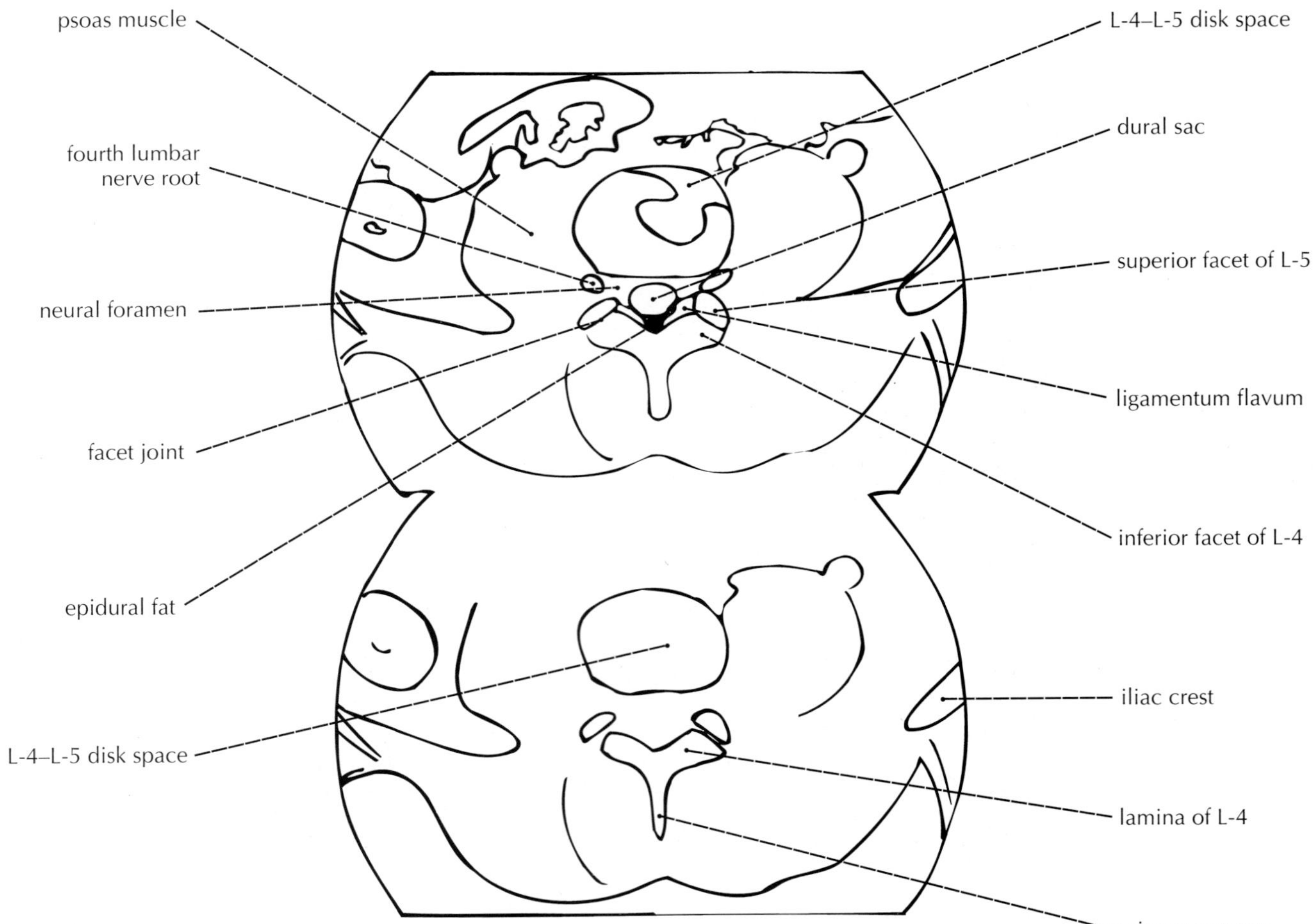

5/Lumbosacral Spine, Sagittal Scout CT and Axial CT

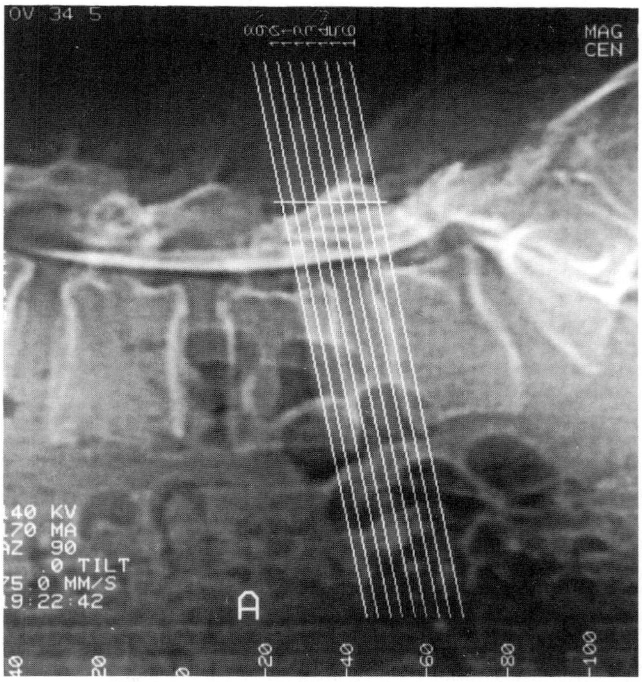

5-9 Sagittal scout CT scan with intrathecal contrast for orientation of axial CT scans through L-4 and through L-4–L-5 disk space. Sections 11, 9 and 12 will be demonstrated in Figs. 5-10, 5-11 and 5-12.

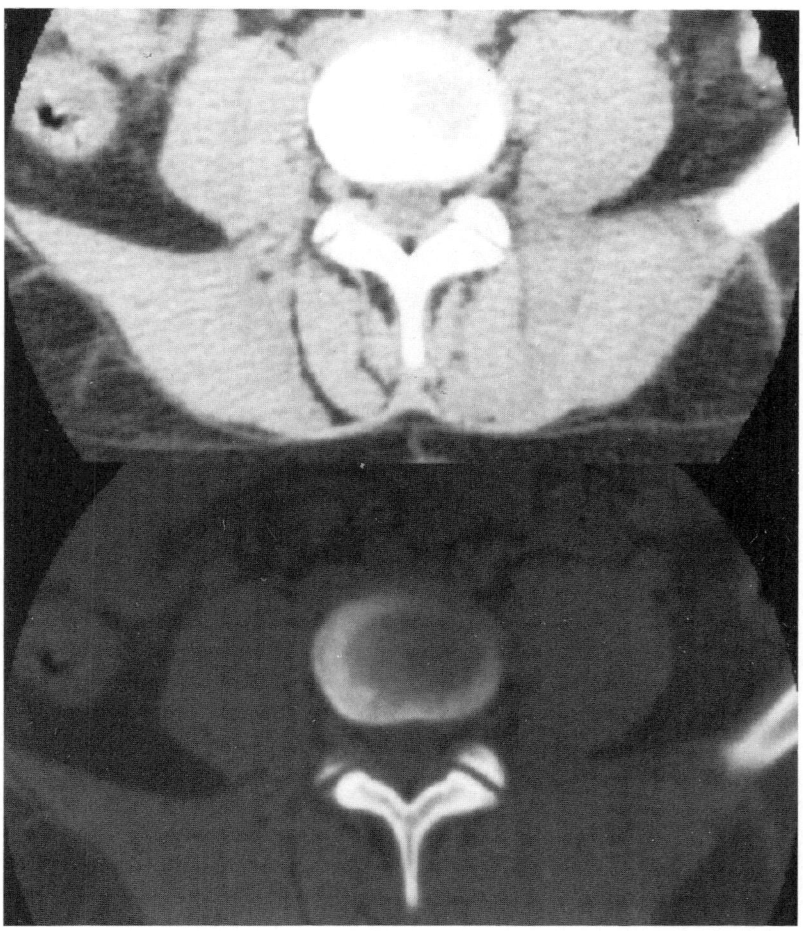

5-10 Axial CT scan through L-4–L-5 disk space (soft-tissue and bone windows). Section 11 in scout 5-10. A noncontrast scan.

5/Lumbosacral Spine, Axial CT

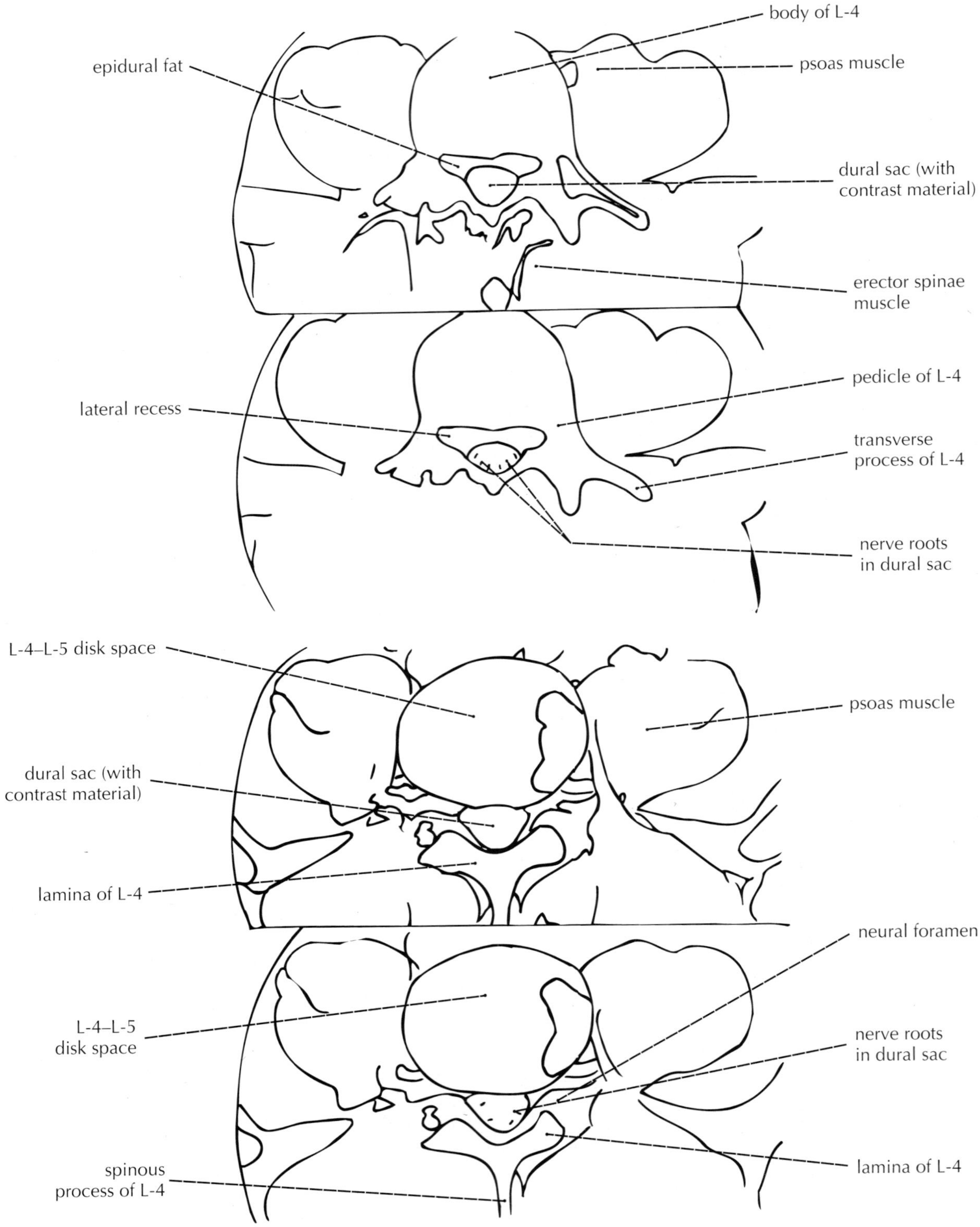

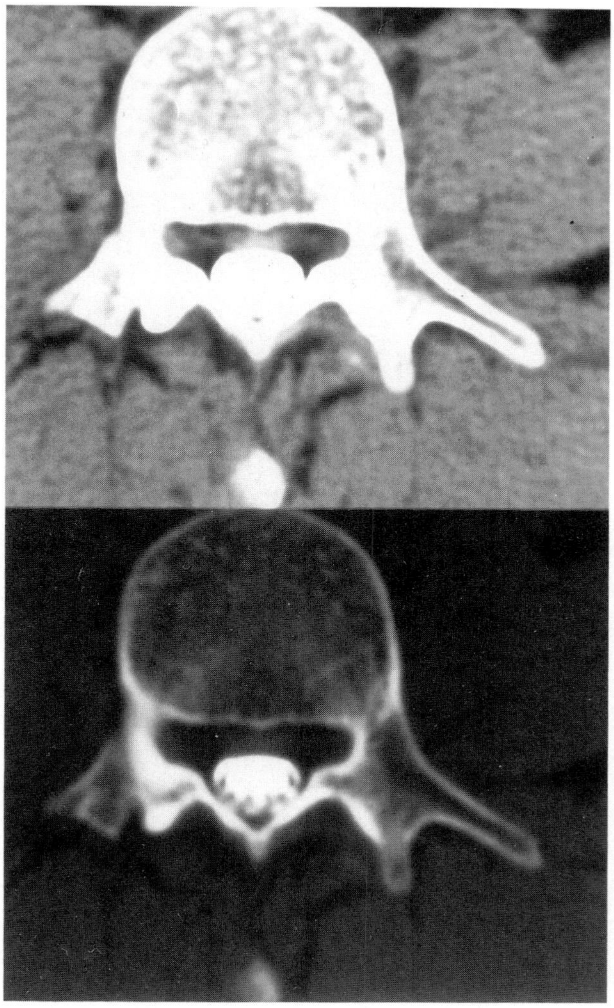

5-11 Axial CT scan through body of L-4 with intrathecal contrast (soft-tissue and bone windows) (section 9 in Fig. 5-9).

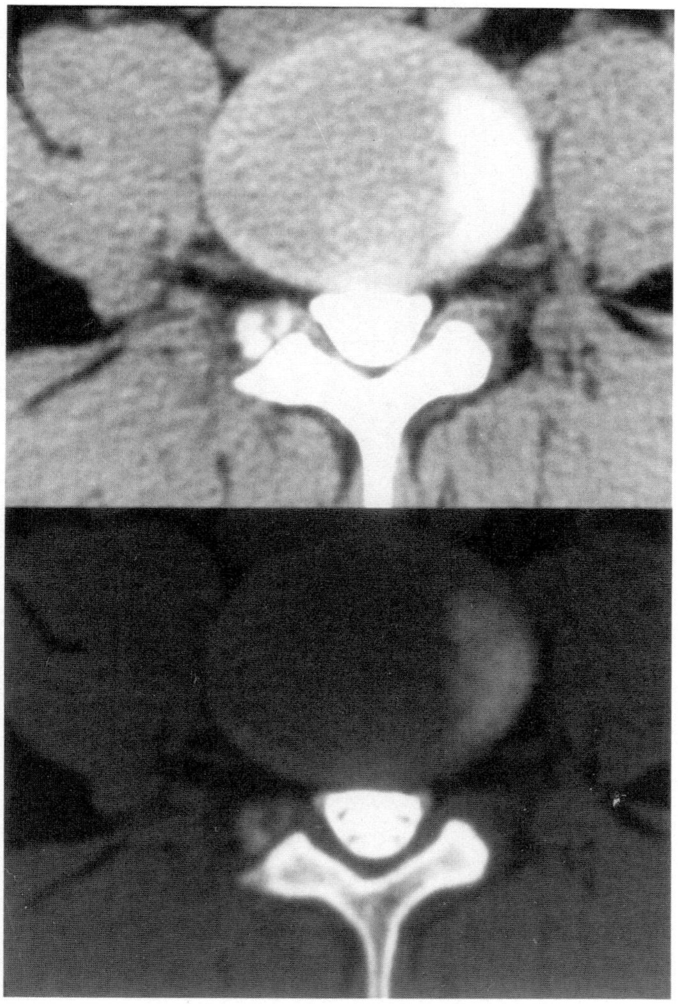

5-12 Axial CT scan through L-4–L-5 disk space with intrathecal contrast (soft-tissue and bone windows) (section 12 in Fig. 5-9).

5/Lumbosacral Spine, Sagittal Scout CT and Axial CT

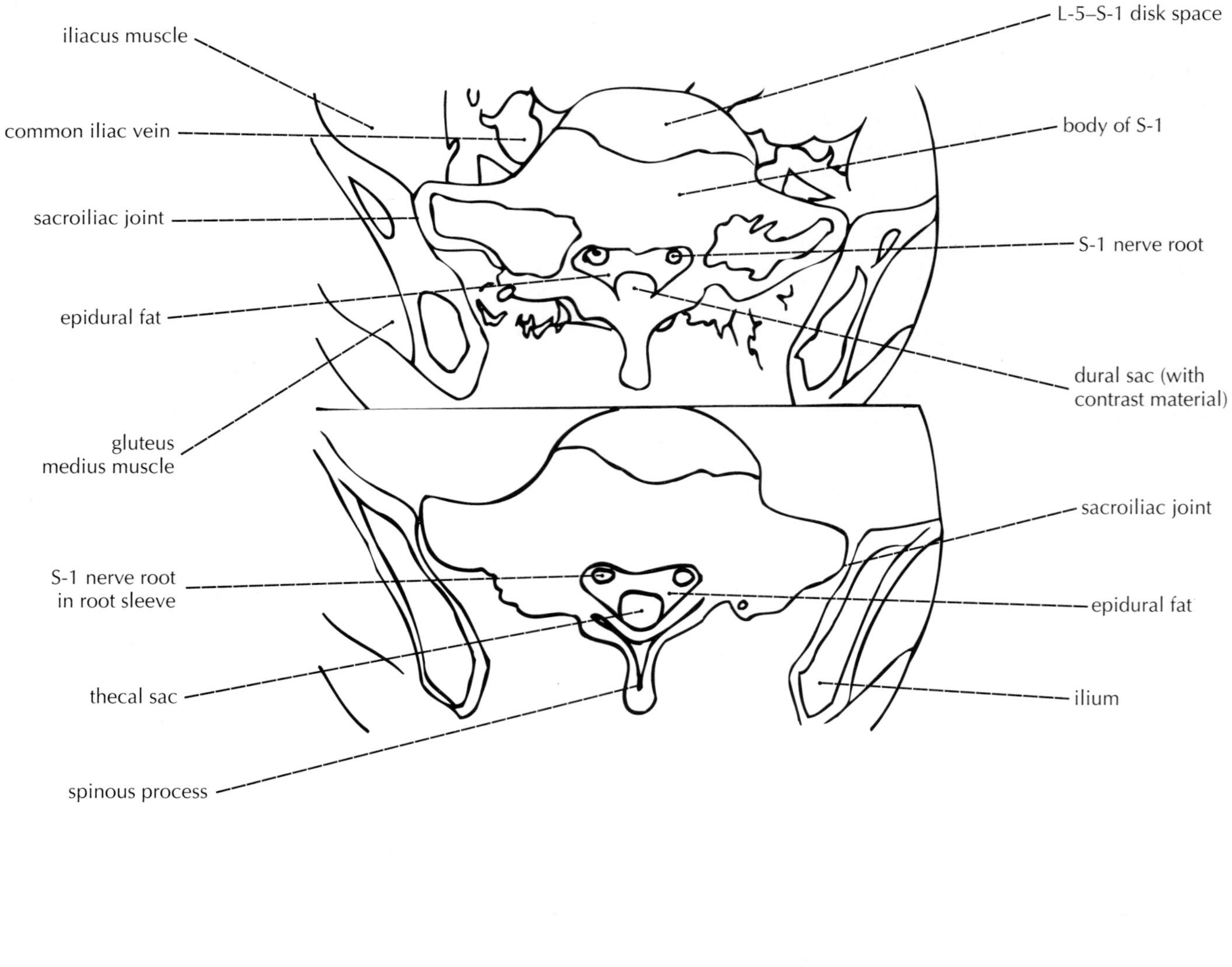

5/Lumbosacral Spine, Sagittal Scout CT and Axial CT

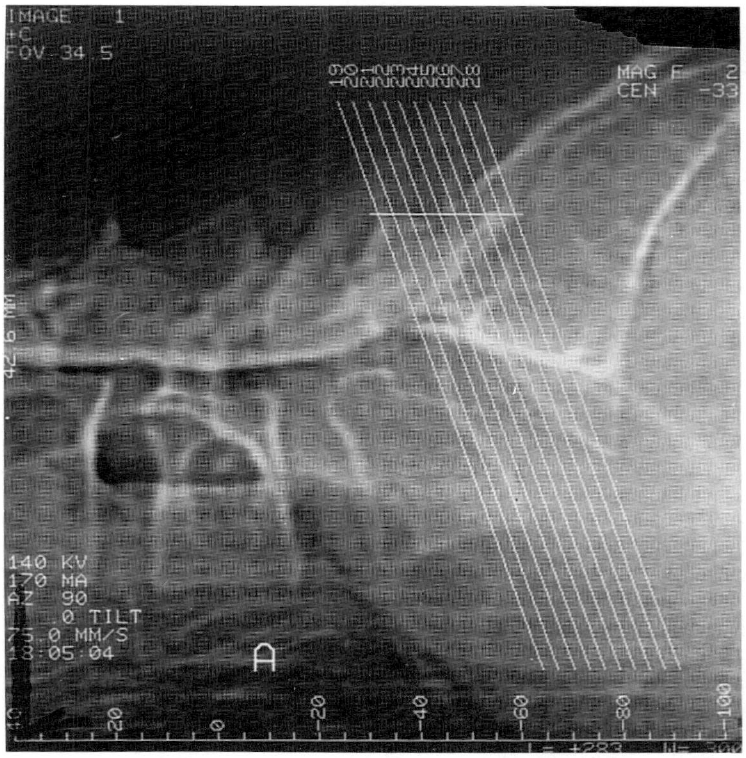

5-13 Sagittal scout CT scan with intrathecal contrast through L-5–S-1 disk space for orientation of axial CT scans. Section 25 will be demonstrated in Fig. 5-14.

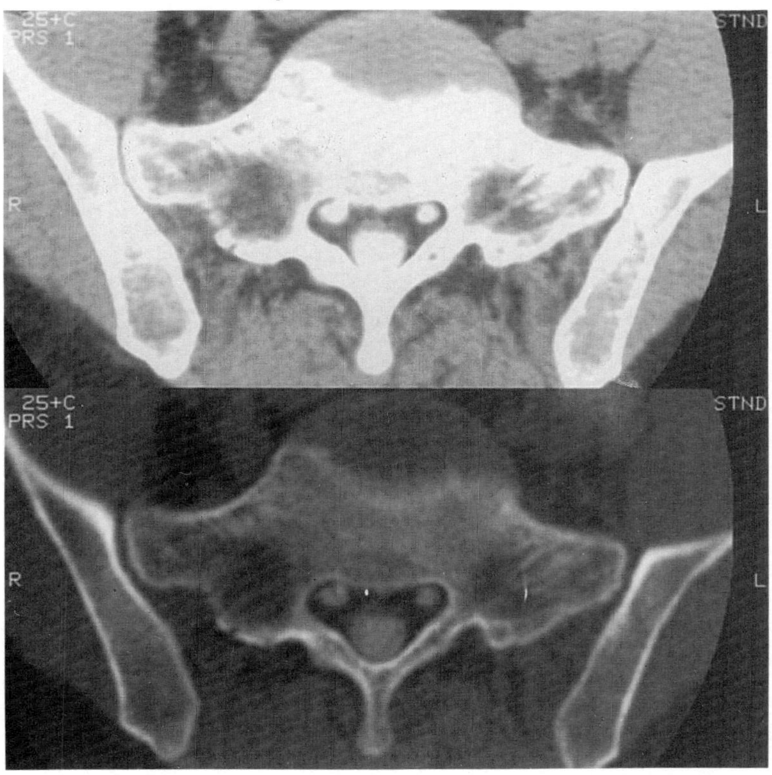

5-14 Axial CT scan through body of S-1 with intrathecal contrast (soft-tissue and bone windows) (section 25 in Fig. 5-13).

5/Lumbosacral Spine, MRI

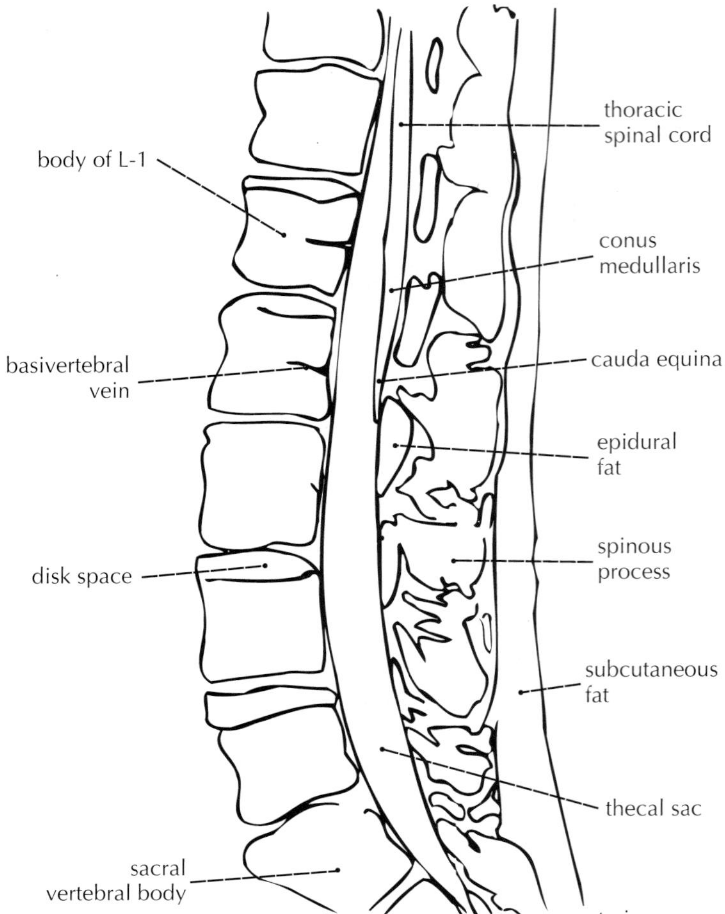

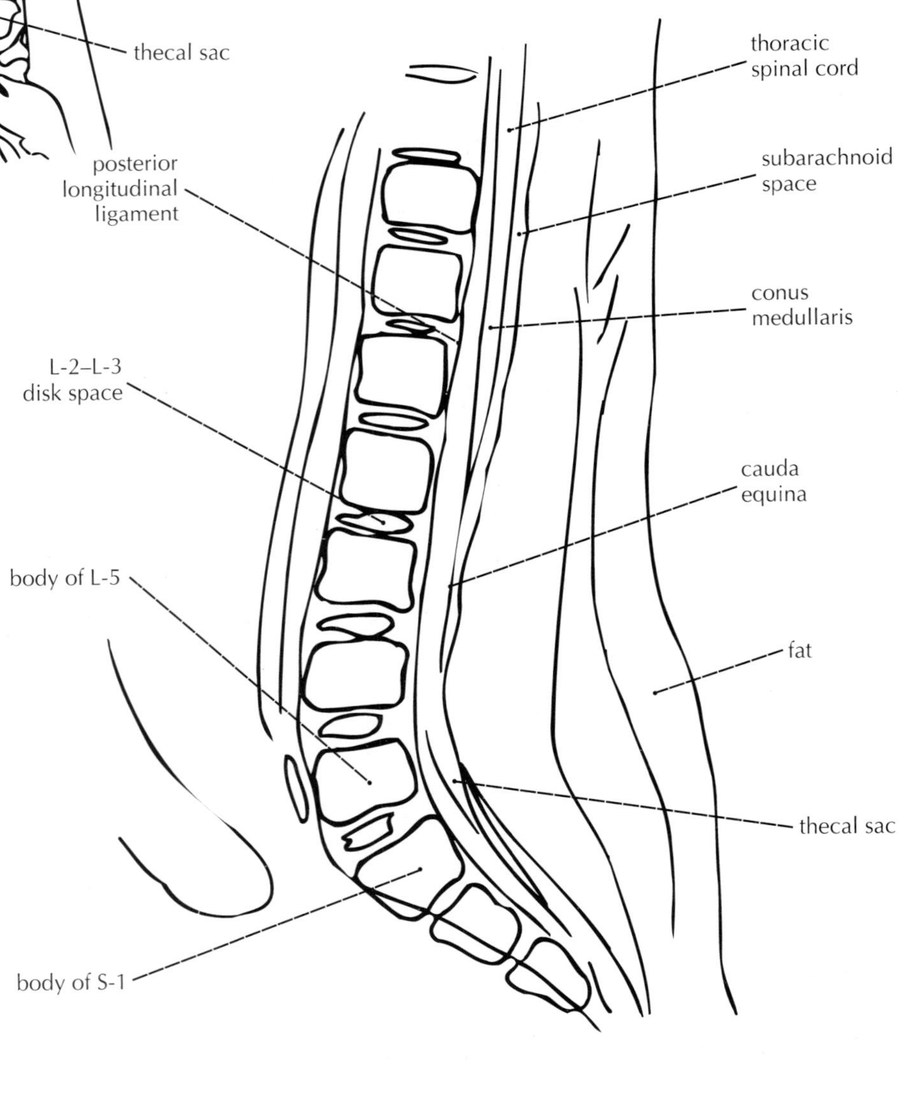

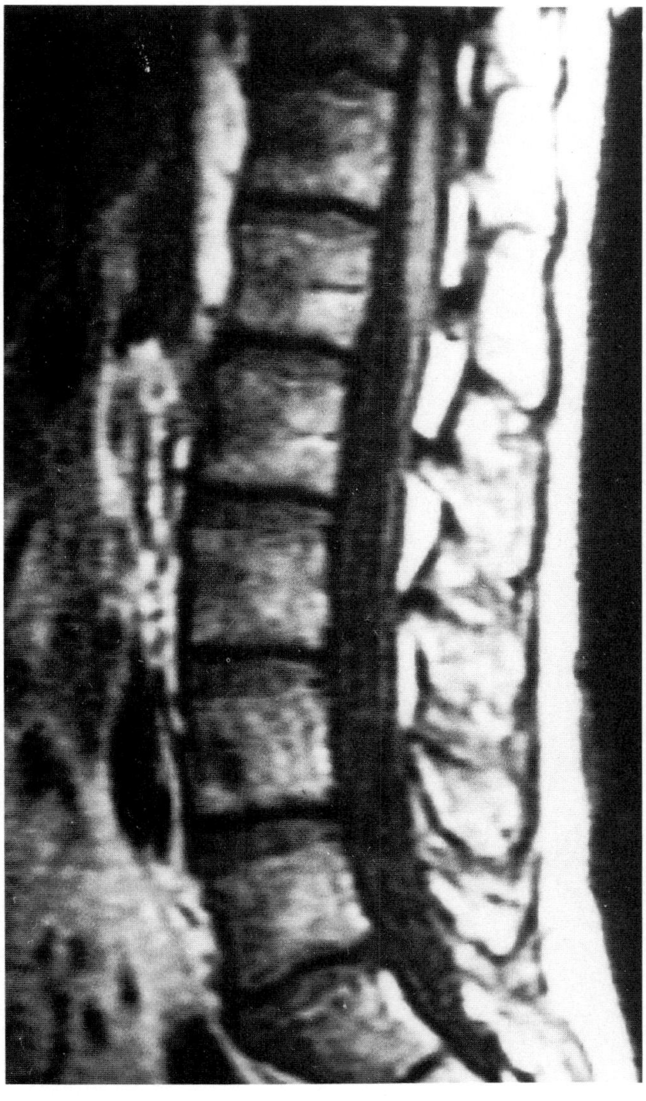

5-15 Midline sagittal MR scan through lumbosacral region (600/20).

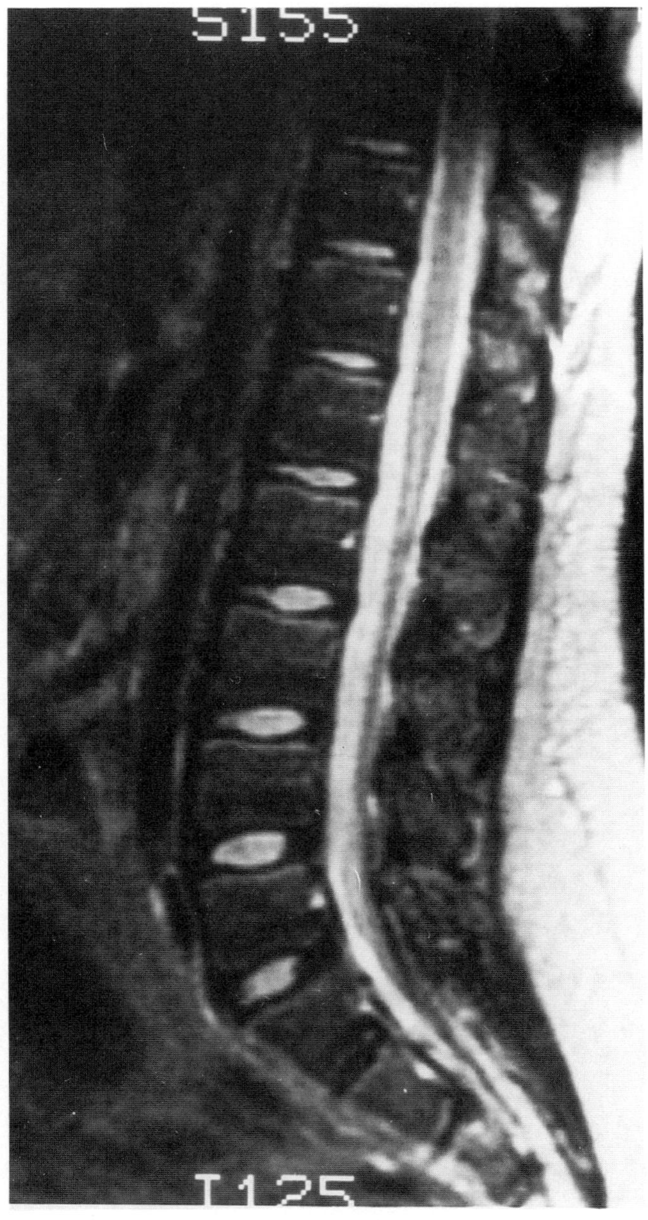

5-16 Midline sagittal MR scan through lumbar region (2000/90).

5/Lumbosacral Spine, MRI

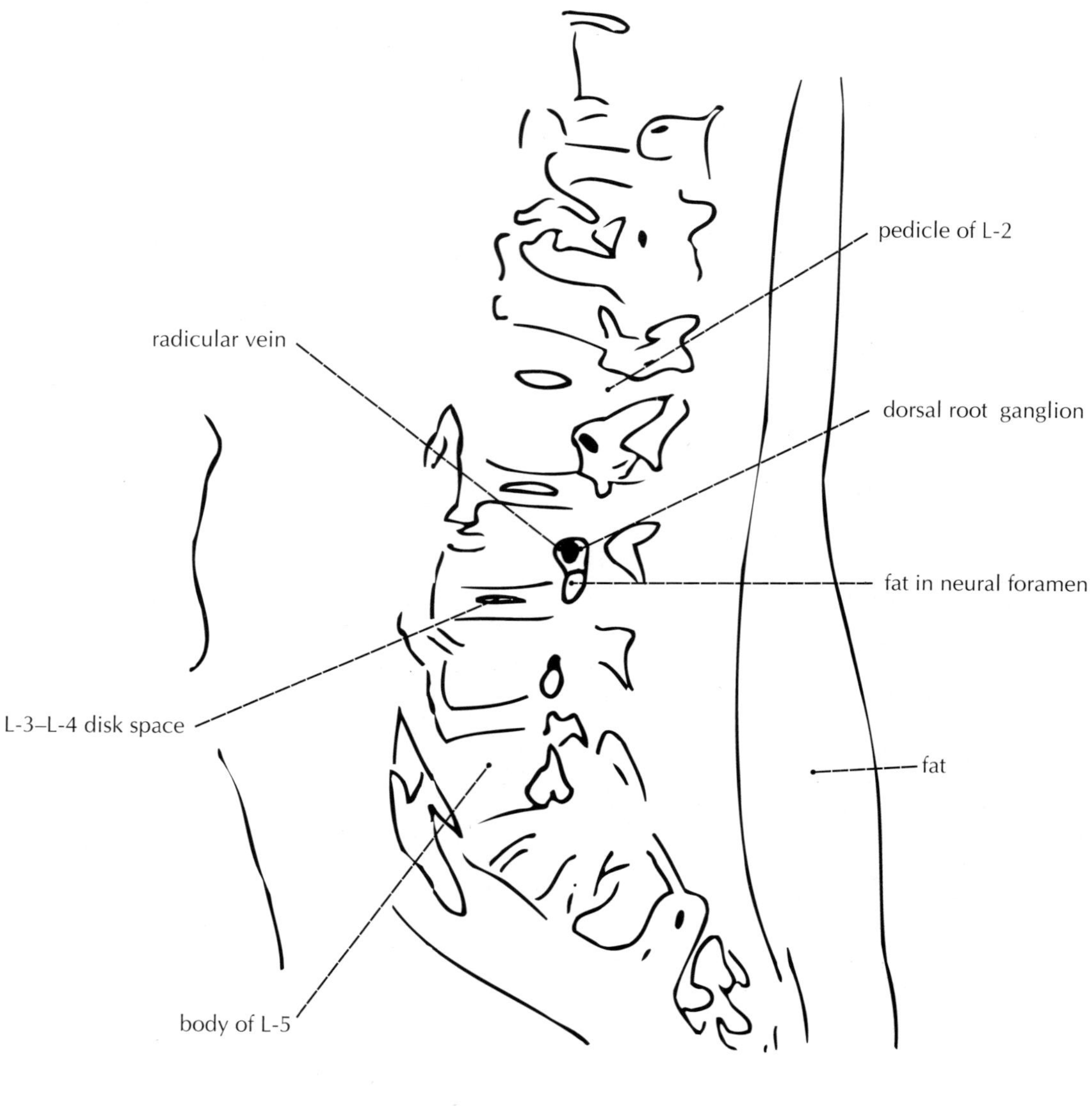

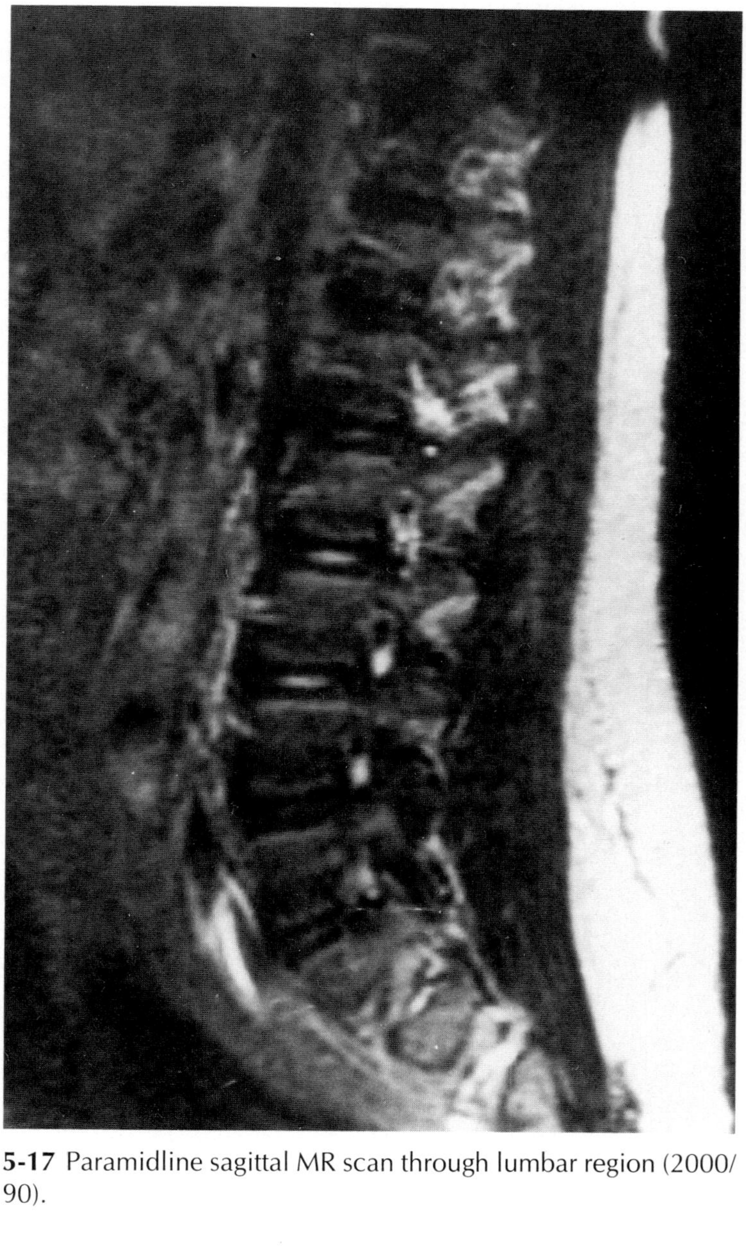

5-17 Paramidline sagittal MR scan through lumbar region (2000/90).

5/Lumbosacral Spine, Sagittal Scout MRI and Coronal MRI

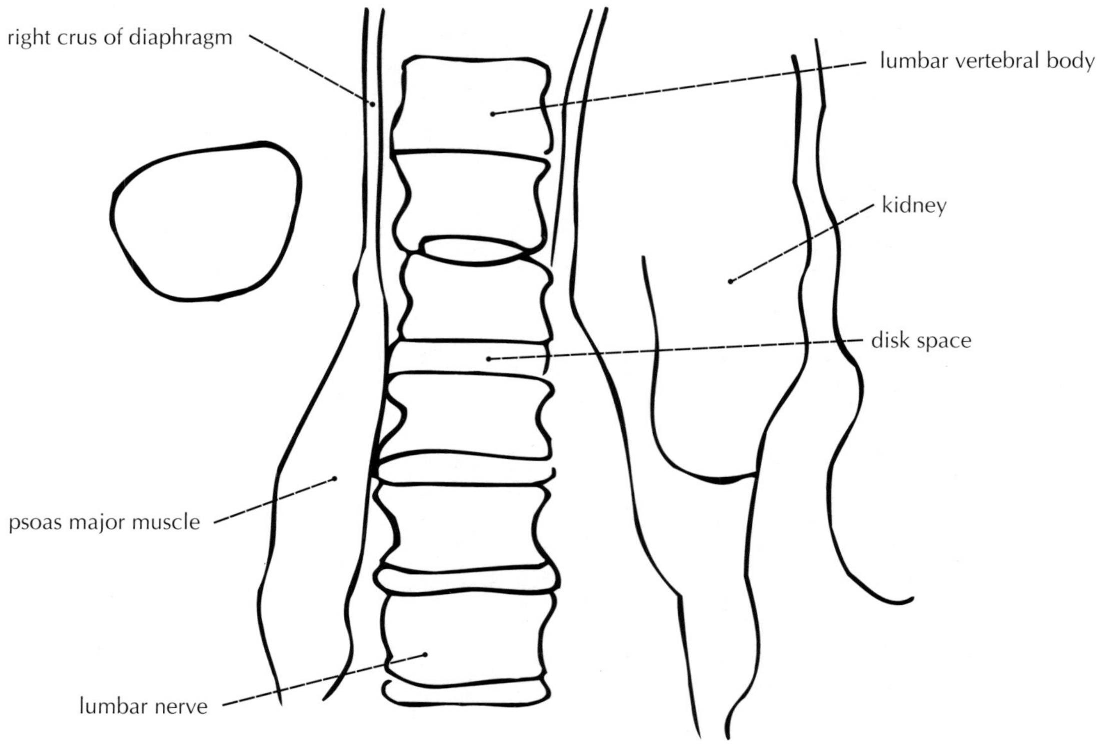

5/Lumbosacral Spine, Sagittal Scout MRI and Coronal MRI

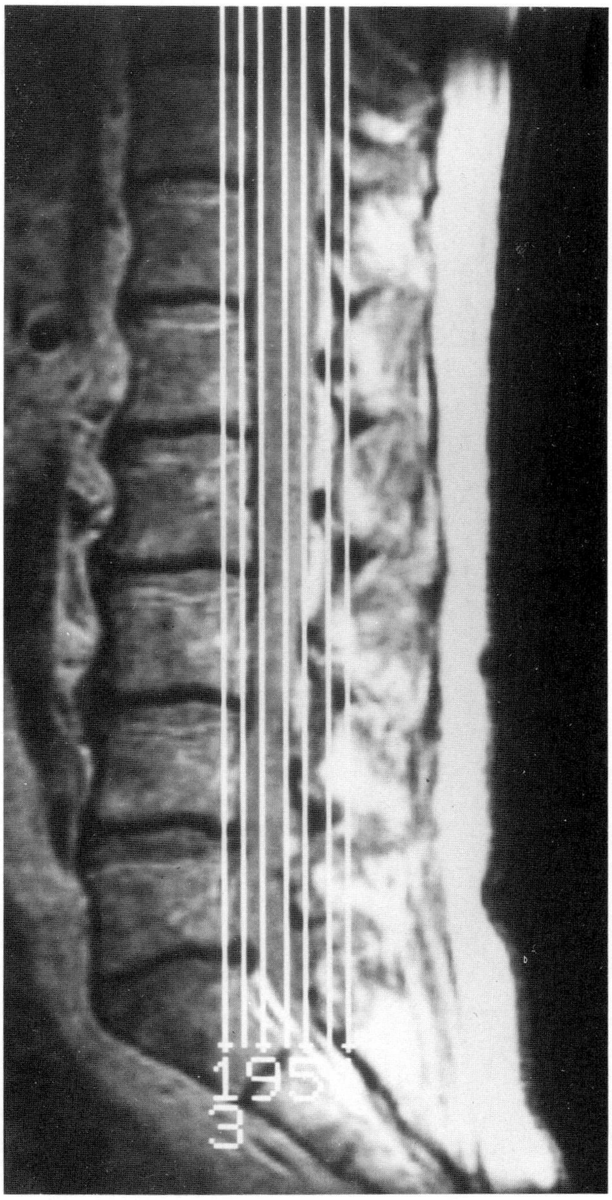

5-18 Sagittal scout MR scan used for demonstration of selected coronal images. Sections 13, 7 and 1 will be shown.

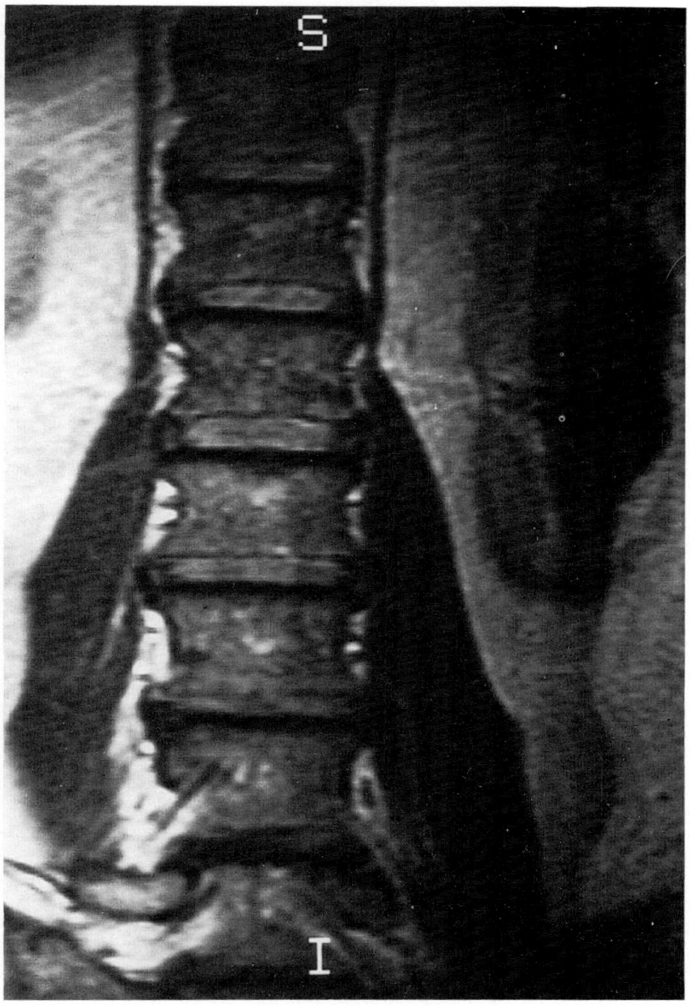

5-19 Coronal MR scan through lumbar spinal canal (2000/30). Section 13 in Fig. 5-18.

5/Lumbosacral Spine, Coronal MRI

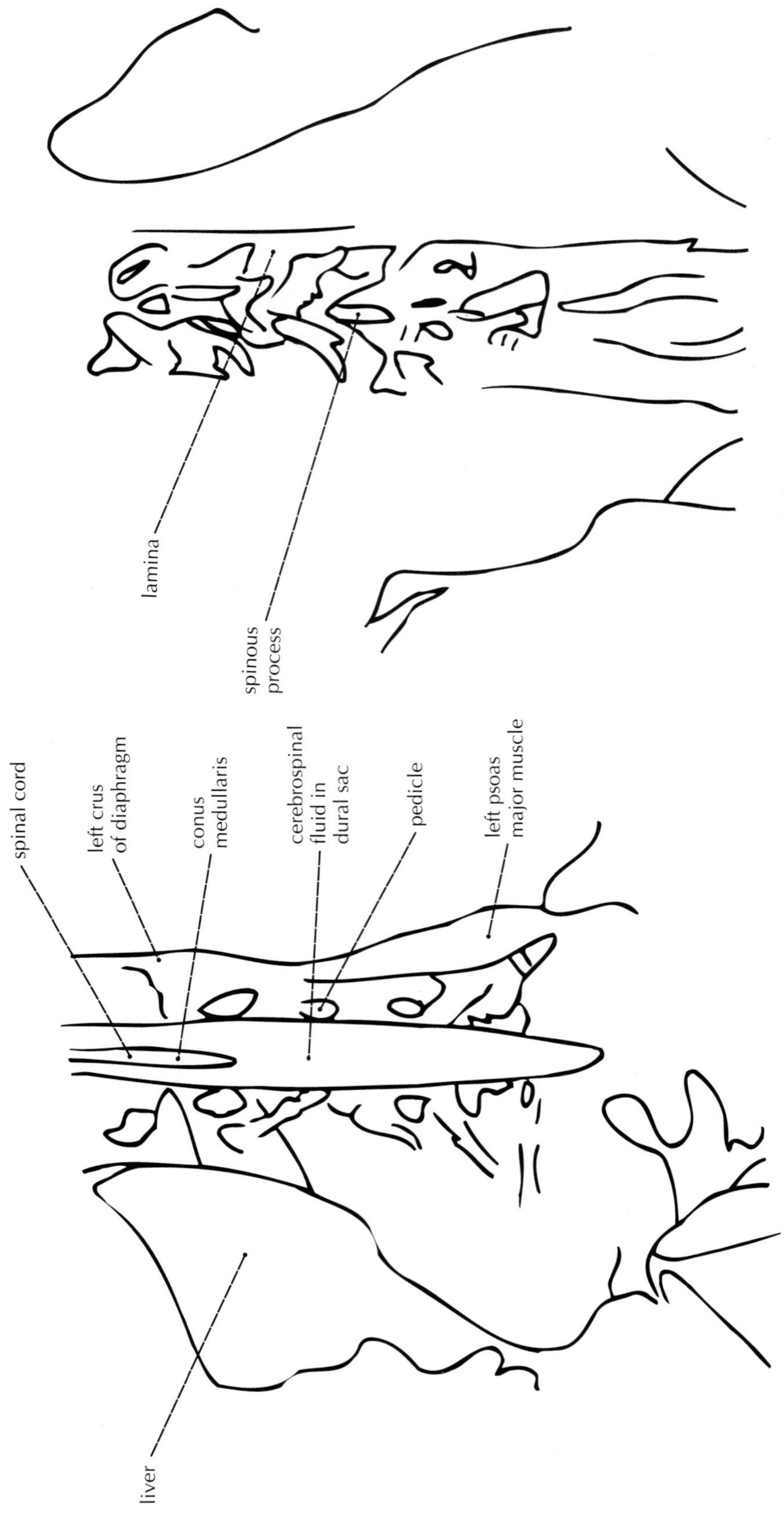

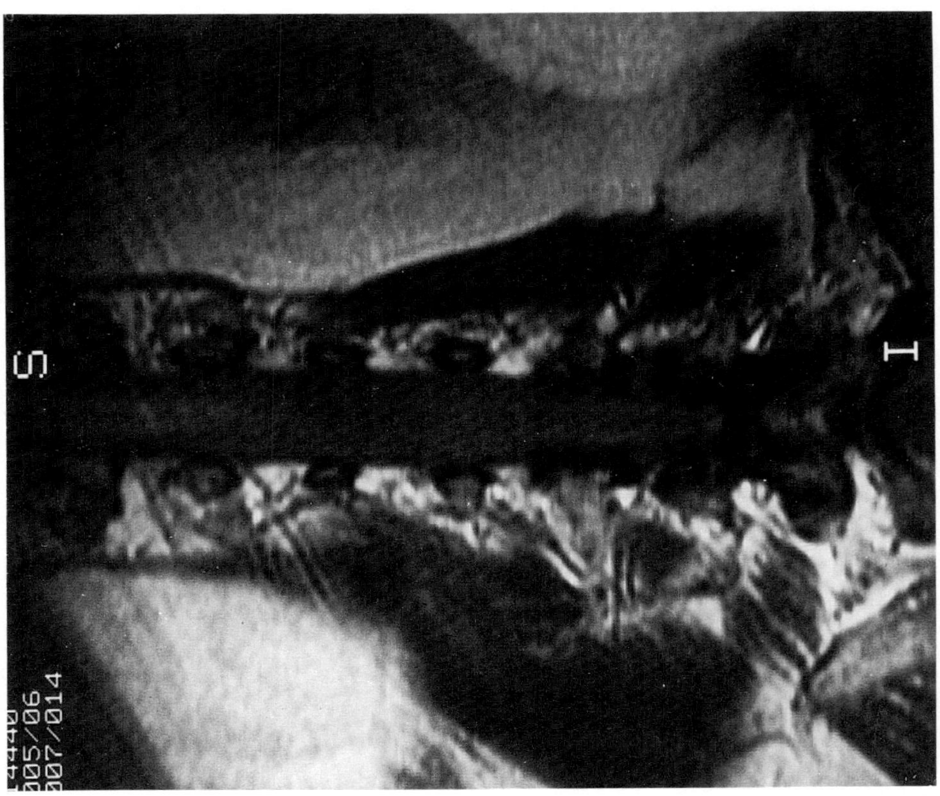

5-20 Coronal MR scan through lumbar spinal canal (2000/30). Section 7 in Fig. 5-18.

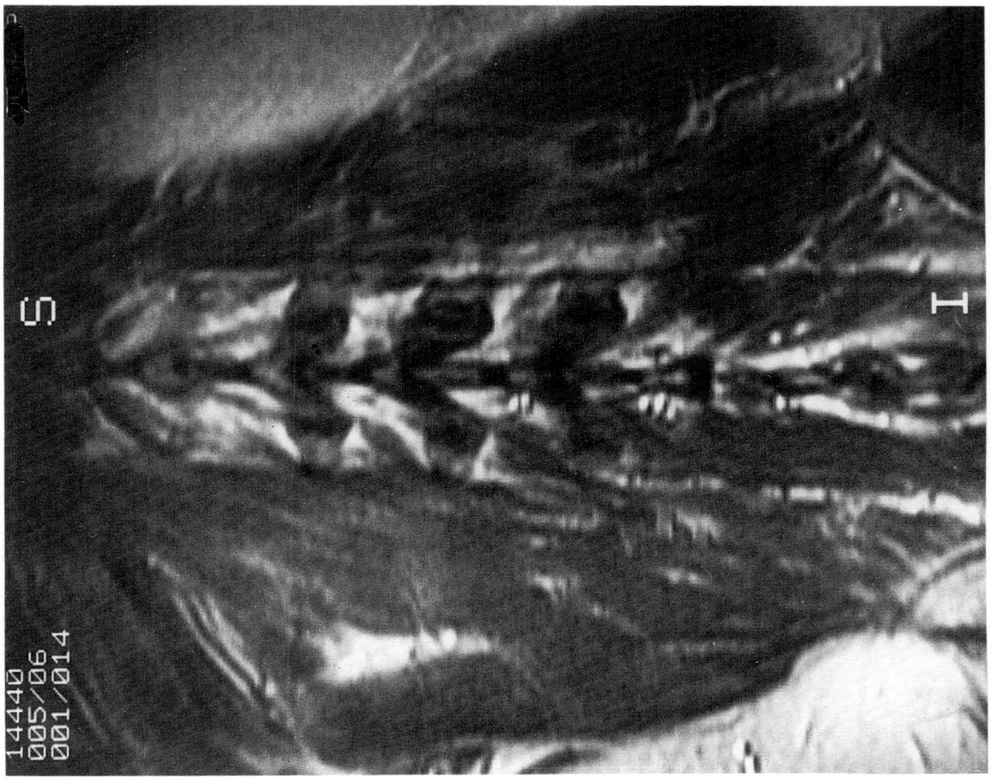

5-21 Coronal MR scan through lumbar spinal canal (2000/30). Section 1 in Fig. 5-18.

5/Lumbosacral Spine, Sagittal Scout MRI and Axial MRI

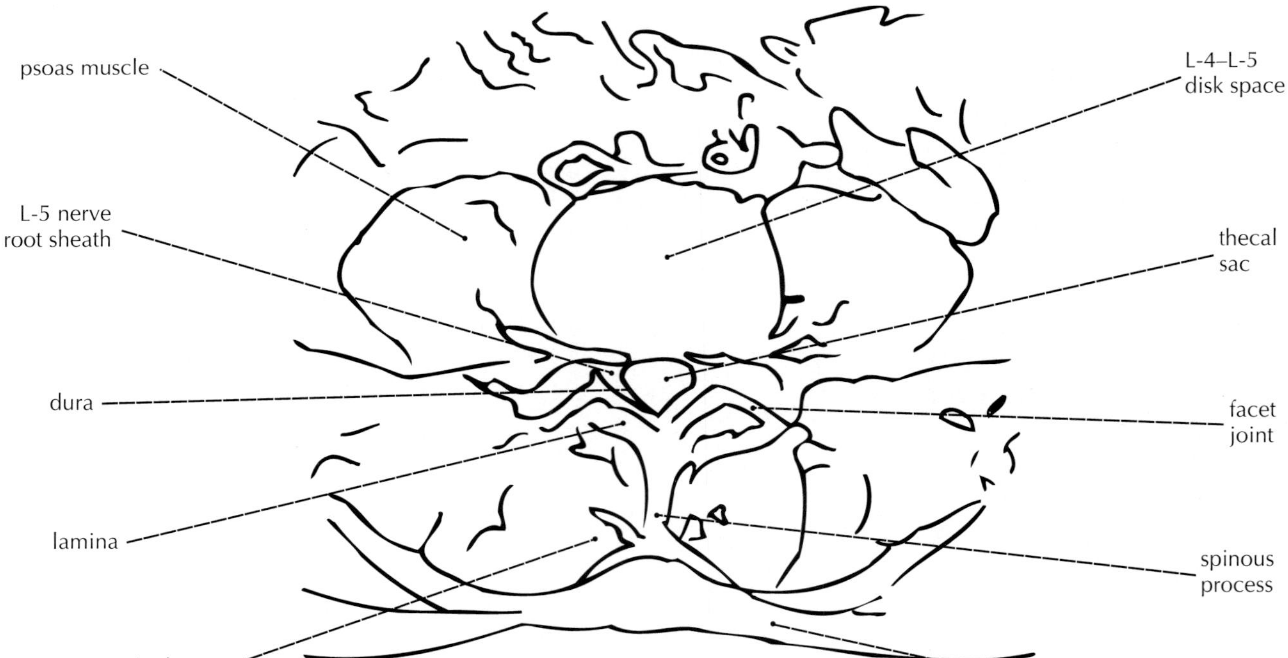

5/Lumbosacral Spine, Sagittal Scout MRI and Axial MRI

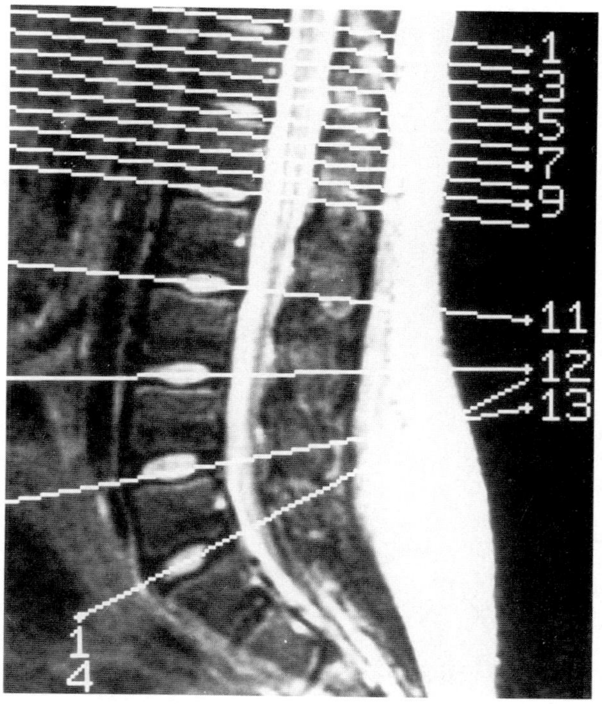

5-22 Sagittal scout MR scan for orientation of axial MR scans of the lumbosacral spine.

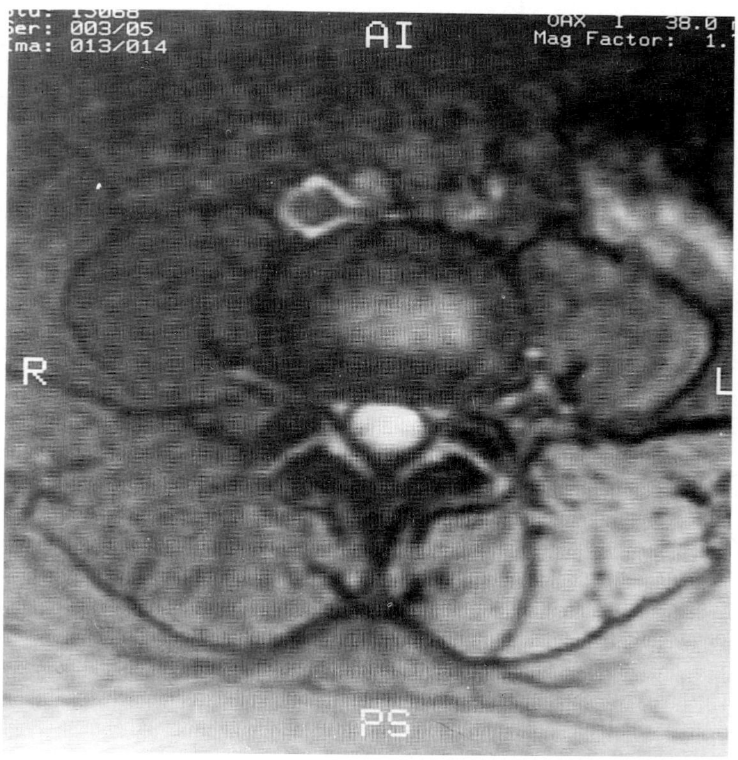

5-23 Axial MR scan through L-4–L-5 disk space (500/18, flip angle 15°) (section 13 in Fig. 5-22).

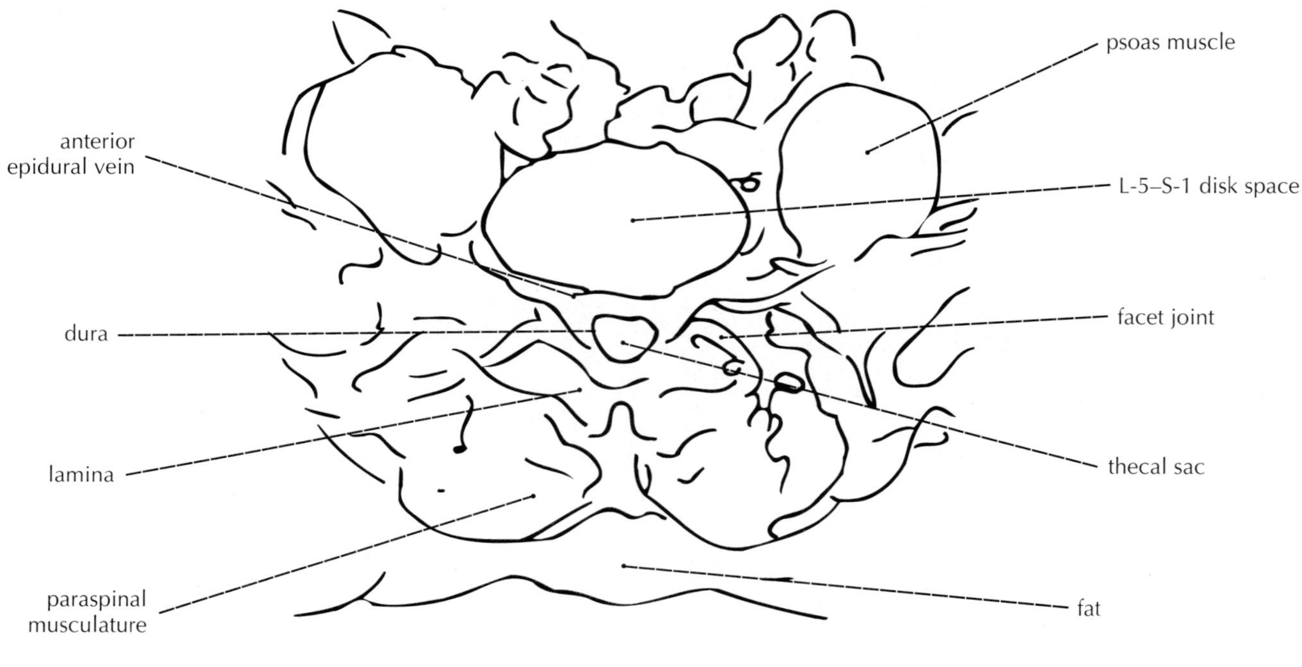
psoas muscle
anterior
epidural vein
L-5–S-1 disk space
dura
facet joint
thecal sac
lamina
paraspinal
musculature
fat

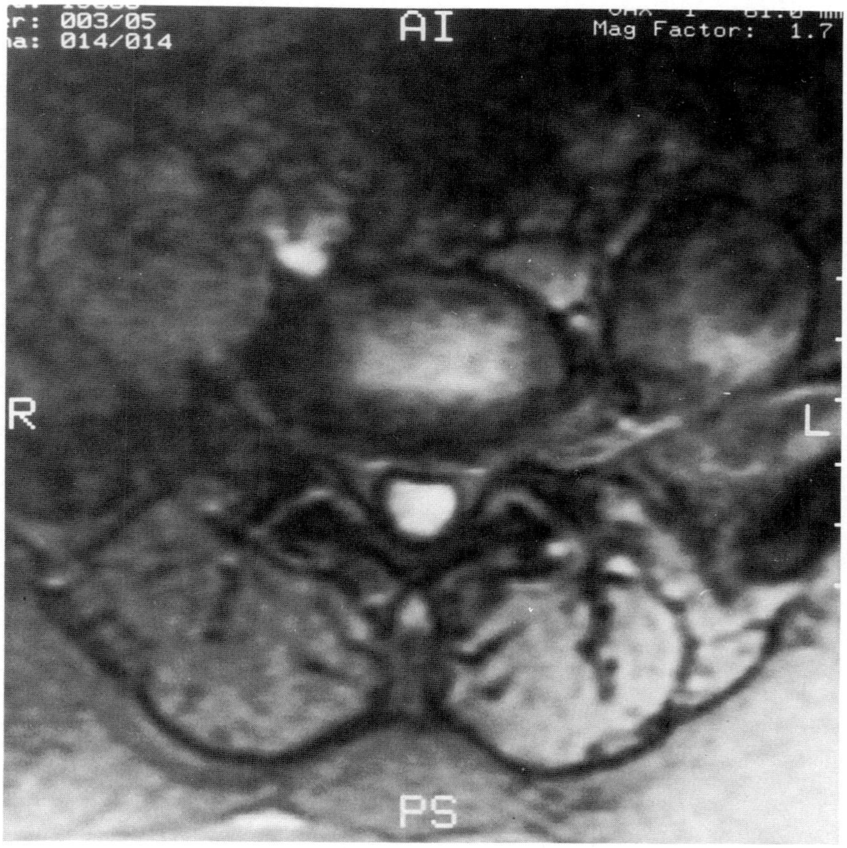

5-24 Axial MR scan through L-5–S-1 disk space (500/18, flip angle 15°) (section 14 in Fig. 5-22).

5/Thoracolumbar Spine, Myelography

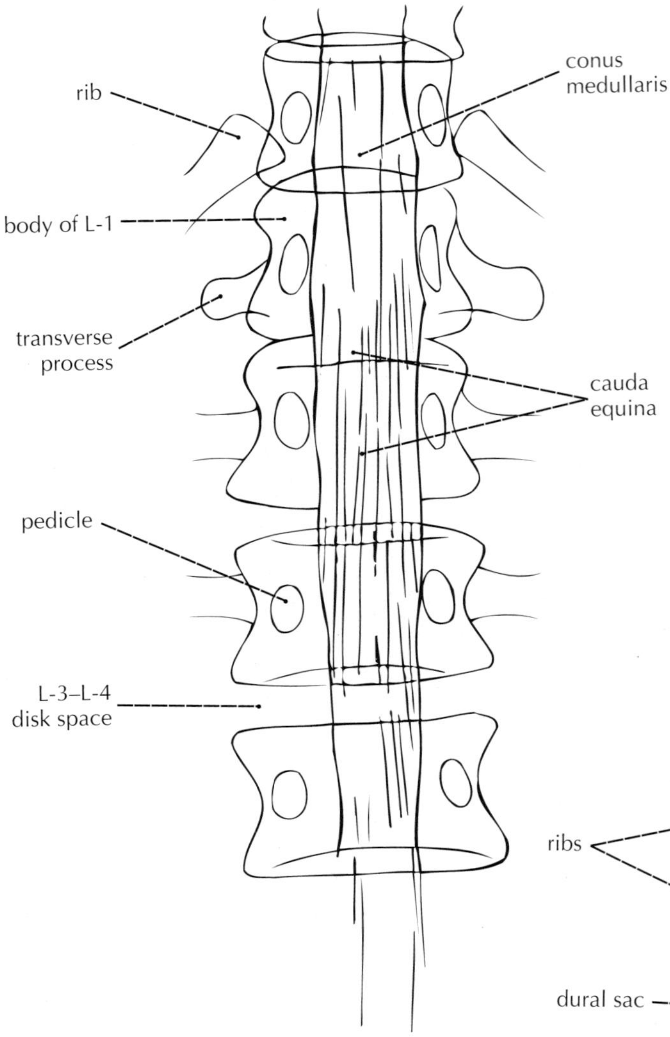

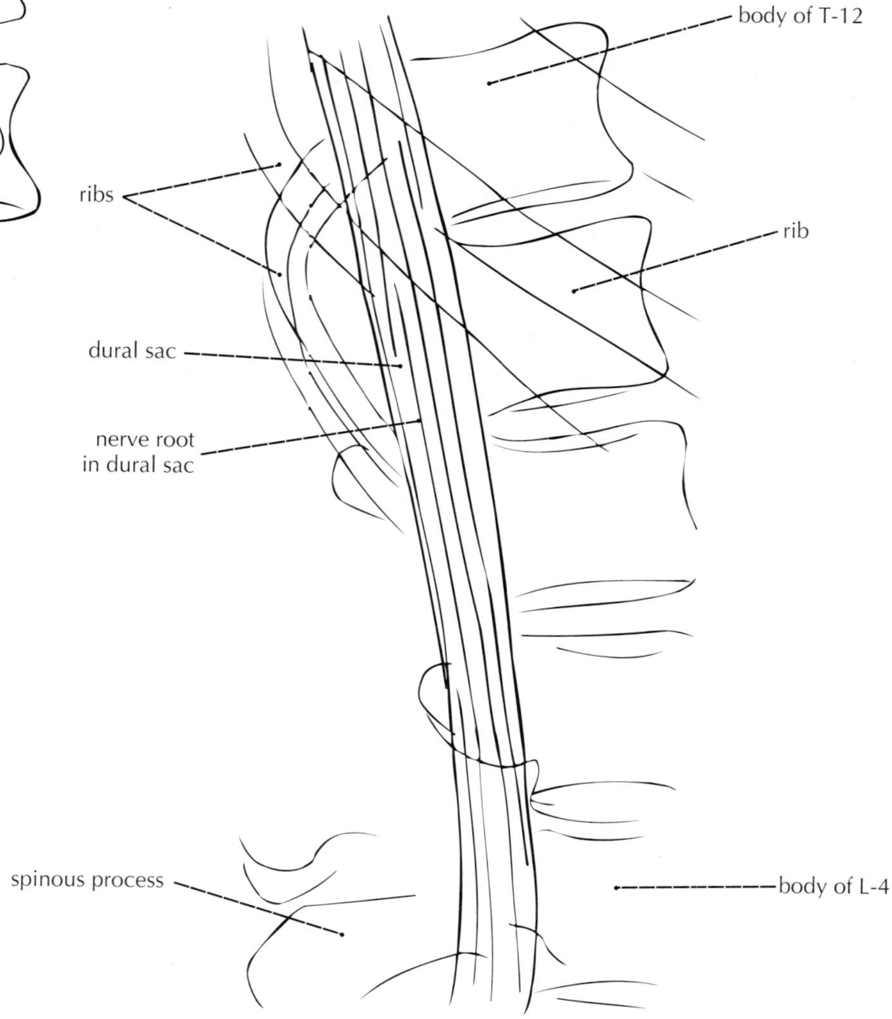

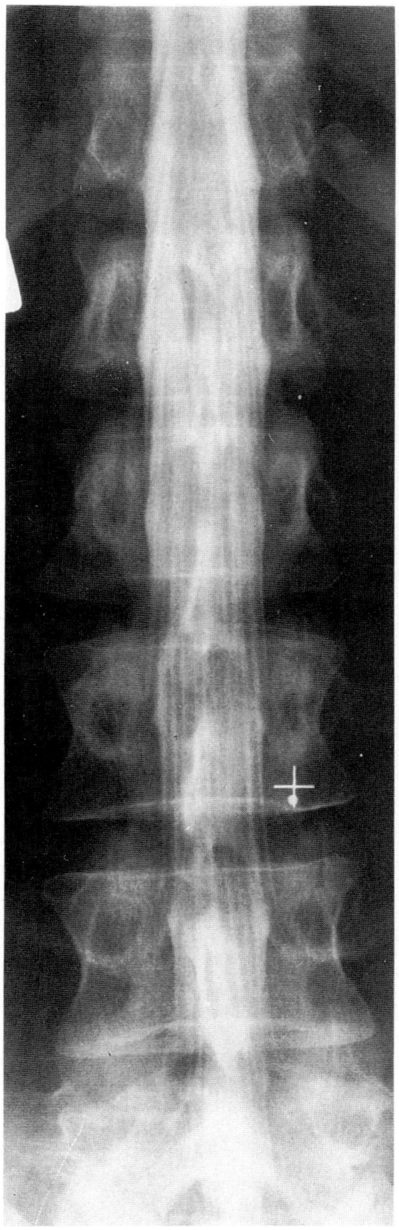

5-25 Myelogram of thoracolumbar region, AP view.

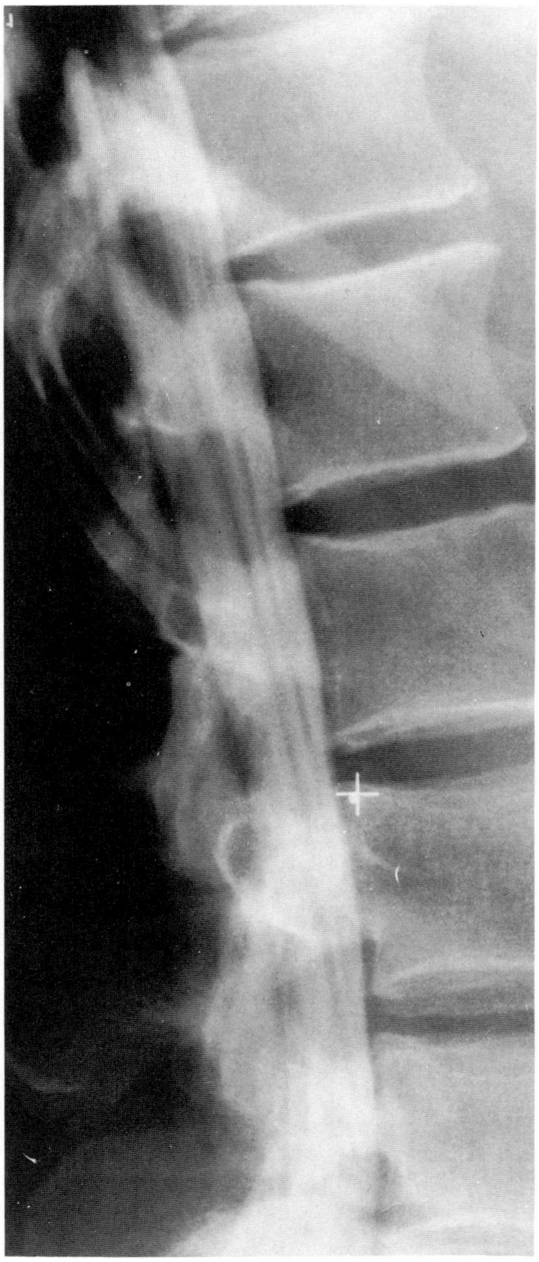

5-26 Myelogram of thoracolumbar region, lateral view.

5/Lumbosacral Spine, Myelography

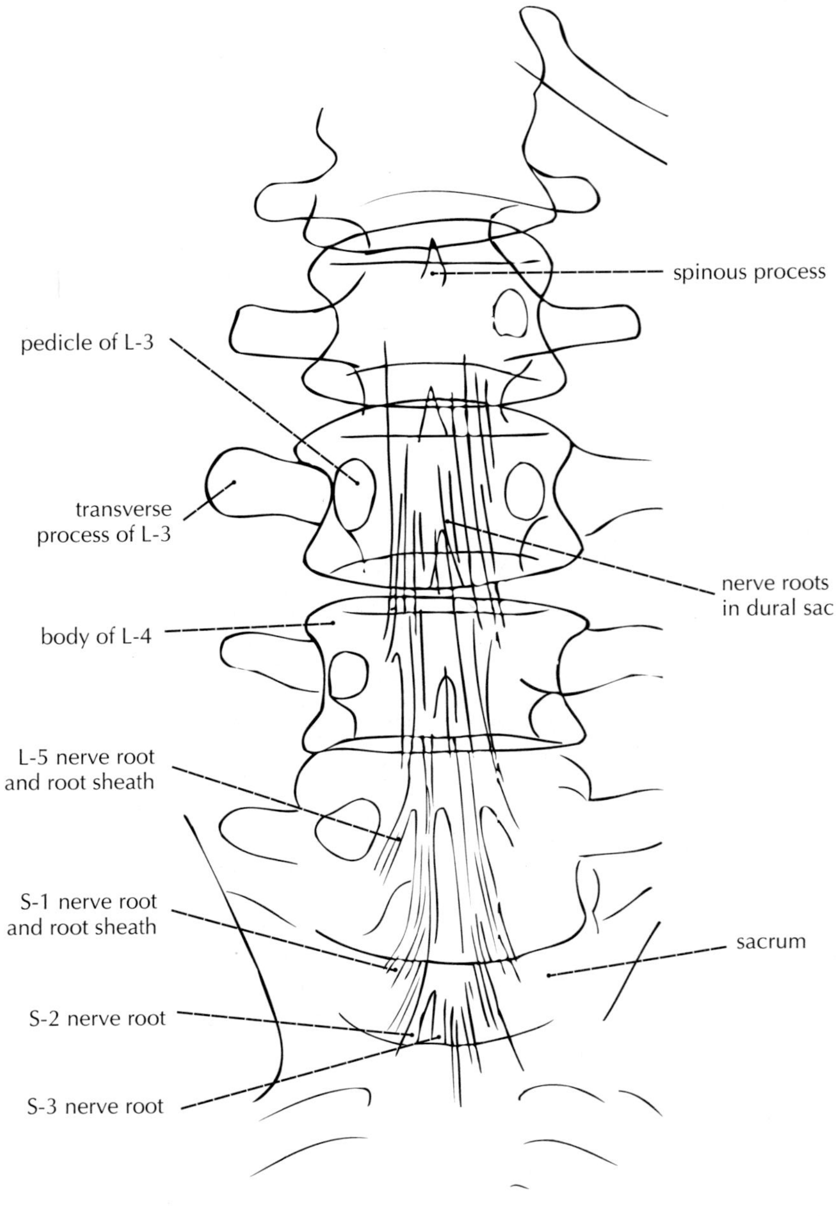

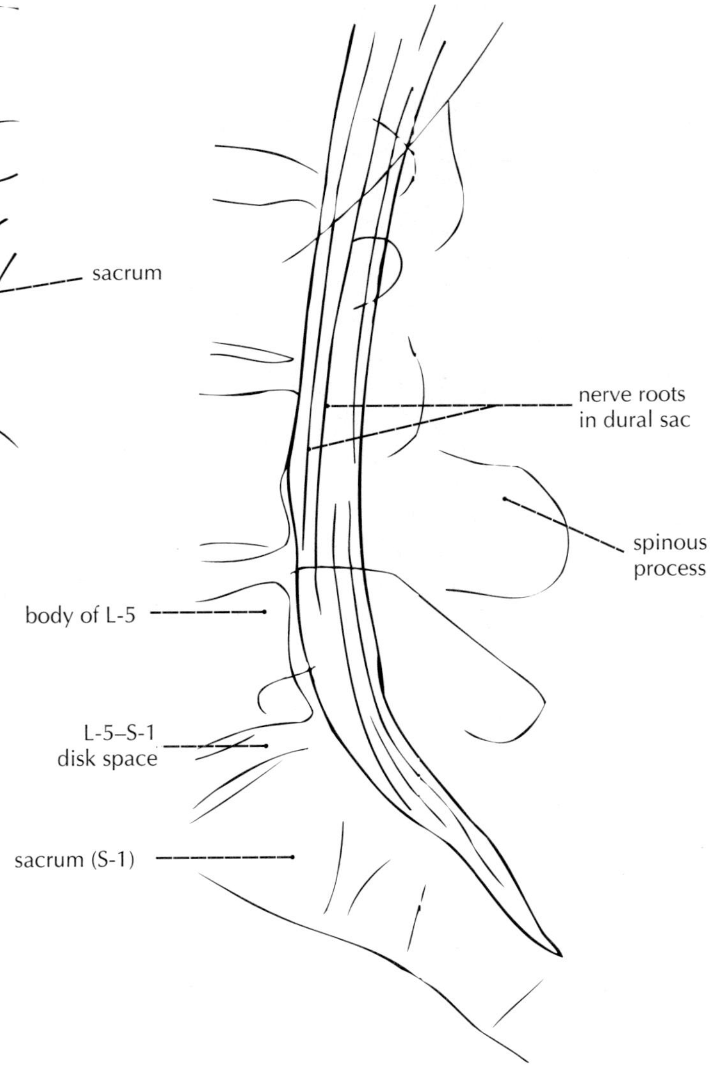

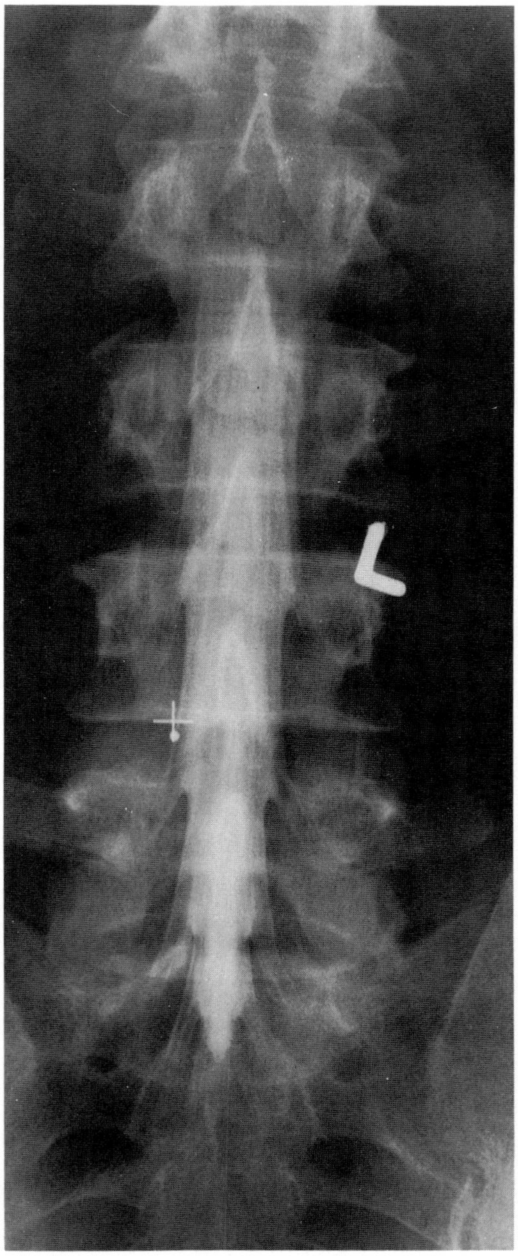

5-27 Myelogram of lumbosacral region, AP view.

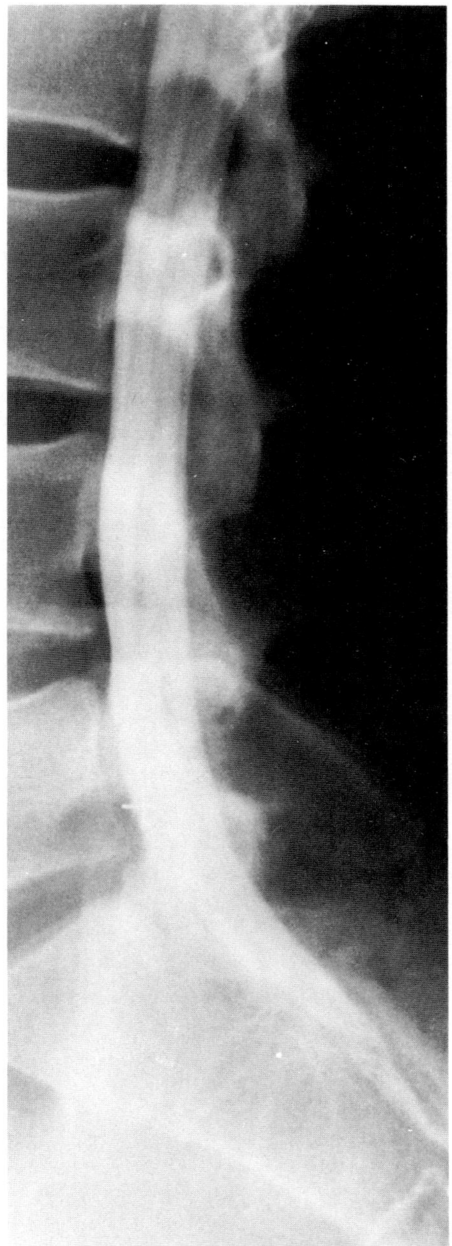

5-28 Myelogram of lumbosacral region, lateral view.

5/Lumbosacral Spine, Myelography

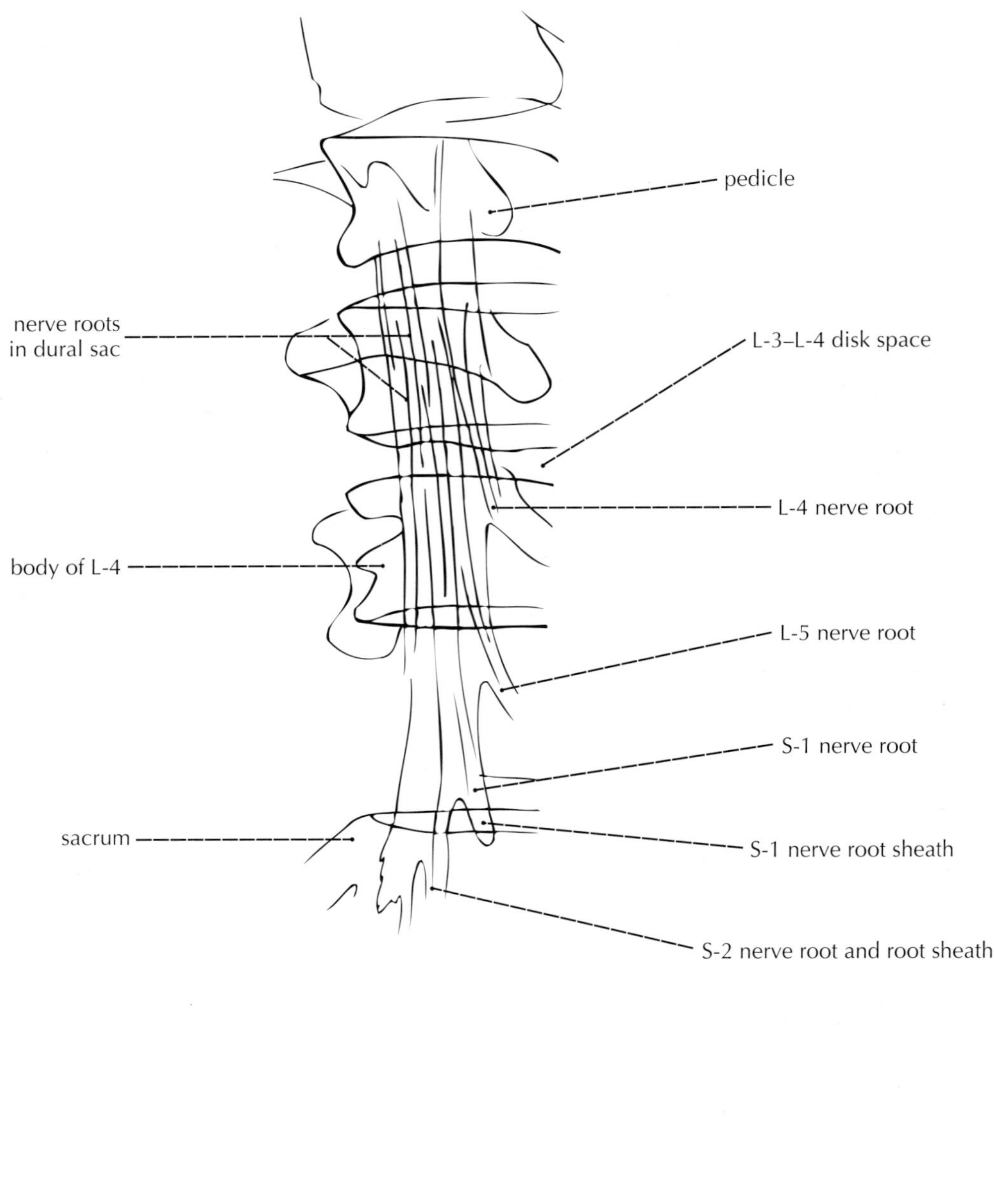

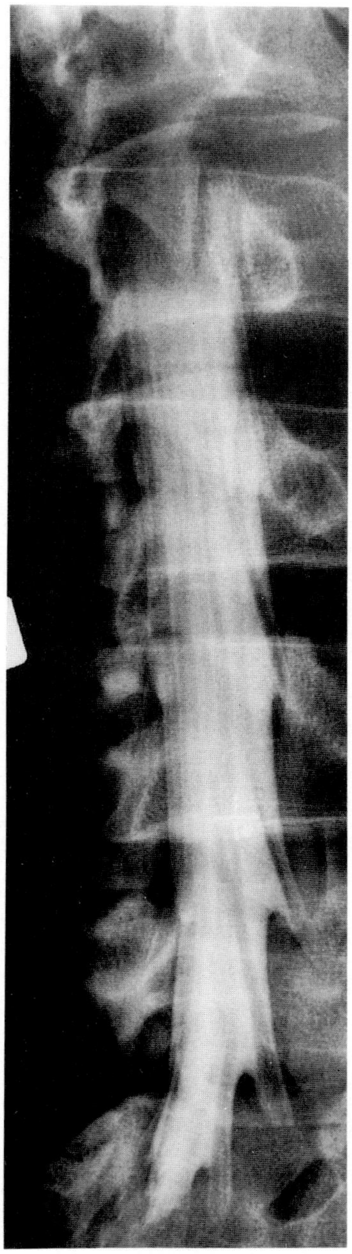

5-29 Myelogram of lumbosacral region, oblique view.